A MATHEMATICAL PRIMER OF MOLECULAR PHYLOGENETICS

A MATHEMATICAL PRIMER OF MOLECULAR PHYLOGENETICS

Xuhua Xia

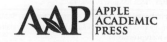

APPLE
ACADEMIC
PRESS

Apple Academic Press Inc.
4164 Lakeshore Road
Burlington ON L7L 1A4
Canada

Apple Academic Press Inc.
1265 Goldenrod Circle NE
Palm Bay, Florida 32905
USA

© 2020 by Apple Academic Press, Inc.

First issued in paperback 2021

Exclusive worldwide distribution by CRC Press, a member of Taylor & Francis Group

No claim to original U.S. Government works

ISBN 13: 978-1-774-63006-8 (pbk)
ISBN 13: 978-1-771-88755-7 (hbk)

Library and Archives Canada Cataloguing in Publication

Title: A mathematical primer of molecular phylogenetics / Xuhua Xia.

Names: Xia, Xuhua, 1959- author.

Description: Includes bibliographical references and index.

Identifiers: Canadiana (print) 20190163291 | Canadiana (ebook) 20190163313 | ISBN 9781771887557 (hardcover) | ISBN 9780429425875 (ebook)

Subjects: LCSH: Phylogeny—Molecular aspects—Mathematics.

Classification: LCC QH367.5 .X53 2020 | 591.3/80151—dc23

Library of Congress Cataloging-in-Publication Data

Names: Xia, Xuhua, 1959- author.

Title: A mathematical primer of molecular phylogenetics / Xuhua Xia.

Description: Oakville, ON ; Palm Bay, Florida : Apple Academic Press, [2020] | Includes bibliographical references and index. | Summary: "This volume, A Mathematical Primer of Molecular Phylogenetics, offers a unique perspective on a number of phylogenetic issues that have not been covered in detail in previous publications. The volume provides sufficient mathematical background for young mathematicians and computational scientists, as well as mathematically inclined biology students, to make a smooth entry into the expanding field of molecular phylogenetics. The book will also provide sufficient details for researchers in phylogenetics to understand the workings of existing software packages used. The volume offers comprehensive but detailed numerical illustrations to render difficult mathematical and computational concepts in molecular phylogenetics accessible to a variety of readers with different academic background. The text includes examples of solved problems after each chapter, which will be particularly helpful for fourth-year undergraduates, postgraduates, and postdoctoral students in biology, mathematics and computer sciences. Researchers in molecular biology and evolution will find it very informative as well. Key features: Provides mathematical background for young mathematicians and computational scientists to understand the expanding field of molecular phylogenetics Includes information for researchers in phylogenetics to understand the workings of existing software packages used in phylogenetics Offers a unique perspective on a number of phylogenetic issues that have not been covered in detail in previous publications Provides support via a comprehensive software package (DAMBE), written by the book's author Aims to act as a middle ground for effective interdisciplinary communication among molecular biologists, mathematics, and computational scientists"-- Provided by publisher.

Identifiers: LCCN 2019034524 (print) | LCCN 2019034525 (ebook) | ISBN 9781771887557 (hardcover) | ISBN 9780429425875 (ebook)

Subjects: LCSH: Phylogeny--Molecular aspects--Mathematical models. | Evolutionary genetics--Mathematical models.

Classification: LCC QH367.5 .X53 2020 (print) | LCC QH367.5 (ebook) | DDC 576.8/8--dc23

LC record available at https://lccn.loc.gov/2019034524

LC ebook record available at https://lccn.loc.gov/2019034525

Apple Academic Press also publishes its books in a variety of electronic formats. Some content that appears in print may not be available in electronic format. For information about Apple Academic Press products, visit our website at **www.appleacademicpress. com** and the CRC Press website at **www.crcpress.com**

About the Author

Dr. Xuhua Xia obtained his Ph.D. in population biology from University of Western Ontario. He became an assistant professor at University of Hong Kong in 1996, and served in 2001 as a senior scientist and head of Bioinformatics Laboratory in the newly established HKU-Pasteur Research Centre. He came back to Canada in 2002 and has been full professor at University of Ottawa since 2009. He serves as an associate editor for several journals, including *Molecular Biology and Evolution, Scientific Reports,* and *Journal of Heredity*. He has published in leading journals in molecular phylogenetics and evolution, including *Systematic Biology, Molecular Biology and Evolution, Genetics,* and *Global Ecology and Biogeography*. Dr. Xia is the author of the widely used software package DAMBE which is freely available at http://dambe.bio.uottawa.ca.

Dr. Xia's current research is on (1) developing bioinformatic algorithms and software to meet the challenge of accurate analysis of high-throughput data, (2) optimization of translation and splicing machinery to facilitate mRNA processing and protein production, and (3) interaction and evolution of macromolecules over time and space to understand the origin and maintenance of biodiversity.

Contents

Abbreviations

BH	Benjamini–Hochberg
BMM	Brown motion model
BY	Benjamini–Yekutieli
DF	degree of freedom
EM	expectation–maximization
FDR	false discovery rate
FM	Fitch–Margoliash
GE	gap extension penalty
GO	gap open penalty
HA	hemagglutinin
HMM	hidden Markov models
IE	independent estimation
IUPAC	International Union of Pure and Applied Chemistry
LGT	lateral gene transfer
lnL	log-likelihood
LRT	likelihood ratio test
LS	least-squares
ME	minimum evolution
ML	maximum likelihood
MM	match-mismatch
MP	maximum parsimony
MSA	multiple sequence alignment
mtDNA	mitochondrial DNA
NC	number of changes
NJ	neighbor-joining
OGT	optimal growth temperature
OLS	ordinary least-squares
OTUs	operational taxonomic units
PhyPA	phylogenetics with pairwise alignment
PSA	pairwise sequence alignment
rRNA	ribosomal RNA
RSS	residual sum of squares

SD	standard deviation
SE	simultaneous estimation
SE	simultaneously estimated
SE	standard error
SM	scoring matrix
SPS	sum-of-pairs score
ssu rRNA	small subunit ribosomal RNA
TL	tree length
WC	weighted contrasts
WLS	weight least-squares

Preface

Molecular phylogenetics is important, and I wish to promote it.

Different people have different ways of promoting their ideas and beliefs. Many would use dramatic or witty titles such as "The Communist Manifesto" or "A pain in the torus." Some would resort to incendiary, but typically audacious or even mendacious claims, such as "What is true in *E. coli* is also true in the elephant, only truer," "Nothing in biology makes sense except in the light of evolution," or "All science is either physics or stamp collecting." Occasionally, some rare authors would adopt even more extreme but less acceptable ways of imposing their views on others, such as Ted Kaczynski the Unabomber.

But I am not capable of dramatizing, and English as my second language prevents me from being witty. Making incendiary or audacious claims seems repugnant to me and to those around me. In particular, I do not wish to impose my views on others just as I am not fond of having others imposing their views on me. So how am I going to promote molecular phylogenetics when all these options are unavailable?

Evangelical preachers often promote their religion by linking their belief to famous people of the past, with the implication that, if such great people have adopted their religion, then you should, too. This has resulted in the creation of fables such as Darwin repenting in his last days and Einstein being God-fearing and deeply religious. Phylogeneticists have often taken the same approach, by highlighting two historical observations. The first is a quote from Aristotle that "He who sees things from the very beginning has the most advantageous view of them," and the second is that the single figure in the 1859 book by the old man in evolutionary biology represents a phylogenetic tree. If bright people such as Aristotle and Darwin were so fond of tracing natural history back to its beginning, then surely you should, too, shouldn't you? Being an empiricist, I have tried this trick multiple times in multiple situations. Unfortunately, it did not work magic.

Some authors, confident in their eloquence and passionate about their beliefs, will simply issue a directive: "Please read the book." This is indeed a simple sentence, but I found it hard and heavy to articulate when my passion is not buttressed by eloquence.

So I will just paraphrase what A. W. F. Edwards said in his lovely little book entitled *Likelihood*. Molecular phylogenetics has been a fertile land for me. I have toiled on it and reaped the harvest. Although I would not claim myself to be a great farmer, I did have the privilege of meeting many great and productive ones on the land who have helped me to settle down comfortably. Given my own positive experience, I have no hesitation to invite you to join me in growing your crops here. This book is the best fruit of my harvest, produced in collaboration with Sandra Sickels and Ashish Kumar of Apple Academic Press. I am presenting it to you, for you to enjoy and to be convinced that it is good fruit from good earth. The book contains many useful advices on how you can grow, and improve upon, the existing crops.

If you are a young mathematics-inclined student interested in phylogenetics, this book is exactly for you. It provides not only a mathematical conceptual framework for molecular phylogenetics, but also algorithmic details and programming tips. However, I wish to take this opportunity to warn you that molecular phylogenetics is not easy and would demand two prerequisites from you. First, you need to have faith in yourself that you can learn molecular phylogenetics well. Second, you should never underestimate the difficulty in gaining proficiency in molecular phylogenetics.

While I generally do not cite religious books in teaching molecular phylogenetics, there happen to be two excellent examples in the Bible to illustrate the paramount importance of the two prerequisites. In the first example, Moses led the Israelites to the edge of their promised land flowing with milk and honey. In order to gather information to facilitate an attack, Moses sent 12 spies to survey the enemy territory. While two spies (Joshua and Caleb) came back with a united voice in favor of an attack, the other 10 were terrified by the giants inhabiting the territory and lost their faith in winning the battle. Their fear quickly spread out of control and the Israelites fled without a fight. Many biology students came to the land of molecular phylogenetics, surveyed its fertile land flowing with milk and honey, but became terrified by just a few symbols and equations that loomed large like giants, and fled without making an effort to gain an entry. Failure is guaranteed when one loses faith in oneself. In the second example, the Israelites came to the edge of Ai, a Canaanite royal city. This time they had in themselves a great deal of faith built up over 40 years of overcoming trials and tribulations. However, they committed the sin of underestimating the difficulty of conquering the city—they sent only about 3000 half-hearted soldiers into the battle against the well-prepared enemy and consequently got beaten and slaughtered. They did learn the lesson and eventually took the city by mobilizing more than 30,000 mighty warriors and careful deployment of their forces. The bottom line is that you should never underestimate the difficulty you are facing. Many students came to the land of molecular phylogenetics half-prepared, thinking that they could master the subject by just going to the class and listening to lectures. This is equivalent to sending 3000 half-hearted soldiers when 30,000 mighty warriors are required. So have faith in yourself and try your best to mobilize the 30,000 mighty warriors in you. Don't run away and wander for another 40 years before circling back.

This book aims to serve three purposes. First, it is a personal invitation to you from a phylogeneticist. I hope that it will spin an invisible link between you and me so that I can be your personal guide. Please contact me whevever you have issues with my presentation of phylogenetic algorithms and applications. Second, it serves as a self-contained textbook that paves the way to ease your entry into the terrain of phylogenetics. Third, it represents a token of appreciation for the logistic support from University of Ottawa, the research grant from the Natural Science and Engineering Research Council of Canada and, in particular, the love and care I received from my wife and my children. One of the most emotionally voiced phrases by Christians is "God of our fathers." I wish that my children and their generation would someday come to explore this rugged terrain of science, and speak softly and emotionally "This land of our parents."

None of these purposes would be well served without your holding the book in your hand. Thank you for reading.

CHAPTER 1

Introduction to Molecular Phylogenetics

ABSTRACT

Molecular phylogenetics has two key objectives: (1) to elucidate the branching pattern of speciation and gene duplication events, and (2) to date the speciation and gene duplication events with a molecular clock. Molecular phylogenetics is instrumental in the discovery of the three domains of life, in providing crucial evidence for the hypothesis of endosymbiosis for the origin of mitochondria and plastids, and in offering a new perspective in a variety of biological research. I illustrate the success of molecular phylogenetics with a few classic and not-so-classic examples.

Although there is only one phylogenetic tree in Charles Darwin's book (Darwin, 1859), that tree has proliferated over years and spawned a jungle of mathematics and computational algorithms. This chapter does not plunge you right into this jungle. Instead, it will just share with you a few legends and landmarks that may entice you to see more of the jungle in subsequent chapters.

1.1 GENETIC MARKERS ARE IDEAL FOR GENEALOGICAL RELATIONSHIPS

Molecular phylogenetics uses genetic markers as building blocks. The most fundamental genetic marker is the genome responsible for the manifestation of life in any living entity. These genetic markers have been imprinted a history of life, its origin, and its diversification on earth. Molecular phylogenetics aims to reconstruct this history of life from these genetic markers.

I once attended, as a graduate student at Western in the 1980s, a seminar by Dr. Shiva Singh on genetic markers after his sabbatical. Shiva showed photos of a number of places he had visited during his sabbatical, and nobody knew where they were. Finally Shiva flashed a picture of Eiffel Tower and everyone knew that he was in Paris.

"You won't get lost if you know the landmarks," Shiva asserted, "and geneticists won't get lost if they have genetic markers," and he proceeded to offer a nice presentation on the development and application of genetic markers in solving practical biological and biomedical problems.

Genetic markers go way beyond science. I came across a story of a farmer and his two sons who lived in Germany in early 1970s. The older son spent most of his time working as a farmer like his father. They are both muscular and robust with copper-colored skin. The younger son, in contrast, disliked manual labor. He was not muscular, had pale skin, and did not look quite manly. The morphological difference between the German farmer and his younger son was so obvious that the father decided to go to court to disinherit his younger son, believing that the boy must have resulted from an extramarital affair. At that time, there was no DNA available, but the method of allozyme electrophoresis and immune responses allowed forensic scientists to reach a rather dramatic and surprising conclusion. The younger son was definitely the biological son of the German farmer, but the older one was quite doubtful. The story highlighted how lost the German farmer was without the guidance of genetic markers.

In retrospect, we can see that the morphological similarity between the German farmer and his older son is a consequence of morphological convergence resulting from working hard in the farm. Such similarities are weak for tracing human relationships. Other examples of convergence include the morphological similarities between certain placental mammals and their marsupial counterpart, e.g., between the placental wolf (*Canis lupus*) and the marsupial Tasmanian wolf (*Thylacinus cynocephalus*), between the placental cat (*Felis catus*) and the marsupial tiger quoll (*Dasyurus maculatus*), and between the placental mouse (*Mus musculus*) and the marsupial fat-tailed mouse opossum (*Thylamys elegans*). All these examples of morphological convergence that are not related to true genetic affinity, together with the peculiar phenomenon of mimicry, remind us of nature's tendency to hide true geological relationships from us.

Genetic markers have been used not only to identify paternity in humans but also in studying multiple paternity in animals. Circumstantial evidence suggests that the white-footed mouse, *Peromyscus leucopus,* may be promiscuous because (1) males do not provide any sort of parental care (Xia and Millar, 1988) based on observations in semi-natural enclosures, and (2) males gather around females in the field only when females are in estrus (Xia and Millar, 1989). When pregnant females were brought back and allowed to give birth to her young, and when the genotype of both mother and offspring were assessed, one obtains clear evidence of multiple paternity in single litters (Xia and Millar, 1991). For example, a mother's genotype at one autosome locus is AA, but three offspring genotypes are AA, AB, and AC. This implies that alleles A, B, and C are from males. Because each male has only two alleles, at least two males must have contributed to the litter of offspring.

Genetic markers can also contribute to resolving national conflicts. Between Canada and the United States, there has been a long-term dispute on the management and harvest of Pacific salmon, in particular the allocation of fishing quotas (Emery, 1997). The most fundamental principle of allocation, the equity principle, is to "ensure that each country receives benefits equivalent to the production of salmon originating in its waters." This principle, rational in its articulation, has one major difficulty in its implementation. That is, how would one know if a salmon caught in the Pacific originated in Canadian or US waters? Fish biologists in the past have studied differences in morphological characters, parasite loads, and many other traits of salmon sampled in Canadian and American rivers, but these traits provide poor resolution for discrimination. Fortunately, sea-type salmons are philopatric and migrate to their natal place to breed. This implies genetic differentiation among salmon populations between Canadian and US river systems. Identification of salmon at species, population, or even individual level is now possible with well-developed DNA markers (Beacham et al., 2017).

1.2 SUCCESS STORIES IN THE APPLICATION OF DNA AND RNA AS GENETIC MARKERS

There are many success stories in the application of molecular phylogenetics, some well-known and some little known. I will present two well-known stories as well as two little known ones, partly because of my conviction that many biological Cinderellas deserve a better fate in real life, and partly because all these stories illustrate the unique insights we can gain only through molecular phylogenetics.

1.2.1   THE DISCOVERY OF THREE KINGDOMS OF LIFE

One of the landmark discoveries in molecular phylogenetics is the discovery of three domains of life (Eubacteria, Archaea, and Eukarya) in 1977. Prior to that discovery, we have two domains, prokaryotes without a cell nucleus and eukaryotes with a nucleus. Based on a similarity index (S_{AB}) derived from sharing of RNA fingerprints between taxa A and B, with $S_{AB} = 2N_{AB}/(N_A+N_B)$, Woese and Fox (1977) showed that the three domains of life are roughly of equal distance from each other. No phylogenetic tree was constructed in that paper, but one can readily derive distances (D) from S_{AB} values and reconstruct a tree (Fig. 1.1a). As the maximum of S_{AB} is 1, we may simply have $D_{AB} = 1 - S_{AB}$. I have replicated such a distance matrix in Figure 1.1b. The resulting distance matrix, when analyzed by a distance-based phylogenetic method such as FastME (Desper and Gascuel, 2002; 2004) which is also implemented in DAMBE (Xia, 2013b; 2017a), would generate the tree in Figure 1.1a with the representatives of the three kingdoms.

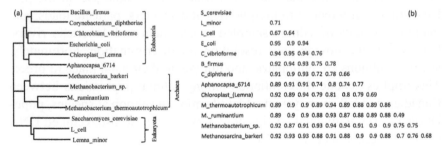

FIGURE 1.1   A distance-based tree (a) with a distance matrix (b) derived from S_{AB} values in Table 1 of Woese and Fox (1977).

While the result in Figure 1.1 by itself is not strong evidence for the three-kingdom trichotomy, it is sufficient to stimulate further investigation by scientists. This has eventually resulted in empirical substantiation of the three-kingdom classification. In today's world with almost every corner of the earth being accessible by human, it would have been quite remarkable to discover just a single new species. Imagine how electrified biologists were when a whole new domain of life was discovered!

The effort to trace history back to its origin has gradually shaped a new scientific consensus of cenancestor (Xia and Yang, 2013), the common ancestor of all forms of life. The cenancestor is neither a single cell nor a single genome, but is instead an entangled bank of heterogeneous genomes with relatively free flow of genetic information. Out of this entangled bank of frolicking genomes arose probably many evolutionary lineages with horizontal gene transfer gradually reduced and confined within individual lineages. Only three of these early lineages (Archaea, Eubacteria, and Eukarya) have known representatives survived to this day.

1.2.2 ORIGIN OF MITOCHONDRION AND PLASTIDS (e.g., CHLOROPLASTS)

One of the most fundamental questions in evolutionary biology is the origin of species, but the origin of species ultimately involves the origin of new traits, especially landmark traits such as the origin of mitochondria and chloroplasts. Mitochondria are powerhouses in eukaryotic cells, and chloroplasts allow life on earth to harvest the energy of the sun. How did eukaryotes gain these fantastic organelles?

The endosymbiosis theory, originally proposed by the Russian botanist Konstantin Mereschkowski (1905) but promoted most vigorously by Lynn Margulis (Lynn Sagan) since 1967 (Margulis, 1970; Sagan, 1967) stipulates that mitochondria and plastids in eukaryotic cells represent formerly free-living prokaryotes engulfed by other prokaryotes and reduced in the process of endosymbiosis, around 1.5 billion years ago. However, there was no direct evidence supporting the theory when Margulis articulated the theory, and her paper was rejected about 15 times before its final appearance in the *Journal of Theoretical Biology* (Margulis, 1995).

The most convincing evidence supporting the endosymbiosis theory came from phylogenetic analysis of conserved segments of small subunit (ssu) ribosomal RNA (rRNA) sequences (Gray, 1989a; 1989b; 1992; 1993) from bacteria, archaea, mitochondria of plants, fungi and animals, and chloroplasts of plants. Mitochondrial sequences from eukaryotic species appear to be monophyletic and their common ancestor clustered with Alphaproteobacteria. Similarly, chloroplast sequences clustered with cyanobacteria. The significant sequence homology represents undisputable coancestry between mitochondria and Alphaproteobacteria, and between chloroplasts and cyanobacteria.

The mitochondrial genome (mtDNA) that perhaps best represents the ancestral state is that of *Reclinomonas americana*, a heterotrophic flagellate. *R. americana* has a large mtDNA of 69,034 bp and 97 genes, including 4 genes specifying a multisubunit eubacterial-type RNA polymerase. Almost all extant mtDNA lineages can be viewed as containing a subset of its genes. It is reasonable to infer that the proto-mtDNA is very similar to that of *R. americana,* and that extant mtDNA lineages were subsequently derived from this proto-mtDNA and now exist as various degenerated forms.

The phylogenetic relationship between the mtDNA in *R. americana* and bacterial species can be reconstructed by using small and large subunit of rRNA. rRNA genes have been termed universal yardstick (Olsen and Woese, 1993) because they are shared among all living organisms and therefore can facilitate the quantification of their phylogenetic relationship. I have reconstructed such a tree based on aligned ssu rRNA from *R. americana* mtDNA and from the genome of a diverse array of bacterial species (Fig. 1.2). It is interesting to note that *R. americana* mtDNA forms a monophyletic group with Rickettsiales, an order of bacteria that are intracellular endosymbionts or pathogens of eukaryotic cells. They all exhibit genome degeneration due to the endosymbiont or parasitic lifestyle. Thus, a mitochondrion is just an extremely degenerated intracellular endosymbiont.

While the original hypothesis of mitochondrial origin by endosymbiosis does not preclude multiple mitochondrial origins through multiple endosymbiotic events, the common consensus is that the protomitochondrion originated only once, through the internalization of a Rickettsia-like bacterium into a host cell which is more likely a prokaryotic cell than a eukaryotic one (Gray, 2012; Lane and Martin, 2010). This ancestral host with the protomitochondrion subsequently diverged into numerous eukaryotic lineages. Only the *R. americana* lineage still has a mitochondrial genome retaining many of the protomitochondrial states.

I should make a point here that a biologically appealing hypothesis, such as the endosymbiosis hypothesis for the single origin of mitochondria, is often accepted without rigorous and critical examination of relevant evidence. rRNA genes, while universal, may have difficulty even for resolving shallow phylogenies such as vertebrate phylogeny (Xia et al., 2003a). If we replace the mitochondrial ssu rRNA sequence from *R. americana* in Figure 1.2 by mitochondrial ssu rRNA sequences from other species, we do not consistently observe these other mitochondrial ssu rRNA sequences clustering with species in Rickettsiales. In fact, most of them cluster with bacterial species remotely related to Rickettsiales, that is, evidence for monophyly of mitochondrial rRNA genes is extremely weak. We thus have at least two hypotheses. First, mitochondrial DNA, after accumulating so many substitutions eroding phylogenetic information, is no longer good genetic markers for reconstructing a deep phylogeny. Accepting this hypothesis would effectively rescind the phylogenetic support for the endosymbiosis hypothesis. Second, the diverse array of mitochondria, with many associated genetic codes, resulted from multiple origins involving multiple endosymbiosis events.

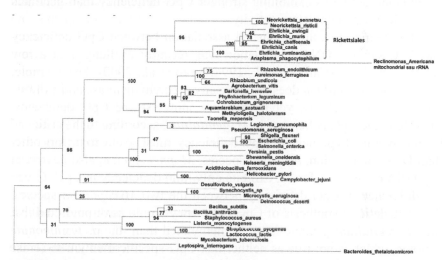

FIGURE 1.2 Phylogenetic relationship of *Reclinomonas americana* mtDNA with bacterial species, based on aligned small subunit ribosomal RNA gene sequences, reconstructed using PhyML (Guindon and Gascuel, 2003; Guindon et al., 2005) with GTR+Γ as substitution model. The values next to internal nodes are support values.

1.2.3 RESOLVING THE CONTROVERSY ON DNA METHYLATION AND CpG DEFICIENCY

CpG deficiency has been documented in a large number of genomes covering a wide taxonomic distribution (Cardon et al., 1994; Josse et al., 1961; Karlin and Burge, 1995; Karlin and Mrazek, 1996; Nussinov, 1984). DNA methylation is one of several hypotheses proposed to explain differential CpG deficiency in different genomes (Bestor and Coxon, 1993; Rideout et al., 1990; Sved and Bird, 1990). This methylation hypothesis of CpG deficiency features a plausible mechanism as follows. Methyltransferases in many species, especially those in vertebrates, appear to methylate specifically the cytosine in CpG dinucleotides, and the methylated cytosine is prone to mutate to thymine by spontaneous deamination (Frederico et al., 1990; Lindahl, 1993). This implies that CpG would gradually decay into TpG and CpA, leading to CpG deficiency, TpG and CpA surplus, and reduced genomic GC%, which has been substantiated numerous times by genomic analysis. Different genomes may differ in CpG deficiency because they differ in methylation activities, with genomes having high methylation activities exhibiting stronger CpG deficiency than genomes with little or no methylation activity.

The seemingly well-established association between CpG deficiency and CpG-specific DNA methylation was recently challenged in a few genomic analyses (Cardon et al., 1994; Goto et al., 2000). For example, *Mycoplasma genitalium* does not have any methyltransferase and exhibits no methylation activity, yet its genome shows strong CpG deficiency. Therefore, the CpG deficiency in *M. genitalium*, according to the critics of the methylation hypothesis of CpG deficiency, must be due to factors other than DNA methylation. A related species, *M. pneumoniae*, also devoid of any DNA methyltransferase, exhibits only mild deficiency in CpG. Given the difference in CpG deficiency between the two *Mycoplasma* species, the methylation hypothesis of CpG deficiency would have predicted that the *M. genitalium* genome is more methylated than the *M. pneumoniae* genome, which is not true as neither has CpG-specific methyltransferase genes. Thus, the methylation hypothesis does not seem to have any explanatory power to account for the variation in CpG deficiency, at least in the two *Mycoplasma* species.

These criticisms are derived from phylogeny-free reasoning and its fallacy is easy to see in a phylogenetic perspective (Xia, 2003). First, several lines of evidence suggest that the common ancestor of *M. genitalium* and *M. pneumoniae* have CpG-specific methyltransferases, and should have evolved strong CpG deficiency and low genomic GC% as a result of the specific DNA methylation. Methylated m^5C exists in the DNA of a close relative, *Mycoplasma hyorhinis* (Razin and Razin, 1980), suggesting the existence of methyltransferases in *M. hyorhinis*. Methyltransferases are also present in *Mycoplasma pulmonis* which contains at least four CpG-specific methyltransferase genes (Chambaud et al., 2001). Methyltransferases are also found in all surveyed species of a related genus, *Spiroplasma* (Nur et al., 1985). These lines of evidence suggest that methyltransferases are present in the ancestors of *M. genitalium* and *M. pneumoniae.*

Second, the methyltransferase-encoding *M. pulmonis* genome is even more deficient in CpG and lower in genomic GC% than *M. genitalium* or *M. pneumoniae,* consistent with the methylation hypothesis of CpG deficiency (Fig. 1.3). It is now easy to understand that, after the loss of methyltransferase in the ancestor of *M. genitalium* and *M. pneumoniae* (Fig. 1.3), both genomes would begin to accumulate CpG dinucleotides and increase their genomic GC%. However, the evolutionary rate is much faster in *M. pneumoniae* than in *M. genitanlium* based on the comparison of a large number of protein-coding genes (Xia, 2003). So *M. pneumoniae* regained CpG dinucleotide and genomic GC% much faster than *M. genitalium* whose slow rate of genomic evolution allows it to retain the ancestral low CpG phenotype better than *M. pneumoniae.* In short, the Mycoplasma genomic data that originally seem to contradict the methylation hypothesis actually provide strong support for the methylation hypothesis when phylogeny-based genomic comparisons are made.

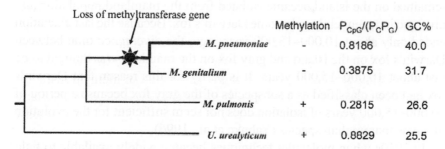

FIGURE 1.3 Phylogenetic tree of *Mycoplasma pneumoniae, M. genitalium,* and their relatives, together with the presence (+) or absence (−) of CpG-specific methylation, $P_{CpG}/(P_C P_G)$ as a measure of CpG deficiency, and genomic GC%. *M. pneumoniae* evolves faster and has a longer branch than *M. genitalium.* Cytosine methylation in *U. urealyticum* is not CpG specific, so it does not reduce CpG dinucleotide but does reduces GC% in the genome.

One might note that *Ureaplasma urealyticum* in Figure 1.3 is not deficient in CpG because its $P_{CpG}/(P_C P_G)$ ratio is close to 1, yet its genomic GC% is the lowest. Has its low genomic GC% resulted from CpG-specific DNA methylation? If yes, then why doesn't the genome exhibit CpG deficiency? It turns out that *U. urealyticum* has C-specific, but not CpG-specific, methyltransferase, so the genome of *U. urealyticum* is expected, and indeed observed, to have low CG% (because of the methylation-mediated C→T mutation) but not a low $P_{CpG}/(P_C P_G)$ ratio. The methyltransferase gene from *U. urealyticum* is not homologous to those from *M. pulmonis*.

1.2.4   CHILOÉ ISLAND AND DARWIN'S FOX

Off the western coast of South America is Chiloé Island on which a special kind of fox, named Darwin's fox (*Dusicyon fulvipes*), was found. On the mainland opposite the island thrives another fox species, the gray fox (*Urocyon cinereoargenteus*). For a long time it has been thought that Darwin's fox has descended from the gray fox. In other words, during the Quaternary glaciation period with a low sea level (because much water was retained on land in the form of ice sheets), Chiloé Island, just slightly north of the northern edge of glaciation, was connected to the mainland. Gray foxes were expected to roam the Chilean Coast Range including Chiloé Island. When glaciation period ended, the ice sheets returned to the ocean and sea level rose to isolate the island from the mainland. Gray foxes that remained on the island became isolated from the mainland population and diverged independently to become Darwin's fox. Because the last glaciation ended only about 10,000–15,000 years ago, the divergence time between Darwin's fox on the island and gray fox on the mainland was thought to be just about 10,000–15,000 years. It is partly for this reason that Darwin's fox had been classified as a subspecies of the gray fox because a period of 10,000–15,000 years of isolation does not seem sufficient for the evolution of a new mammalian species (Yahnke et al., 1996).

   In 1980s when molecular techniques became widely available to field biologists, researchers began to reconstruct phylogenetic trees for various fox species and to date their speciation events. They were surprised to find that the divergence time between Darwin's fox and the gray fox was about a million years, much longer than the originally hypothesized 10,000–15,000 years. This is clearly incompatible with the original hypothesis that Darwin's fox evolved from gray fox after the isolation of Chiloé Island from the mainland at the end of last glaciation period.

   One possible hypothesis is that Darwin's fox had diverged from the gray fox for a long time on the mainland, long before the geographic separation of Chiloé Island from the mainland. During the last glaciation period, some Darwin's foxes, not gray foxes, remained on the island and became isolated from the mainland population of Darwin's fox. Meanwhile, the mainland population of Darwin's fox had gone extinct in competition against the gray fox.

This is a bold hypothesis. It predicted the existence of a species on the mainland that nobody had seen. However, researchers had faith in the prediction and went on looking for historical footprints (e.g., fossils) of Darwin's fox left on the mainland. It is in search of these footprints that researchers were pleasantly surprised to find a living population of Darwin's fox on the mainland. This discovery, in my opinion, rivals the success of predicting the existence of an unseen planet based on the orbits of other visible planets in astrophysics.

You might be thinking privately that the researchers, out of desperation to support their hypothesis, might have sneaked onto the island, caught some Darwin's foxes, transported them to the mainland, and then declared "Lo and behold ..." However, the molecular clock can again come to their rescue. If they were indeed guilty of the crime, then there would be no genetic variation between the island population and the mainland population. However, if the island population has been isolated from the main population for 1,000–15,000 years, then there should be genetic variation consistent with such isolation.

The dating evidence that Darwin's fox diverged from the gray fox for about a million years immediately raised Darwin's fox not only from subspecies to species, but also to a high conservation status because the population has only about 500 individuals. Keep in mind that species conservation has two essential criteria. The first is that the species is indeed endangered. The second is genetic uniqueness. If Darwin's fox diverged from gray fox for only 10,000–15,000, then it will not be considered genetically unique enough for a high conservation status. A divergence time of a million years makes all the differences. While the exact sequence of events related to the phylogenetic research on Darwin's fox is difficult to reconstruct, the potential of molecular phylogenetics in science and in species conservation is clearly visible.

1.3 TWO KEY OBJECTIVES OF MOLECULAR PHYLOGENETICS

Molecular phylogenetics has two objectives (Fig. 1.4): (1) characterizing the branching patterns (cladogenic events, specifically the speciation and gene duplication events) in evolution and (2) dating of these speciation or gene duplication events that may help us understand origin of species and functional divergence of duplicated genes (Vlasschaert et al., 2017; Vlasschaert et al., 2015). Phylogenetics can also help us to identify common ancestors such as the mitochondrial "Eve" (because mitochondrial genomes in mammals are maternally inherited) or the Y-chromosome "Adam" (because human Y-chromosome is passed down from father to son). The universal common ancestor for all living organisms is termed cenancestor which is assumed to exist on the basis of extensive sharing of inferred homologous characters among representatives of living cellular organisms, such as the near universal genetic code, the concordance of phylogenetic trees from different genes, the sharing of fundamental biochemical processes, and the existence of numerous transitional fossils. Cenancestor is a logical necessity if the cellular structure originated only once, and if we assume to be true the cell theory stating that new cells are created only by old cells dividing into two. One early concept of cenancestor is a genome that codes a minimal set of core genes essential for cellular life (the minimal genome) and from which all other genomes are derived. However, few genes are shared universally because a biological function can often be performed by unrelated genes. Even if such a set of core genes can be identified, the identification and dating of the cenancestor is difficult because of the lack of a universal global molecular clock and the rampant horizontal gene transfer.

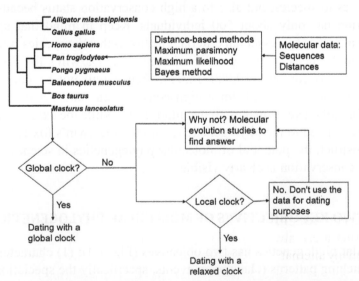

FIGURE 1.4   High-level summary of molecular phylogenetics: defining branch patterns and dating internal nodes.

Note that the first objective of molecular phylogenetics, i.e., characterizing the branching patterns (cladogenic events, specifically the speciation and gene duplication events) in evolution involves two types of genes, orthologous and paralogous genes. Paralogous genes arose by gene duplication within a lineage, e.g., α-globin and β-globin genes in a mouse genome, but orthologous genes are more difficult to define. In this book, I impose a strong definition of orthologous genes, that is, they are single-copy genes in different genomes resulting from speciation, descending from a common ancestral genome, and having never undergone gene duplication, that is, their "single-copy" is an ancestral character that does not result from gene duplication and then gene loss leading to the survival of a single copy. The *ERN1* gene from human and mouse are orthologous because the gene has no paralogues not only among mammals, but also among vertebrates, suggesting an extremely low likelihood of the gene ever being duplicated. Species trees should only be inferred from orthologous genes, while gene duplication events are inferred from paralogous genes by studying genes in a gene family (which is a collection of all homologous genes in one genome) from multiple lineages, ideally with one or more lineages that branched out before any gene duplication events and consequently retain the single-copy ancestral status.

Both species events and gene duplication events contribute to biodiversity and represent parts of natural history. Molecular phylogenetics aims to trace natural history as close as possible to the cenancestor and to reconstruct what experiments nature has performed over billions of years. Such knowledge will not only enlighten us on the origin and evolution of biodiversity, but also guide us toward a more profitable and more harmonious way of life. This last sentence I borrowed from an Evangelical preacher because it sounds very profound.

Molecular phylogenetics almost always start with compilation of homologous sequences from OTUs (optional taxonomic units such as species), alignment of the sequences to identify homologous sites and inference of phylogenetic relationships among the OTUs represented by the sequences. There could be many multiple sequence alignments and phylogenetic trees from even a single set of homologous sequences, so some criteria are always necessary for us to choose the best alignment among many alternative alignments, and the best tree among many possible trees. One may go so far as to claim that the entire field of molecular phylogenetics is about formulating, justifying, and applying these criteria. Pay particular attention to these criteria in reading the following chapters.

KEYWORDS

- **three kingdoms**
- **endosymbiosis**
- **mitochondria**
- **DNA methylation**
- **Darwin's fox**

CHAPTER 2

Sequence Alignment Algorithms

ABSTRACT

Accuracy of molecular phylogenetic analysis depends on correct identification of homologous sites. Sequence alignment serves two purposes: Global alignment is mainly for identifying site homology between sequences to facilitate the inference of ancestral-descendant relationships and local alignment mainly for identifying sequence similarities that may be due to either coancestry or convergence. I illustrate, with published data, how misalignment can distort phylogenetic signal. Sequences can be aligned in many different ways, so a criterion is needed for choosing the best alignment. Operationally, the best alignment is one with highest alignment score for a given scoring scheme. Dynamic programming algorithm guarantees to find the best alignment with the highest alignment score. It is illustrated in detail for pairwise alignment and profile alignment with both constant gap penalty and affine function gap penalty, followed by progressive multiple sequence alignment using a guide tree, and by how to align protein-coding nucleotide sequences against aligned amino acid sequences. PAM and BLOSUM matrices, which are typically derived from protein alignments, are derived from both nucleotide and amino acid sequences. The effect of mutation, selection, and amino acid dissimilarities on substitution frequencies were illustrated and discussed.

Almost all molecular phylogenetic studies start with sequence alignment of homologous sequences. Global sequence alignment (Needleman and Wunsch, 1970) and local sequence alignment (Smith and Waterman, 1981) by dynamic programming represent the core algorithms for sequence alignment. Dynamic programming algorithms constitute a general class of algorithms not only used in sequence alignment but also in many other applications. For example, the Viterbi algorithm and the forward algorithm used in hidden Markov models (HMM), which were numerically illustrated in detail (Xia, 2018a, Chapter 7) are also dynamic programming algorithms, so are Fitch and Sankoff algorithms for maximum parsimony (MP) and the pruning algorithm for maximum likelihood (ML) reconstruction of phylogenetic trees. We will cover MP and ML algorithms in great numerical detail latter. Learning the dynamic programming algorithms used in sequence alignment paves the way for more advanced applications in later chapters.

This chapter covers (1) pairwise global and local alignment by dynamic programming with different scoring schemes, from the simplest scoring scheme with two-valued match/mismatch scores and constant gap penalties, to the more useful scoring schemes with match-mismatch (MM) matrices and affine function gap penalties, (2) detailed derivation of PAM and BLOSUM matrices, (3) profile alignment between one sequence and a set of aligned sequences which is essential for practical implementation of multiple sequence alignment (MSA), and (4) multiple alignment that is reduced to pairwise alignment and profile alignment by using a guide tree. Most textbooks on bioinformatics omit the dynamic programming algorithm using affine function gap penalty (Gotoh, 1982) and no textbook I know of includes any detailed explanation of profile alignment. This chapter is intended to fill the gap.

The objective of sequence alignment is to identify homologous sites among sequences so that functional and phylogenetic inferences can be made. For example, the multiple alignments of FoxL2 protein (Fig. 2.1) show a highly conserved and positively charged domain (the forkhead domain, with many positively charged residues, such as R and K) which should have strong electrostatic interactions with negatively charged molecules such as nucleic acids. It was found that FoxL2 is indeed a nuclear transcription factor with the forkhead domain being DNA-binding (Baron et al., 2004; Cocquet et al., 2003). Another feature standing out from the alignment is the conserved polyalanine tract of exactly 14 residues (Fig. 2.1). Indeed, lengthening the polyalanine tract is frequently associated with the blepharophimosis syndrome (De Baere et al., 2002). From a phylogenetic point of view, one can immediately see the difference between the mammalian sequences (first seven in Fig. 2.1) and the fish sequences (the last three in Fig. 2.1).

While biological insights can often be derived directly from MSA, the main objective of MSA is to build phylogenetic trees so as to make phylogeny-based inferences. Inaccurate multiple alignments can introduce not only phylogenetic noise but also distort phylogenetic signals. This I illustrate below based on a reanalysis by Noah et al. (2020) of aligned sequences from a paper published in the journal *Nature*.

```
M AEKRLTLSGIYQYIIAKFPFYEKNKKGWQNSIRHNLSLNECFIKVPREGGGERKGNYWTLDPACEDMFEKGNYRRRRRMKRPFRP
R AEKRLTLSGIYQYIIAKFPFYEKNKKGWQNSIRHNLSLNECFIKVPREGGGERKGNYWTLDPACEDMFEKGNYRRRRRMKRPFRP
B AEKRLTLSGIYQYIIAKFPFYEKNKKGWQNSIRHNLSLNECFIKVPREGGGERKGNYWTLDPACEDMFEKGNYRRRRRMKRPFRP
C AEKRLTLSGIYQYIIAKFPFYEKNKKGWQNSIRHNLSLNECFIKVPREGGGERKGNYWTLDPACEDMFEKGNYRRRRRMKRPFRP
S AEKRLTLSGIYQYIIAKFPFYEKNKKGWQNSIRHNLSLNECFIKVPREGGGERKGNYWTLDPACEDMFEKGNYRRRRRMKRPFRP
H AEKRLTLSGIYQYIIAKFPFYEKNKKGWQNSIRHNLSLNECFIKVPREGGGERKGNYWTLDPACEDMFEKGNYRRRRRMKRPFRP
O AEKRLTLSGIYQYIIAKFPFYEKNKKGWQNSIRHNLSLNECFIKVPREGGGERKGNYWTLDPACEDMFEKGNYRRRRRMKRPFRP
F SEKRLTLSGIYQYIISKFPFYEKNKKGWQNSIRHNLSLNECFIKVPREGGGERKGNYWTLDPACEDMFEKGNYRRRRRMKRPFRP
T SEKRLTLSGIYQYIISKFPFYEKNKKGWQNSIRHNLSLNECFIKVPREGGGERKGNYWTLDPACEDMFEKGNYRRRRRMKRPFRP
D SEKRLTLSGIYQYIISKFPFYEKNKKGWQNSIRHNLSLNECFIKVPREGGGERKGNYWTLDPACEDMFEKGNYRRRRRMKRPFRP
  ************* **********************************************************************

M PPAHFQPGKGLFGSGGAAGGCGVPGAGADGYGYLAPPKYLQSGFLNNSWPLPQPPSPMPYASCQMAAAAAAAAAAAAAAGPGSPG
R PPAHFQPGKGLFGSGGGAGGCGVPGAGADGYGYLAPPKYLQSGFLNNSWPLPQPPSPMPYASCQMAAAAAAAAAAAAAAGPGSPG
B PPAHFQPGKGLFGAGGAAGGCGVAGAGADGYGYLAPPKYLQSGFLNNSWPLPQPPSPMPYASCQMAAAAAAAAAAAAAAGPGSPG
C PPAHFQPGKGLFGAGGAAGGCGVAGAGADGYGYLAPPKYLQSGFLNNSWPLPQPPSPMPYASCQMAAAAAAAAAAAAAAGPGSPG
S PPAHFQPGKGLFGAGGAAGGCGVAGAGADGYGYLAPPKYLQSGFLNNSWPLPQPPSPMPYASCQMAAAAAAAAAAAAAAGPGSPG
H PPAHFQPGKGLFGAGGAAGGCGVAGAGADGYGYLAPPKYLQSGFLNNSWPLPQPPSPMPYASCQMAAAAAAAAAAAAAAGPGSPG
O PPAHFQPGKGLFGAAGAAGGCGVAGAGADGYGYLAPPKYLQSGFLNNSWPLPQPPSPMPYASCQMAAAAAAAAAAAAAAGPGSPG
F PPTHFQPGKSLFG--------------GDGYGYLSPPKYLQSSFMNNSWSLGQPPAPMSYTSCQMASGNVSPVN----------
T PPTHFQPGKSLFG--------------GDGYGYLSPPKYLQSSFMNNSWSLGQPPPPMSYTSCQMASGNVSPVN-----------
D PPTHFQPGKSLFG--------------GEGYGYLSPPKYLQSGFINNSWS----PAPMSYTSCQVSSGSVSPVN-----------
  ** ********    ***** ******* * ****    * ** *.***
```

FIGURE 2.1 Partial multiple alignments of partial FoxL2 protein of 10 vertebrate species. M: *Mus musculus*, mouse (GenBank AI: AF522275); R: *Rattus norvegicus*, rat (AI: AC105826); B: *Bos taurus*, cow (AI: AY340970); C: *Capra hircus*, goat (AI: AY112725); S: *Sus scrofa*, pig (AI: AY340971); H: *Homo sapiens*, human (AI: AF301906); O: *Oryctolagus cuniculus*, rabbit (AI: AY340972); F: *Fugu rubripes*, pufferfish (AI: Scaffold_8165/Prot JGI_24134); T: *Tetraodon nigroviridis*, tetraodon; and D: *Danio rerio*, zebrafish. Shown are the part of the highly conserved and positively charged forkhead domain and its downstream polyalanine tract (in bold) which is missing in the three fish species.

2.1 POOR ALIGNMENT INTRODUCES NOT ONLY NOISE BUT ALSO PHYLOGENETIC BIAS

Reliable MSA is difficult to obtain with divergent lineages because of erosion of homology over time (Blackburne and Whelan, 2013; Edgar and Batzoglou, 2006; Herman et al., 2014; Kumar and Filipski, 2007; Lunter et al., 2008; Wong et al., 2008; Xia, 2016). A poor alignment typically leads to bias and inaccuracy in phylogenetic estimation (Blackburne and Whelan, 2013; Kumar and Filipski, 2007; Wong et al., 2008; Xia et al., 2003a). There are many publications with poor MSA. The examples of alignment errors shown here are taken from the Online Supplemental file nature08742-s2.nex in Regier et al. (2010).

2.1.1   PHYLOGENETIC NOISE INTRODUCED BY POOR ALIGNMENT

A sample of the alignment from Regier et al. (2010) is shown in Figure 2.2a, together with an alternative alignment (Fig. 2.1b) which is clearly more preferable. The phylogenetic impact of a poor alignment is often unpredictable. If a phylogenetic analysis includes the poorly aligned region in Figure 2.2a, then the evolutionary distance among the species or branch length in the tree will be overestimated. If one excludes this poorly aligned region, then the distances and branch lengths may be underestimated. Regier et al. (2010) kept the poorly aligned region in nucleotide-based phylogenetic analysis, which generated their main results in their Figure 2.1, but excluded the region in amino acid-based analysis. While the alignment in Figure 2.2b is visibly better than that in Figure 2.2a, we do need to have a sensible criterion for evaluating different alignments. We will learn to use pairwise alignment score and its derivatives to evaluate the quality of sequence alignment.

```
(a)              190        200        210
                ---|----|----|----|----|----...
FauNEOPT      GAUGUUCCACCUCCAGUA---GAAUUUU...
ApaukNEOPT  GGGCGCCUCCCGGUA--------GAACUGU...
CpoNEOPT   GGC GGCAAGCAACCUGUG------GAACUGU...
PquNEOPT      AACGGUCGCGCGCCGGUC---GAGCUGU...
PamNEOPT      GACACACCACCUCCAGUG---GAAUUCU...
AdoNEOPT      AAUUUGCCACCUCCA---GUGGAGUUUU...

(b)
FauNEOPT      GAUGUUCCACCUCCAGUAGAAUUUU...
ApaukNEOPT    ---GGYCGCCUCCCGGUAGAACUGU...
CpoNEOPT      GGCGGCAAGCAACCUGUGGAACUGU...
PquNEOPT      AACGGUCGCGCGCCGGUCGAGCUGU...
PamNEOPT      GACACACCACCUCCAGUGGAAUUCU...
AdoNEOPT      AAUUUGCCACCUCCAGUGGAGUUUU...
```

FIGURE 2.2   Part of multiple alignments for a subset of six species (a) taken from the supplementary file (nature08742-s2.nex) in Regier et al. (2010). Realignment by MAFFT with the optimized options is shown in (b). Note that the two codons highlighted in red (coding for amino acids Pro and Val) are identical among the six species. Dots in (b) represent nucleotides not present in (a).

2.1.2 POOR ALIGNMENT CAN INTRODUCE PHYLOGENETIC BIAS

The original alignment in Regier et al. (2010) in the left panel of Figure 2.3 suggests a phylogenetic similarity between the first nine species and the last two species, with the two Archeognatha species (PsaARCHEO for *Pedetontus saltator* and MbaARCHEO for *Machiloides banksi*) and a copepod (A369COPE for *Acanthocyclops vernalis*) being different. However, the last codon in red (Fig. 2.3) is a lysine codon in all sequences, and the second last is a threonine codon in all but one sequence (A369COPE). The evidence of homology is strong among these codon sites that they should really be aligned as shown in the right panel of Figure 2.3. Thus, the difference of the three species (PsaARCHEO, MbaARCHEO, A369COPE) from the rest in the original alignment (left panel of Fig. 2.3) is an alignment artifact. Of course, if these three species happen to be phylogenetically more closely related to each other than to the rest, then the wrong alignment will in fact be more efficient in recovering the true tree, just as the MP method will be more efficient in recovering the true tree if two sister lineages happen to have long branches. However, as I emphasized before (Xia, 2014), such efficiency is purchased with illegal phylogenetic currency.

A similar situation is shown in the top panel of Figure 2.4 where the alignment from Regier et al. (2010) introduced an alignment artifact increasing the distance between the first pycnogonid species (TorPYCNO for *Tanystylum orbiculare*) and the three other pycnogonid species. The 3-nt deletion in the first sequence (TorPYCNO) is misplaced, with the alignment in the bottom of Figure 2.4 having high alignment scores by any reasonable scoring scheme. The "big data" approach is disastrous for science because authors often do not have enough resources for data validation, neither do reviewers.

```
PamNEOPT    AGAACACGAGUUACCAAA---AUGUUGUGCAU   PamNEOPT    ...AGAACACGAGUUACCAAAAUGUUGUGCAU
MayEPHEM    AGAUCUCGCGUCACCAAA---AUGUUAUGUCA   MayEPHEM    ...AGAUCUCGCGUCACCAAAAUGUUAUGUCA
EinEPHEM    AGAACCAGAGUUACCAAA---AUUUUAUGUAU   EinEPHEM    ...AGAACCAGAGUUACCAAAAUUUUAUGUAU
IveODONAT   AGAAGGACUCUCACUAAA---AUGCUUUGUAU   IveODONAT   ...AGAAGGACUCUCACUAAAAUGCUUUGUAU
LlyODONAT   CGGAGGAAUAUAACUAAG---AUGCUUUGUUU   LlyODONAT   ...CGGAGGAAUAUAACUAAGAUGCUUUGUUU
StuREMI     AGGAAAAGACUUACCAAA---AUGCUGUGUAU   StuREMI     ...AGGAAAAGACUUACCAAAAUGCUGUGUAU
CliZYGEN    AGGACGAGAGUCACUAAA---AUGCUUUGCAU   CliZYGEN    ...AGGACGAGAGUCACUAAAAUGCUUUGCAU
NmeZYGEN    AGAUCAAGGGUCACAAAG---AUGUUGUGUAU   NmeZYGEN    ...AGAUCAAGGGUCACAAAGAUGUUGUGUAU
JapDIPLUR   AGGACGACAGUGACCAAG---CUCCUGUGCCA   JapDIPLUR   ...AGGACGACAGUGACCAAGCUCCUGUGCCA
PsaARCHEO   GCCAGAACAAGAGUAACAAAAAUGCUGUGUAU   PsaARCHEO   GCCAGAACAAGAGUAACAAAAAUGCUGUGUAU
MbaARCHEO   GCCAGAACGAGAGUAACAAAAAUGUUGUGUAU   MbaARCHEO   GCCAGAACGAGAGUAACAAAAAUGUUGUGUAU
A369COPE    AGCGUAACCAGGCGGAGCAAGCUGUUGUGCAA   A369COPE    AGCGUAACCAGGCGGAGCAAGCUGUUGUGCAA
DtyMYSTACO  AGGAGAAGGUGCACCAAA---CUACUCUGUCA   DtyMYSTACO  ...AGGAGAAGGUGCACCAAACUACUCUGUCA
NamDIPLO    AGGAAAAGAUUUACAAAA---UUAUUAUGCCA   NamDIPLO    ...AGGAAAAGAUUUACAAAAUUAUUAUGCCA
```

FIGURE 2.3 Poor alignment can distort phylogenetic signals. The left alignment, taken from the supplementary file (nature08742-s2.nex) in Regier et al. (2010), confers undue similarity between the first nine and the last two sequences (DtyMYSTACO and NamDIPLO). An alternative alignment is shown at right, which is better by any alignment criterion.

```
TorPYCNO    GCTGTTTTAGGTAAGGTAGCAGCCGAAAAA---TGGGCTGATGTGGTCATTGCT
AeliPYCNO   TCTATAATAGGAAAAGTTTCT---TCTGAAAAATGGGCAGATGTTGTAATTGCA
AhiPYCNO    GCCGTTACCGGAAAGGTTTCT---TCCGATAAGTGGGCAGATGTTGTCATTGCA
Col2PYCNO   GCAATAATTGGTAAGATTCCA---GATAGCAAGTGGAGTGAAGTTGTCCTTGCA

TorPYCNO    GCTGTTTTAGGTAAGGTAGCAGCCGAAAAATGGGCTGATGTGGTCATTGCT
AeliPYCNO   TCTATAATAGGAAAAGTTTCTTCTGAAAAATGGGCAGATGTTGTAATTGCA
AhiPYCNO    GCCGTTACCGGAAAGGTTTCTTCCGATAAGTGGGCAGATGTTGTCATTGCA
Col2PYCNO   GCAATAATTGGTAAGATTCCAGATAGCAAGTGGAGTGAAGTTGTCCTTGCA
```

FIGURE 2.4   Poor alignment at the top, taken from the supplementary file (nature08742-s2. nex) in Regier et al. (2010), unnecessarily increase the distance between TorPYCNO and the three other Pycnogonid species, with the improved alignment at the bottom.

2.1.3   POOR ALIGNMENT LEADS TO UNNECESSARY LOSS OF PHYLOGENETIC SIGNALS

Because of the poor alignment illustrated above, some parts in the MSA were deemed unalignable by Regier et al. (2010) and removed from the translated amino acid sequences for phylogenetic analysis based on amino acid sequences. For example, the shaded segment in Figure 2.5a was deleted. This deletion is unnecessary because sequence homology is identifiable as shown in Figure 2.5b. Deleting phylogenetically significant signals reduces the phylogenetic resolution. However, the deletion of unalignable segments by Regier et al. (2010) is not consistent. While the shaded segment in Figure 2.5a is deleted, the undesirable alignment in Figure 2.2a remains in their degenerated sequence file (nature08742-s3Degen1.nex) used to generate their main phylogenetic results in their Figure 1.

I finally wish to make two points. First, the data set with the many alignment problems is still often incorporated into still larger data set without realignment, a common practice in today's phylogenetic reconstruction that erodes the credibility of published phylogenetic results and degrades this branch of science that used to be more rigorous. Second, scientists are deprived of the responsibility of being the custodians of their own science by academic journals, so fewer and fewer scientists really care much about their academic home. What matters today is to create a data set that is big, really big, and so big that reviewers will never be able to find time to check the quality of the data or details of the analysis.

(a)
```
                10        20        30        40        50        60
     ----|----|----|----|----|----|----|----|----|----|----|----|--
FauNEOPT   RHASNMGWLNFTFSLQKSFKSLFGEKLEVVRTHQQQENLKFMAHFKRQFVIHQGKRKEILPS
ApaukNEOPT RRAPNMGWLTFTFGLERKFKQLCK-RLEVVRTHQQQETLKFMSHFHRRRFIIKDGKRNDKPEG
CpoNEOPT   RRAPNMGWLTFTFGLERKFKQLCK-RLEVVRTHQQQESLKFMSHFHRRRFIIRDGKRNQPPEG
PquNEOPT   RHAPNMGWLTFTFGLERKFKSLCT-RLEVVRTHQQQENLKFMAHFNRRFIIKEGKRNGDNKV
PamNEOPT   REASNMGWLTFTFSLQKKFKSLFGEKLEVVRTHQQQENLKFMAHFKRKFIIHQGKRKETLPR
AdoNEOPT   REASNMGWLTFTFSLQKKFKSLFGEKLEVIRTHQQQENLKFMAHFKRKFVIHQGKRKEIPDP
           * *  ***** *** *    ** *    *** ******* **** ** * * *  ***
```

```
                70        80        90       100       110       120
     --|----|----|----|----|----|----|----|----|----|----|----|----
FauNEOPT   DVPPPV-EFYHLRSNGSALCTRLIQIRPDASALNSQFCYILKVPLNNQEEEPSGIVYVWIGS
ApaukNEOPT RLPV---ELFELRSNGSALCTRLIQVKADATQLNSAFCYILNVPLEGNSDTSSAIVYAWIGS
CpoNEOPT   GKQPV--ELFELRSNGSALCTRLVQVKADAAQXNSAFCYILNVPLEGANDTSSAIVYAWIGS
PquNEOPT   NGRAPV-ELYELRSNGSALCTRLVQVRADAAQLNSCFCYILNVPLEGADDTXSAIVYVWVGS
PamNEOPT   DTPPPV-EFYHLRSNGSPLCTRLIQIKPDATALNPAFTYILKVPFDNEEQ--SGIVYVWIGS
AdoNEOPT   NLPPP-VEFYHLRSNSSSLCTRLIQIKPDAAALNSAFCYILKVPLNKEEQ--TGIVYVWIGS
           *    **** * ***** *   **  *  * *** **     *** * **
```

(b)
```
FauNEOPT   LKFMAHFKRQFVIHQGKRKEILPSDVPPPVEFYHLRSNGSALCTRLIQIRPDASALNSQFCY
ApaukNEOPT LKFMSHFHRRRFIIKDGKRNDKPE--GRLPVELFELRSNGSALCTRLIQVKADATQLNSAFCY
CpoNEOPT   LKFMSHFHRRRFIIRDGKRNQPPE-GGKQPVELFELRSNGSALCTRLVQVKADAAQXNSAFCY
PquNEOPT   LKFMAHFNRRFIIKEGKRNGDNKVNGRAPVELYELRSNGSALCTRLVQVRADAAQLNSCFCY
PamNEOPT   LKFMAHFKRKFIIHQGKRKETLPRDTPPPVEFYHLRSNGSPLCTRLIQIKPDATALNPAFTY
AdoNEOPT   LKFMAHFKRKFVIHQGKRKEIPDPNLPPPVEFYHLRSNSSSLCTRLIQIKPDAAALNSAFCY
           **** ** * * *  ***       ***   **** * ***** *   **    *  * *
```

FIGURE 2.5 Unnecessary deletion of phylogenetically informative data. (a) Partial amino acid sequences translated from the codon sequences in the supplementary file (nature08742-s2.nex) in Regier et al. (2010). The shaded segments, including the amino acid Eat labeled site 70, were deemed by Regier et al. (2010) as unalignable and removed in the final amino acid sequence alignment for phylogenetic analysis. (b) Realigned sequences.

2.2 PAIRWISE ALIGNMENT

Given two strings S ($=s_1s_2...s_n$) and T ($=t_1t_2...t_m$), a pairwise alignment of S and T is defined as an ordered set of pairings of (s_i, t_j) and of gaps $(s_i,-)$ and $(-,t_j)$, with the constraint that the alignment is reduced to the two original strings when all gaps in the alignment are deleted. A prefix of S, specified here as S_i, is a substring of S equal to $s_1s_2...s_i$, where $i \le n$. Figure 2.6 shows two different alignments from the same set of two sequences.

```
Alignment 1:  ACCCAGGGCTTA
              |||| ||   |
              ACCCGGGCTTAG

Alignment 2:  ACCCAGGGCTTA-
              ||||  |||||||
              ACCC-GGGCTTAG
```

FIGURE 2.6 Two sequences in two different alignments implying different homology sites, e.g., A and G at the 5th site in the Alignment 1 is assumed to be homologous but the same A and G are not homologous in Alignment 2.

An optimal alignment is operationally defined as the pairwise alignment with the highest alignment score for a given scoring scheme. For this reason, an optimal alignment is meaningless without specifying the scoring scheme. A scoring scheme has two components. One is the score for the two matching characters, e.g., we may give 2 to a match nucleotide pair, e.g., A/A in the first site of the two sequences and −1 to a mismatched nucleotide pair, e.g., A and G at 5th site in Alignment 1. Thus, for a match score of 2 and a mismatch score of −1, Alignment 1, with 7 matches and 5 mismatches, would have an alignment score of $7 \times 2 + 5 \times (-1) = 9$. The other component of a scoring scheme is gap penalty, which we need in order to obtain an alignment score for Alignment 2 in Figure 2.6. Suppose we take the simplest approach with constant gap penalty and penalize a gap with −2. With the previous match score of 2, mismatch score of −1, and a constant gap penalty of −2, the alignment score for Alignment 2, which has 11 matches, 0 mismatch, and 2 gaps, is $11 \times 2 + 0 \times (-1) + 2 \times (-2) = 18$. Thus, with the given scoring scheme, Alignment 2 is better than Alignment 1. Note that which alignment is better depends on scoring scheme. The scoring scheme we used favors Alignment 2 against Alignment 1. However, if we have a scoring scheme that penalizes gaps heavily, e.g., −7 for a gap, then Alignment 1 will have higher alignment score than Alignment 2. Therefore, when we use a criterion for making a choice, we often need to justify our criterion.

Alignment by dynamic programming guarantees that for a given scoring scheme the resulting alignment has the highest alignment score, or one of the highest alignment scores when there are equally optimal alignments. We will first illustrate the global pairwise alignment (Needleman and Wunsch, 1970) followed by a brief outline of the differences between global and local pairwise alignment (Smith and Waterman, 1981). Local sequence alignment is for searching local similarities between sequences, e.g., homeobox genes which are not similar globally but all share a very similar homeodomain motif.

Here we will first learn a simple dynamic programming algorithm for pairwise alignment using a simple scoring scheme with constant gap penalty. The simple scoring scheme is then extended in two ways, first by introducing a similarity matrix to replace match and mismatch scores and second by introducing the affine function to better approximate the origin of the insertion and deletion during sequence evolution. My experience is that an average student can understand pairwise alignment with constant gap penalty but only a very good student can understand the two extensions.

2.2.1 GLOBAL ALIGNMENT WITH CONSTANT GAP PENALTY

Suppose we want to align two sequences S and T with $S = \text{ACGT}$ and $T = \text{ACGGCT}$. Practical sequence alignment typically involves sequences that are much longer, but the computation is the same. If you learned how to align these two short sequences, you know how to align sequences of any lengths.

Dynamic programming for sequence alignment needs a scoring scheme. We will use a simple one with a constant gap penalty (G) of -2, a match score (s_{ii}, where the subscript 'ii' indicates two identical nucleotides) of 2 and a mismatch score (s_{ij}, where the subscript ij indicates two different nucleotides) of -1. Global alignment with the dynamic programming approach is illustrated numerically in Figure 2.7. One of the two sequences occupies the top row and will be referred to hereafter as the row sequence (sequence S in our example). The other sequence occupies the first column and will be referred to hereafter as the column sequence (sequence T in our example).

We need to fill in two matrices. The first is the scoring matrix (SM) to obtain the alignment score, with the dimensions ($n+1$, $m+1$). A value in row i and column j in the scoring matrix ($SM_{i,j}$) is the alignment score between prefixes S_j and T_i. The second is the backtrack matrix needed to obtain the actual alignment, with the dimensions (n,m). In Figure 2.7A, the two matrices are superimposed, with the scoring matrix being the numbers and the backtrack matrix being made of arrows. The backtrack matrix is sometimes called the traceback matrix.

The first row ($SM_{0,j}$) and the first column ($SM_{i,0}$) of the scoring matrix is filled with $i \times G$ (where $i = 0, 1, ..., n$) and $j \times G$ (where $j = 0, 1, ..., m$), respectively. They represent consecutive insertion of gaps. For example,

$SM_{0,4} = -8$ (Fig. 2.7) implies the alignment of S against four consecutive gaps, so you get an alignment score of -8 (with gap penalty of -2). Similarly, $SM_{6,0} = -12$ (Fig. 2.7) implies the alignment of T with six consecutive gaps.

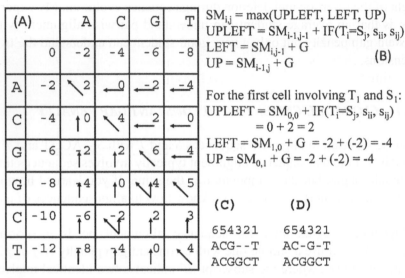

FIGURE 2.7 Aligning sequences S (Top row) and T (left column) by dynamic programming, with the score and the backtrack matrices superimposed (A). The scoring scheme has a match score of 2, mismatch score of -1 and constant gap penalty of -2. Other than the first row and first column, each cell involves computing three values and filling the cell by the maximum of the three (B). The backtrack matrix, made of all arrows in (A), is for obtaining sequence alignments (C and D), where the numbers in the first row show the order of obtaining the alignment site by site from the last to the first by backtracking.

For each of the other $SM_{i,j}$ values, we need to compute three values designated as UPLEFT, LEFT, and UP specified in Figure 2.7B. The first cell corresponds to T_1 and S_1 (Fig. 2.7B), both being A, with its UPLEFT, LEFT, and UP values being 2, -4, and -4, respectively. The maximum of these three values is UPLEFT ($=2$), so $SM_{1,1} = 2$, and we put an upleft arrow in the cell (Fig. 2.7). If LEFT (or UP) happened to be the maximum of the three, we would have put the LEFT (or UP) value in the cell and add a left-pointing (or up-pointing) arrow in the corresponding cell in the backtrack matrix.

The calculation of $SM_{1,2}$ is illustrated in Figure 2.8, with the maximum of the three values (UPLEFT, LEFT, UP) being 0 (Fig. 2.8A). So, we put

0 in the cell together with a left arrow (because LEFT is the maximum of the three). The three values (UPLEFT, LEFT, UP in Fig. 2.8) correspond to the three alignments in Figure 2.8B. You might wonder why we need to calculate the alignment score for the poorest alignment (with an alignment score of –6). Indeed, for highly similar homologous sequences with few indels, we can get away with calculating alignment scores for only a few cells flanking the diagonal of the matrices.

We continue the computation from left to right and from top to bottom until we reach the bottom right cell to obtain $SM_{6,4} = 4$ (Fig. 2.7A). This is the optimal alignment score for aligning S and T given the scoring scheme. You may note that the cell corresponding to the nucleotide G in the row sequence and the second G in the column sequence is special with two arrows (Fig. 2.7A). You will find that the UPLEFT and UP values are both equal to 4 in this cell, hence both the upleft and the up-pointing arrows in this cell. Such a cell implies the existence of equally optimal alignments. Keep in mind that $SM_{i,j}$ is the optimal alignment score between prefixes T_i and S_j. For example, $SM_{1,1} = 2$ is the optimal alignment score for aligning T_1 (=A) and S_1 (=A) so the alignment score is 2.

```
(A)  UPLEFT=-2-1=-3
     LEFT   = 2-2= 0
     UP     =-4-2=-6
```

(B) UPLEFT	LEFT	UP
AC	AC	AC-
-A	A-	--A
-3	0	-6

FIGURE 2.8   Obtaining the alignment score and the backtrack arrow for the second cell in the scoring matrix $SM_{1,2}$. (A) Calculate the three values and choose the maximum (which is 0 corresponding to LEFT). (B) The three alignment scores correspond to three alternative ways of aligning sequence "AC" against sequence "A."

The aligned sequences are obtained directly from the backtrack matrix without any reference to the scoring matrix. We start from the bottom-right cell and follow the direction of the arrow in the cell. The upleft arrow in the bottom-right cell (Fig. 2.7A) means that we should stack the two corresponding nucleotides (T and T) in the row and column sequences (Fig. 2.7C) regardless of whether they are the same or different. A left-pointing or up-pointing arrow in the cell means a gap in the column sequence or row sequence, respectively.

The upleft arrow in the bottom-right cell leads us to the cell containing an up-pointing arrow, meaning a gap in the row sequence S, that is, we stack a gap character "-" over the corresponding nucleotide (C) in the column sequence T (Fig. 2.7C). This up-pointing arrow brings us to the special cell with two arrows, one pointing upleft and the other up (Fig. 2.7A). This leads to alternative construction of the sequence alignment. If we choose the up-pointing arrow, we will stack a gap character over the corresponding nucleotide (G) in the column sequence and proceed to the cell with a value of 6 and an upleft arrow. This ultimately leads to the sequence alignment in Figure 2.7C. Alternatively, we may choose to follow the upleft arrow and stack the two nucleotides (G in both sequences) as shown in Figure 2.7A. This ultimately leads to the alternative sequence alignment in Figure 2.7D.

Both alignments in Figure 2.7C and D have four matches, two gaps, and zero mismatch. So the alignment score is $4 \times s_{ii} + 2 \times G + 0 \times s_{ij} = 4$, which we already know after completing the scoring matrix whose bottom-right cell contains the alignment score.

When sequences are long, there might be many equally optimal alignments and few computer programs would try to find and output all of them. Instead, only one path is followed, leading to the output of only one of the potentially many equally optimal alignments. It is for this reason that manual adjustment is often required after we obtain the alignment output.

Dynamic programming guarantees that the resulting alignment is optimal given the scoring scheme. In other words, there is no alignment that can have an alignment score greater than 4 given the two sequences and the scoring scheme of $s_{ii} = 2$, $s_{ij} = -1$ and $G = -2$. However, an optimal alignment may change when the scoring scheme is changed, as we have already illustrated in Figure 2.6.

Students often wonder what scoring scheme is the right one to use. Keep in mind that an alignment score is an index of homology. The higher the alignment score, the stronger the evidence of homology. Mismatches and gaps reduce the alignment score because their presence weakens the evidence of homology. Thus, any difference that strongly weakens evidence of homology is assigned a high penalty score. Because point substitutions typically occur more frequently than indels in functional genes, an indel is typically penalized more than a point substitution. Among point substitutions, transitions occur more frequently than transversions and consequently are penalized less than transversions.

Because there is no exact way of choosing the right scoring scheme, it is therefore important to keep in mind that sequence alignment is a method of data exploration instead of an analytical method that will lead to a single best solution. For this reason, nearly all computer programs for sequence alignment allow the user to try various scoring schemes and post-alignment manual editing.

2.2.2 LOCAL ALIGNMENT

Local sequence alignment (Smith and Waterman, 1981) is similar to the global alignment presented above, with only three major differences. First, the first row and the first column of the scoring matrix is filled with zero instead of $i \times G$. Second, whenever the cell value becomes negative (i.e., the maximum of the three values is smaller than 0), the cell value is set to 0. Thus, when two sequences have a short but perfect local match, and little similarity elscwherc, thc alignment score of the short but perfect match is not ncgativcly affcctcd by thc low similarity elsewhere. Third, because a local alignment can end anywhere in the matrix, we will not trace back from the cell in the bottom-right corner of the scoring matrix. Instead, we find the maximal score in the matrix and trace back from that point until we reach a cell with a value of 0, which indicates the start of the local alignment.

2.3 MATCH-MISMATCH MATRICES: PAM AND BLOSUM

Each scoring scheme has two components, the match and mismatch scores, and the gap penalty. The simple scoring scheme that we have used so far, specified by only three values: constant gap penalty and match and mismatch scores, needs to be extended in two ways to approximate biological reality. The constant gap penalty will be replaced by affine function gap penalty which distinguishcs gap opcn (G_O) from gap extension (G_E), and the two-valued match and mismatch scores will be replaced by a match-mismatch (MM) matrix (or a series of matrices for sequences of difference divergence). This section details the derivation of MM matrices for nucleotide and amino acids used in practical sequence alignment. The emphasis is on understanding the rationale and mathematical details underlying the PAM and BLOSUM matrices. The next section deals with alignment algorithms using affine function gap penalty. These two sections demand significant effort in your part. One incentive to learn the derivation of MM matrices is that you will gain an excellent perspective into molecular phylogenetics, especially in understanding substitution models and evolutionary distances.

There are three reasons for replacing the two-valued match and mismatch scores by a matrix. For nucleotide sequences, transitions (A↔G or C↔T) generally occur more frequently than transversions (R↔Y). This suggests that we should not treat transitional differences and transversional differences with the same mismatch score. Instead, transitions should be penalized less than transversions. Second, nucleotide frequencies often differ. If A is more frequent than C, then a C:C match is a stronger indication of homology than an A:A match and therefore should be given a higher match score than the latter.

The same line of reasoning also applies to amino acid sequences. Some amino acids (e.g., Ala, Gly) are typically more frequent than others (e.g., Trp, Cys), so the match score for Ala:Ala should be smaller than that for Trp:Trp. Also, substitutions between some amino acids (e.g., between Lys and Arg, or between Glu and Asp) replace each other quite frequently while others (e.g., between Trp and Gly) rarely, so a mismatch score between Lys and Arg should be smaller than that between Trp and Gly. Thus, the ability to understand currently used MM matrices and, in particular, to generate good MM matrices for your own particular data is an essential skill for any bioinformatician.

The second reason for extending the two-valued match and mismatch scores by a matrix is that the likelihood of amino acids replacing each other changes with time. With a very short time, Gly is very unlikely to be replaced by Arg or Trp but the probability increases with increasing length of time, so different match/mismatch scores should be used for sequences of different divergence. Readers who have done practical amino acid sequence alignment would have already encountered Dayhoff (Dayhoff et al., 1978) or BLOSUM (Henikoff and Henikoff, 1992) matrices that aim to accommodate differences in amino acid frequencies and in substitution rates. Each type is represented by a series of matrices (e.g., PAM1, PAM100, PAM120, ..., PAM250, or BLOSUM90, BLOSOM80, ..., BLOSUM45). How to know which matrix is good for aligning your sequences? Should you use PAM1 or PAM100 or PAM250 for aligning your amino acid sequences? Generally, a reasonable MM matrix should give you a positive alignment score for two properly aligned homologous sequences. If your amino acid sequences differ by only 1% of the sites, then PAM1 will give you a positive alignment score. However, if your amino acid sequences are highly diverged, then even using PAM100 may generate a negative alignment score even if the two sequences still have significant signal of homology, suggesting that PAM250 or any MM matrix for more divergent sequences should be used. Note that a PAM matrix suffixed with a larger number, or a BLOSUM matrix suffixed with a smaller number, is for more divergent sequences.

The third reason for extending the two-valued match and mismatch scores is that there are often ambiguous bases in input sequences, e.g., R for A or G and Y for C or T. An A:R pair is neither a strict match nor a strict mismatch but has a probability of 0.5 being a match and a probability of 0.5 being a transition. A MM matrix offers an explicit way of handling ambiguous codes.

2.3.1 MATCH-MISMATCH MATRICES FOR NUCLEOTIDE SEQUENCES

One example of a similarity matrix is the "transition bias matrix" (Table 2.1). The meaning of the top 4×4 matrix (bolded values in Table 2.1) is for the four resolved nucleotides. The first four diagonal values of 30 are equivalent to the match score. A mismatch score involving a transversion or a transition is −30 or 0, respectively, because transitions in general occur much more frequently than transversions and consequently penalized less (Table 2.1). The rest of the matrix (Table 2.1) involves ambiguous codes specified in Table 2.2, according to the Nomenclature Committee of the International Union of Biochemistry (1985).

TABLE 2.1   A similarity matrix accommodating the transition bias frequently observed in nucleotide substitutions.

A	C	G	U	R	Y	M	W	S	K	D	H	V	B	N
30														
−30	30													
0	−30	30												
−30	0	−30	30											
15	−30	15	−30	15										
−30	15	−30	15	−30	15									
0	0	−15	−15	−8	−8	0								
0	−15	−15	0	−8	−8	−8	0							
−15	0	0	−15	−8	−8	−8	−15	0						
−15	−15	0	0	−8	−8	−15	−8	−8	0					
0	−20	0	−10	0	−15	−10	−5	−10	−5	−3				
−10	0	−20	0	−15	0	−5	−5	−10	−10	−10	−3			
0	−10	0	−20	0	−15	−5	−10	−5	−10	−7	−10	−3		
−20	0	−10	0	−15	0	−10	−10	−5	−5	−10	−7	−10	−3	
−8	−8	v8	−8	−8	−8	−8	−8	−8	−8	−8	−8	−8	−8	−8

TABLE 2.2   IUB codes of nucleotides.

Code	Meaning	Complement
A	A	T
C	C	G
G	G	C
T/U	T	A
M	A or C	K
R	A or G	Y
W	A or T	W
S	C or G	S
Y	C or T	R
K	G or T	M
V	A or C or G	B
H	A or C or T	D
D	A or G or T	H
B	C or G or T	V
X/N	G or A or T or C	X
–	Gap (not G or A or T or C)	–

The coding scheme in Table 2.2 is often referred to as the IUB code or IUB notation. For example, R represents either A or G, so an A/R pair has a probability of 0.5 being an A/A match and a probability of 0.5 being an A/G transition. The corresponding score (=15 in Table 2.1) is consequently the average score of (1) a perfect match with a match score of 30, and (2) a transition with a score of 0. In contrast, Y stands for either C or T/U and an A/Y pair is always a transversion, with a score of −30 (Table 2.1).

What is the justification of a match score of 30, a transition score of 0 and a transversion score of −30? In the default BLAST, a match score is 1 and a mismatch score is −3. What is the justification of such scores and their relative magnitude? There is a mathematical approach to derive MM matrices based on Markov chain models, which we will cover in the chapter on substitution models. Here we will first follow the empirical approach used for deriving MM matrices for amino acid sequences developed by Dayhoff and her colleagues (Dayhoff et al., 1978), although the approach is equally applicable to nucleotide sequences. The BLOSUM approach (Henikoff and Henikoff, 1992) will follow. Keep in mind that PAM and BLOSUM matrices are typically associated with amino acid substitutions and protein sequence alignment. However, the principle can be applied to nucleotide sequences (and indeed can be more easily explained with nucleotide sequences).

Table 2.3 represents an empirical substitution matrix between nonredundant sequence pairs that differ at less than 1 site out of 100 sites. The reason for using sequence pairs of low divergence is to approximate the assumption of few multiple substitutions. A column nucleotide represents the state of one sequence and a row nucleotide the state of the other sequence. Because the sequences are from extant species and we do not know the ancestral state, the two corresponding off-diagonal elements are averaged so that the matrix is symmetrical. The large values in the diagonals mean that most sequence sites between the two sequences are identical. Among sites where the two sequences differ, most are C↔T transitions, followed by A↔G transitions. Transversions are rare relative to transitions. The pattern is suggestive of the TN93 model (Tamura and Nei, 1993) that we will explain in the chapter on substitution models.

TABLE 2.3 Empirical substitution matrix (often referred to as matrix A) from closely related nucleotide sequences with divergence smaller than 1%. Nucleotide frequencies π and mutability (m, which measures the propensity of a nucleotide being replaced by others) are also shown.

	A	G	C	T	N_i	π	M
A	7335	20	10.5	12.5	7378	0.3686	0.0058
G	20	4815	10	12.5	4857.5	0.2427	0.0087
C	10.5	10	3778	39.5	3838	0.1917	0.0156
T	12.5	12.5	39.5	3878	3942.5	0.1970	0.0164

It is helpful to first define the notations. The values in the 4×4 empirical substitution matrix is often referred to as $A(i,j)$, and the number of nucleotides i ($i =$A, G, C, or T) as N_i, $N = \Sigma N_i$. Given these, we have

$$\pi_i = \frac{N_i}{N}$$

$$m_i = \frac{\displaystyle\sum_{i=1, j=1, i \neq j}^{4} A(i,j)}{N_i} \tag{2.1}$$

where m_i is the proportion of nucleotide i involved in observed nucleotide replacement and is often referred to as the index of mutability.

2.3.1.1 PAM MATRIX FOR NUCLEOTIDE SEQUENCES

We will follow the convention and define one PAM time unit as the time needed for one nucleotide substitution to occur in 100 nucleotide sites. The transition probability matrix (M_1, where the subscript 1 indicates one PAM unit of time) can be derived from matrix A. We only need to obtain the off-diagonal elements because the diagonal elements of a transition probability matrix are constrained by each row summing up to 1, that is, a nucleotide can either remain the same or replaced by another nucleotide). The off-diagonal elements of M are

$$M_1(i,j) = \frac{\lambda A(i,j)}{N_i} \tag{2.2}$$

where λ is obtained from the following equation, assuming that multiple substitutions at the same site are negligible:

$$\lambda = \frac{0.01}{\sum_{i=1}^{4} \pi_i m_i} = 0.0953 . \tag{2.3}$$

Note that the denominator in Eq. (2.3) is the summation of all substitutions averaged over the four nucleotides (in other words, weighted by nucleotide frequencies), and that λ is to scale this substitution to a sequence divergence of 1%. Because M is a transition probability matrix with each row values summing up to 1, the diagonal elements of M is simply 1 minus the three off-diagonal elements on the same row. The result M_1 matrix is shown in Table 2.4. M_1 specifies the probability of a nucleotide staying the same or being replaced by another after one PAM unit of time.

Each transition probability matrix can be used to obtain an associated PAM matrix. The PAM matrix associated from M_1 is computed as

$$PAM1(i,j) = 10 \lg \frac{M_1(i,j)}{\pi_j} \tag{2.4}$$

where lg stands for base-10 logarithm (which should be standard notation). The resulting PAM1 matrix is shown in Table 2.4, although PAM matrices used in sequence alignment are typically rounded to integers to speed up computation.

TABLE 2.4 Transition probability matrix (M_I) with a time interval of one nucleotide substitution per 100 nucleotide sites, together with PAM1 matrix.

	Matrix M_I				PAM1 matrix			
	A	G	C	T	A	G	C	T
A	0.9944	0.0026	0.0014	0.0016	4.3102	−19.7283	−21.5036	−20.8631
G	0.0039	0.9917	0.0020	0.0025	−19.7283	6.1133	−19.9003	−19.0478
C	0.0026	0.0025	0.9851	0.0098	−21.5036	−19.9003	7.1075	−13.0279
T	0.0030	0.0030	0.0095	0.9844	−20.8631	−19.0478	−13.0279	6.9878

One may note that the PAM1 matrix in Table 2.4 is symmetrical which is characteristic of a time-reversible substitution model in which $\pi_i M_{ij} = \pi_j M_{ji}$. This time-reversibility is a necessary consequence of our not knowing the root between the two aligned sequences and our averaging the off-diagonal elements in matrix A (Table 2.3).

A few points are worth highlighting in PAM1 (Table 2.4). First, among the four match scores on the diagonal, an A/A match has the smallest score and a C:C match the largest. This is because A is the most frequent and C is the rarest nucleotide in the compiled sequences used to generate PAM1. Thus, an A/A match is more likely to arise by random chance than a C/C match and consequently is a weaker indication of homology than a C/C match. Second, a C/T mismatch is not penalized as much as an A/G match because C↔T transitions occur more frequently than A↔G transitions. In general, the rare the substitution, the heavier the penalty. Third, the average mismatch score is −19, and the average match score is 6. This may be taken as the justification in BLAST default with mismatch penalty three times greater as the match score (e.g., match score = 1 and mismatch score of −3 as in BLAST default).

PAM1 is useful as a MM matrix only for sequences of low divergence. For example, if two sequences have diverged by 25%, then the alignment score (S_a) for the two sequences of length L, given average match score of 6 and mismatch score of −19, will be approximately

$$S_a = L[0.25 \times (-19) + 0.75 \times 6] = -0.25L \qquad (2.5)$$

A negative S_a suggests either that the two sequences have no homology or that the MM matrix is faulty. With the PAM approach, we would take M_1 in Table 2.4 to generate M_{100}, M_{150}, etc., and obtain PAM100, PAM150, ..., etc., for increasingly divergent sequences. M_n is obtained by multiplying M_1 n times, that is $M_n = M_1^n$, and a PAM matrix for n PAM units of time is computed as

$$PAM_n(i,j) = 10 \lg \frac{M_n(i,j)}{\pi_j}. \tag{2.6}$$

M_{100} and PAM100 obtained in this way are shown in Table 2.5. The average match score is 2.677925 and the average mismatch score is -1.49345. The expected alignment score (S_a) per site calculated using the same approach as in Eq. (2.5) would be $0.25*(-1.49345)+0.75*2.677925 = 1.635081$. In fact, even two sequences with 60% divergence will still have positive alignment scores with PAM100.

TABLE 2.5   Transition probability matrix (M_{100}) and the associated PAM100 matrix.

	Matrix M_{100}				PAM100 matrix			
	A	G	C	T	A	G	C	T
A	0.6306	0.1592	0.1012	0.1090	2.3319	−1.8319	−2.7755	−2.5680
G	0.2418	0.4931	0.1269	0.1382	−1.8319	3.0793	−1.7910	−1.5401
C	0.1945	0.1607	0.3636	0.2812	−2.7755	−1.7910	2.7792	1.5458
T	0.2041	0.1702	0.2737	0.3520	−2.5680	−1.5401	1.5458	2.5213

Contrasting M_1 and M_{100}, we note that a nucleotide A will have a probability of 0.9944 of remaining as A after one PAM unit of time but only 0.6306 after 100 PAM units of time. This is why we need different PAM matrices for aligning sequences of different divergence. We also notice that the difference between the four match scores and the 12 mismatch scores is larger in PAM1 than in PAM100. The difference will be even smaller with PAM250. The values in a PAM matrix will eventually all approach zero when homology is completely lost due to substitution saturation. Keep in mind that one PAM unit of time (resulting in 1% sequence divergence) may mean millions of years, so 100 or 250 PAM units of time could be billions of years.

Because M_n is obtained by extrapolation of M_1 through $M_n = M_1^n$, any error inherent in M_1 will be compounded in M_n. For this reason, PAM250, derived from M_{250} and used for highly diverged sequences, may not perform as well as BLOSUM45 which is not extrapolated but derived directly from comparison of sequences being no more than 45% identical.

2.3.1.2   BLOSUM MATRIX FOR NUCLEOTIDE SEQUENCES

The BLOSUM approach (Henikoff and Henikoff, 1992) is based on empirical sets of sequences with different degrees of divergence. For example, those sequences being no more than 45% identical are used to generate BLOSUM45 matrix, the sequence pairs being no more than 52% identical are used to generate BLOSUM52 matrix, and so on for BLOSUM62 all the way to BLOSUM90 for aligning sequences of little divergence. Keep in mind that a PAM matrix suffixed with a larger number is for more divergent sequences, whereas a BLOSUM matrix suffixed with a larger number is for less divergent sequences. While ideally one should use different PAM or BLOSUM matrices for sequences of different divergence, a multiple alignment often involves a number of sequences with different degrees of divergence. If one has to use a single BLOSUM matrix to align them all, then BLOSUM62 is a good compromise and is consequently used as default in sequence alignment programs. Aligning closely related sequences are easy and almost any PAM or BLOSUM matrix can work well.

The same empirical substitution data in Table 2.3, $A(i,j)$, can also be used to derive a BLOSUM matrix. We could call it BLOSUM95 matrix because the sequence pairs used to generate the data in Table 2.3 all have sequence identity approaching 95%. We first compute the expected value of $A(i,j)$, denoted by $E(i,j)$, as illustrated below:

$$E(i, j) = \frac{N_i N_j}{N}$$

$$E(A, A) = \frac{N_A N_A}{N} = \frac{7335^2}{20016} = 2719.569$$

$$E(A, G) = \frac{N_A N_G}{N} = \frac{7335 \times 4857.5}{20016} = 1790.499$$

(2.7)

We next compute the log-odds (Table 2.6), with two numerical illustrations below:

$$\ln\left(\frac{p_{ij}}{p_i p_j}\right) = \ln\left(\frac{A(i,j)}{E(i,j)}\right)$$

$$\ln\left(\frac{p_{AA}}{p_A p_A}\right) = \ln\left(\frac{A(A,A)}{E(A,A)}\right) = \ln\left(\frac{7335}{2719.569}\right) = 0.9922$$

$$\ln\left(\frac{p_{AG}}{p_A p_G}\right) = \ln\left(\frac{A(A,G)}{E(A,G)}\right) = \ln\left(\frac{20^{\cdot}}{1790.499}\right) = -4.4945 \tag{2.8}$$

Note that the $E(i,j)$ is computed by assuming independence of the two nucleotides occurring at the same site between two sequences. It is calculated in the same way as in the test of independence in contingency table analysis. Existence of homology tends to result in $\ln[A(i,i)/E(i,i)]$ > 0 and $\ln[A(i,j)/A(i,j)]$ <0. The likelihood ratio chi-square statistic, $2*sum\{A(i,j)*\ln[A(i,j)/E(i,j)]\}$, can be used to test against the null hypothesis of no homology between two sequences.

Finally, the resulting log-odds (Table 2.6) are scaled and rounded to integers to generate the final BLOSUM matrix. The scaling factor (λ) is to allow the log-odds to be well represented by integers. If we round the original log-odds, then the rounding error will be large. If we multiply the values by 100 before rounding, then the rounding error would be small but the values would take too much space. A good compromise is to use some value in between. BLOSUM62 divides log-odds by $\lambda = \ln(2)/2$ (half-bit units) and BLOSUM50 by $\lambda = \ln(2)/3$ (third-bit units). The rule of thumb is to use a scaling factor so that the difference between the average match score and the average mismatch score is about 30. The BLOSUM matrix in Table 2.6 is produced by dividing the log-odds by $\lambda = \ln(2)/3$ and then rounded to integers.

TABLE 2.6 Deriving BLOSUM matrix with log-odds and scaled BLOSUM matrix by $\lambda=\ln(2)/3$ and rounded to integers.

	Log-odds				BLOSUM			
	A	G	C	T	A	G	C	T
A	0.9922	-4.4945	-4.9033	-4.7558	4	-19	-21	-21
G	-4.4945	1.4072	-4.5341	-4.3378	-19	6	-20	-19
C	-4.9033	-4.5341	1.6358	-2.9517	-21	-20	7	-13
T	-4.7558	-4.3378	-2.9517	1.6082	-21	-19	-13	7

The values in the BLOSOM matrix in Table 2.6 and those in the PAM1 matrix in Table 2.4 are essentially perfectly correlated (r = 0.999998). However, because all PAM matrices are extrapolated from M_1 while each BLOSUM matrix results from separate compilation of empirical substitution matrix, BLOSUM matrices are likely more robust than PAM matrices for highly diverged sequences.

Note that, if we know the frequencies of the nucleotides and the BLOSUM matrix, we could infer λ with the following equation (Xia, 2018a, p 11):

$$\sum_{i=1}^{4}\sum_{j=1}^{4} \pi_i \pi_j e^{s_{ij}\lambda} = 1 \qquad (2.9)$$

where s_{ij} refers to entries in the BLOSUM. Given the π values in Table 2.3 and BLOSUM matrix in Table 2.6. We can obtain $\lambda = 0.2368$, which is not exactly $\ln(2)/3$ (=0.2310). This discrepancy between the estimated λ and the true λ is because the values in the BLOSUM matrix in Table 2.6 have been rounded, otherwise the two would be identical. The "lambda" in the BLAST output is the same λ as defined in Eq. (2.9).

2.3.2   MATCH-MISMATCH MATRICES FOR PROTEINS

2.3.2.1   AMINO ACID PROPERTIES AND SUBSTITUTION FREQUENCIES

Amino acids (Table 2.7) differ from each other in volume, charge, polarity and many other properties (Fig. 2.9) and amino acid residues in a protein confer to the protein different properties. For example, proteins with long half-life (>1 day) typically have glycine, valine or methionine at their N-terminus, whereas those with a short half-life (a few minutes) typically have positively charged residues (arginine, lysine) at their N-terminus. A small amino acid residue, such as glycine and alanine at the penultimate site (the second amino acid site in the nascent peptide) allows the initiator methionine to be efficiently cleaved, whereas a large and/or charged residue will not (Moerschell et al., 1990). Although the word "penultimate" is explained as meaning "second to the last" in English dictionaries, it has become standard in protein literature to mean the amino acid right after the initiation methionine.

TABLE 2.7 IUB letter codes of amino acids, proposed by the Nomenclature Committee of the International Union of Biochemistry (1985). These codes are now universally adopted by the scientific community. also listed are molecular weight (MW), hydropathy index (HI, Kyte and Doolittle, 1982), and usage in *E. coli* K12 (*E. coli*) and *Saccharomyces cerevisiae* (Yeast).

1-letter	3-letter	Meaning	Codon[a]	HI	MW	*E. coli*	Yeast
A	Ala	Alanine	GCT, GCC, GCA, GCG	1.8	89.094	125332	160810
R	Arg	Arginine	CGT, CGC, CGA, CGG, AGA, AGG	−4.5	174.203	72502	130068
N	Asn	Asparagine	AAT, AAC	−3.5	132.119	51075	179836
D	Asp	Aspartic	GAT, GAC	−3.5	133.104	67349	171072
C	Cys	Cysteine	TGT, TGC	2.5	121.154	15188	37093
Q	Gln	Glutamine	CAA, CAG	−3.5	146.146	58360	115741
E	Glu	Glutamic	GAA, GAG	−3.5	147.131	75786	191267
G	Gly	Glycine	GGT, GGC, GGA, GGG	−0.4	75.067	96701	145433
H	His	Histidine	CAT, CAC	−3.2	155.156	29751	63505
I	Ile	Isoleucine	ATT, ATC, ATA	4.5	131.175	78845	191677
L	Leu	Leucine	TTG, TTA, CTT, CTC, CTA, CTG	3.8	131.175	140571	277988
K	Lys	Lysine	AAA, AAG	−3.9	146.189	57620	214842
M	Met	Methionine	ATG	1.9	149.208	37093	60672
F	Phe	Phenylalanine	TTT, TTC	2.8	165.192	51131	129516
P	Pro	Proline	CCT, CCC, CCA, CCG	−1.6	115.132	58293	128177
S	Ser	Serine	TCT, TCC, TCA, TCG, AGT, AGC	−0.8	105.093	75661	263096
T	Thr	Threonine	ACT, ACC, ACA, ACG	−0.7	119.119	70494	173084
W	Trp	Tryptophan	TGG	−0.9	204.228	20060	30387
Y	Tyr	Tyrosine	TAT, TAC	−1.3	181.191	37134	98746
V	Val	Valine	GTT, GTC, GTA, GTG	4.2	117.148	93061	162642
*	End	Terminator	TAA, TAG, TGA				

[a]Assuming the standard genetic code.

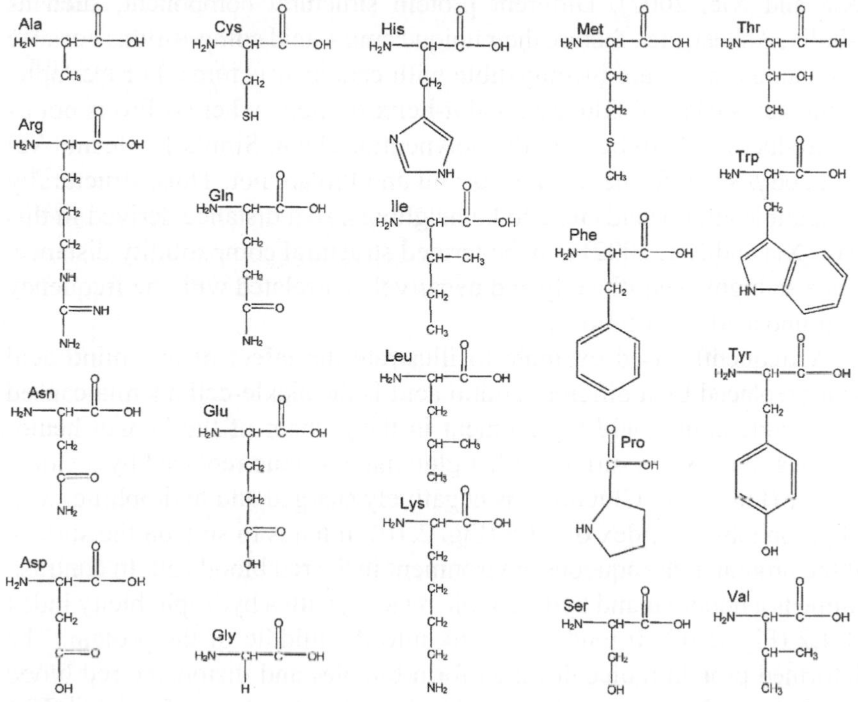

FIGURE 2.9 Structural formula of 20 amino acids.

Hydropathy index (Table 2.7) as a good measure of amino acid polarity and molecular weight (Table 2.7) as a measure of amino acid size have been used for deriving amino acid dissimilarity indices of which two kinds are used frequently. Grantham's distance (Grantham, 1974) is based on polarity, size, and chemical composition of amino acid residues, whereas Miyata's distance (Miyata et al., 1979) is based on polarity and size only. These distances are typically evaluated against empirical amino acid substitution matrix because a good index of amino acid dissimilarity should be negatively correlated with the frequency of amino acid substitution. Paradoxically, Miyata's distance generally performs better than Grantham's distance in predicting the frequency of amino acid substitutions, presumably because the chemical composition of the side chain is a messy variable that probably contributes more noise than information.

Another amino acid dissimilarity, based not on physiochemical properties of amino acid but on structural consideration, has also been proposed

(Xia and Xie, 2002). Different protein structural component, such as α-helix, β-sheet, etc., feature their unique amino acid compositions because some amino acids are incompatible with certain structures. For example, amino acids Ala and Glu are good α-helix formers, whereas Pro is not as it introduces a sharp bend in the polypeptide chain. Similarly, Ile and Val are good β-sheet formers, whereas Glu and Pro are not. Thus, structurally compatible amino acids tend to be neighbors, so a distance derived in this way (Xia and Xie, 2002) may be termed structural compatibility distance. It is also highly significantly and negatively correlated with the frequency of amino acid substitutions.

A frequently used example to illustrate the effect of an amino acid being replaced by a different amino acid is the sickle-cell anemia caused by a single amino acid replacement in the β-chain of the human hemoglobin at the sixth position, with a glutamate residue replaced by a valine residue (Fig. 2.10). Glutamate is negatively charged and hydrophilic, with a hydrophobicity index of −3.5 (Fig. 2.10). It tends to stay on the surface of the protein in the aqueous environment in the red blood cell. In contrast, valine is a nonpolar and hydrophobic residue, with a hydrophobicity index of 4.2 (Fig. 2.10). It tends to shrink into the middle of the protein. The deformed protein molecules then form bundles and distort the red blood cell that carries them, resulting in the characteristic shape of a sickle (Fig. 2.10). It is generally true that amino acids of different polarity rarely replace each other (Xia and Li, 1998), whereas amino acids with similar polarity can replace each other quite often (Xia and Kumar, 2006).

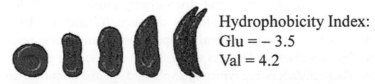

Hydrophobicity Index:
Glu = − 3.5
Val = 4.2

Hb-A: Val-His-Leu-Thr-Pro-**Glu**-Glu......
Hb-S: Val-His-Leu-Thr-Pro-**Val**-Glu......

FIGURE 2.10 Sickle-cell anemia is caused by a single amino acid replacement of a glutamate residue at the sixth position (Hb-A allele) by a valine residue (Hb-S allele). The mutant deformed hemoglobin molecules distort the red blood cell which progresses from the normal disk-like shape to the sickle-like shape. The hydrophobicity index is taken from Table 2.7.

TABLE 2.8 Empirical substitution matrix A from aligned HIV-1gag protein sequences with about 85% identity. Amino acid pairs replacing each other frequently are in bold.

	Ala	Arg	Asn	Asp	Cys	Gln	Glu	Gly	His	Ile	Leu	Lys	Met	Phe	Pro	Ser	Thr	Trp	Tyr	Val
Ala	792	1.5	5.5	4	0.5	1.5	5.5	9	0.5	4	0.5	6	1	1.5	6	10.5	**24**	0.5	0.5	12
Arg	1.5	670	6.5	1	1	8.5	6	12.5	2	1	1.5	**55.5**	2	0.5	2	5.5	7.5	1	0.5	2
Asn	5.5	6.5	645	**16.5**	0.5	2	6.5	6.5	5.5	5.5	1.5	14	2	1	1.5	**34.5**	20	0.5	1.5	2.5
Asp	4	1	**16.5**	426	0.5	0.5	**30.5**	8.5	2	1	1	5	0.5	0.5	1	7	4.5	0.5	1	1.5
Cys	0.5	1	0.5	0.5	346	0.5	0.5	0.5	0.5	0.5	0.5	0.5	0.5	1.5	0.5	1	0.5	1	2	1.5
Gln	1.5	8.5	2	0.5	0.5	715	6.5	1	6.5	0.5	5	**17.5**	1	0.5	9.5	2.5	2.5	0.5	1	0.5
Glu	5.5	6	6.5	**30.5**	0.5	6.5	724	16	1	1	1.5	**18**	0.5	0.5	2	3	6.5	0.5	1	3.5
Gly	9	12.5	6.5	8.5	0.5	1	16	865	1	1	0.5	3.5	3	0.5	1	13	3.5	3.5	1.5	1
His	0.5	2	5.5	2	0.5	6.5	1	1	255	0.5	2	1.5	0.5	1	1.5	1.5	1.5	0.5	7	0.5
Ile	4	1	5.5	1	0.5	0.5	1	1	0.5	741	**31.5**	5.5	13	3.5	1	5	17.5	0.5	1.5	**47**
Leu	0.5	1.5	1.5	1	0.5	5	1.5	0.5	2	**31.5**	1031	1	10	8.5	6	4	3.5	3	1	11
Lys	6	**55.5**	14	5	0.5	17.5	18	3.5	1.5	5.5	1	695	2.5	0.5	0.5	4.5	7	0.5	0.5	1.5
Met	1	2	2	0.5	0.5	1	0.5	3	0.5	13	10	2.5	344	0.5	0.5	1.5	4	0.5	0.5	1.5
Phe	1.5	0.5	1	0.5	1.5	0.5	0.5	0.5	1	3.5	8.5	0.5	0.5	372	0.5	2.5	1	1	9	1
Pro	6	2	1.5	1	0.5	9.5	2	1	1.5	1	6	0.5	0.5	0.5	636	7.5	5.5	1	0.5	0.5
Ser	10.5	5.5	**34.5**	7	1	2.5	3	13	1.5	5	4	4.5	1.5	2.5	7.5	627	**22**	1	1	1
Thr	**24**	7.5	20	4.5	0.5	2.5	6.5	3.5	1.5	17.5	3.5	7	4	1	5.5	**22**	677	0.5	1	6
Trp	0.5	1	0.5	0.5	1	0.5	0.5	3.5	0.5	0.5	3	0.5	0.5	1	0.5	1	0.5	367	1.5	0.5
Tyr	0.5	0.5	1.5	1	2	1	1	1.5	7	1.5	1	0.5	0.5	9	0.5	1	1	1.5	299	1
Val	12	2	2.5	1.5	0.5	0.5	3.5	1	0.5	**47**	11	1.5	1.5	1	0.5	1	6	0.5	1	645

2.3.2.2   PAM AND BLOSUM MATRICES FOR AMINO ACID SUBSTITUTIONS

Frequently used MM matrices for aligning protein sequences are of two types, the PAM matrix (Dayhoff et al., 1978) and the BLOSUM matrix (Henikoff and Henikoff, 1992). While these MM matrices can be used for nucleotide sequences as we have shown in the previous section, they are originally developed for protein sequences. The Derivation of PAM and BLOSUM matrices for amino acid sequences is exactly the same as what we have used for nucleotide sequences in the previous section, except that now the matrix is 20×20 instead of 4×4. The same steps are involved in generating the matrices. For PAM, we (1) compile an empirical substitution matrix from closely related sequences, (2) obtain λ, (3) compute M_1, and (4) generate M_n as M_1^n and the associated PAM matrices. For BLOSUM, we compile sets of sequences with different degrees of divergence and use them to generate respective BLOSUM matrices.

Suppose we have an empirical substitution matrix A (Table 2.8) obtained from comparing HIV-1 gag sequences with about 85% similarity. The numbers are just small enough to fit the page and are for illustration purposes only because a representative matrix A would need significantly more data. From this empirical substitution matrix, we can obtain a series of PAM matrices and a BLOSUM85 matrix (so named because the sequence similarity is about 85%.

Amino acid frequencies (π) and mutability (m), shown in Table 2.9, vary much among the 20 amino acids. In general, two factors strongly affect the frequency of amino acid replacement. The first is amino acid similarity in physiochemical properties (Grantham, 1974; Miyata et al., 1979; Xia and Li, 1998). Almost all high-replacement amino acid pairs are polar ones (Xia and Kumar, 2006). A polar amino acid tends to stay on the protein surface whereas a nonpolar one tends to shrink into the center. For this reason, polar residues are rarely replaced by nonpolar ones and one of the deleterious consequences of a polar amino acid by a nonpolar one is illustrated in Figure 2.10. The second factor is similarity in their codons (Xia, 1998b). Arg and Lys have the highest $A(i,j)$ value (Table 2.8) among mismatched amino acids, although the two have only close to average frequencies (Table 2.9). Such a high replacement rate can be attributed to both amino acids (1) being positively charged and (2) differing only at the 2nd codon site (AAR for Lys and AGR for Arg). Similarly, Asp and Glu also replace each other frequently, both being negatively charged and differing only at the 3rd codon site (GAY for Asp and GAR for Glu). Another example is Val and Ile, both being nonpolar, similar in size and differing mainly at the first codon site (AUH for Ile and GUN for Val). The genetic code has evolved in such a way that nonsynonymous mutations often lead to similar amino acids with little phenotypic effect on protein function. We should also note that the two factors affecting amino acid replacement with different time scales. When divergence time is short, the similarity in two families of nonsynonymous codons strongly affects the frequency of amino acid replacement. However, with long divergence time, multiple nucleotide substitutions would have happened and the similarity in physiochemical properties becomes a key predictor of the frequencies of amino acid replacement. For this reason, we expect a mismatch between Arg and Lys to have negative mismatch score with a short time interval but to have a positive mismatch score with a long time interval. In other words, a mismatch score between Arg and Lys may be negative for PAM1 matrix, but positive for PAM250 matrix.

TABLE 2.9 Amino acid frequencies (π) and mutabilities (m) computed from Table 2.8.

AA	π	m	AA	π	m
Ala	0.0654	0.1066	Leu	0.0830	0.0831
Arg	0.0582	0.1497	Lys	0.0621	0.1731
Asn	0.0575	0.1720	Met	0.0288	0.1168
Asp	0.0379	0.1696	Phe	0.0301	0.0871
Cys	0.0265	0.0376	Pro	0.0505	0.0702
Gln	0.0578	0.0868	Ser	0.0558	0.1701
Glu	0.0616	0.1329	Thr	0.0602	0.1698
Gly	0.0703	0.0914	Trp	0.0284	0.0468
His	0.0216	0.1267	Tyr	0.0246	0.1021
Ile	0.0651	0.1599	Val	0.0546	0.1284

To obtain the series of PAM matrices from the A matrix in Table 2.8, we can obtain $\lambda = 0.08096$ from Table 2.9 by using Eq. (2.3), and then compute M_1 as previously illustrated with nucleotide sequences. We can then obtain M_{100}, M_{200}, ..., M_{250} and their associated PAM100,

TABLE 2.10 PAM250 derived from the A matrix in Table 2.8. Scaled by dividing the values from Eq. (2.6) by $\lambda = \ln(2)/2$.

	Ala	Arg	Asn	Asp	Cys	Gln	Glu	Gly	His	Ile	Leu	Lys	Met	Phe	Pro	Ser	Thr	Trp	Tyr	Val
Ala	12	-3	1	0	-11	-6	-1	0	-5	-1	-6	-2	-4	-6	0	2	4	-10	-7	2
Arg	-3	10	1	0	-8	3	2	2	-1	-6	-9	8	-3	-9	-4	0	-1	-7	-7	-6
Asn	1	1	7	4	-9	-3	2	1	1	-3	-6	1	-3	-5	-3	5	3	-9	-3	-3
Asp	0	0	4	10	-9	-3	8	4	0	-5	-9	1	-5	-7	-5	2	1	-8	-4	-5
Cys	-11	-8	-9	-9	36	-10	-10	-11	-3	-10	-10	-10	-8	4	-10	-8	-10	1	7	-11
Gln	-6	3	-3	-3	-10	17	0	-5	5	-8	-5	5	-6	-8	4	-3	-4	-10	-3	-9
Glu	-1	2	2	8	-10	0	11	4	-2	-6	-9	3	-6	-9	-5	0	-1	-9	-5	-5
Gly	0	2	1	4	-11	-5	4	14	-4	-7	-11	0	-4	-9	-7	2	-1	-11	-5	-7
His	-5	-1	1	0	-3	5	-2	-4	20	-5	-4	-1	-5	3	-1	-1	-2	-4	12	-6
Ile	-1	-6	-3	-5	-10	-8	-6	-7	-5	10	7	-5	6	6	-6	-2	1	-8	-4	9
Leu	-6	-9	-6	-9	-10	-5	-9	-11	-4	7	14	-8	6	5	-2	-5	-3	-2	-3	5
Lys	-2	8	1	1	-10	5	3	0	-1	-5	-8	8	-3	-9	-5	0	0	-9	-6	-5
Met	-4	-3	-3	-5	-8	-6	-6	-4	-5	6	6	-3	18	-2	-6	-3	0	-6	-5	3
Phe	-6	-9	-5	-7	4	-8	-9	-9	3	6	5	-9	-2	24	-7	-4	-5	0	15	-2
Pro	0	-4	-3	-5	-10	4	-5	-7	-1	0	-2	-5	-6	-7	21	3	-1	-10	-7	-7
Ser	2	0	5	2	-8	-3	0	2	-1	-2	-5	0	-3	-4	3	7	3	-7	-4	-3
Thr	4	-1	3	1	-10	-4	-1	-1	-2	1	-3	0	0	-5	-1	3	6	-9	-5	1
Trp	-10	-7	-9	-8	1	-10	-9	-11	-4	-8	-2	-9	-6	0	-10	-7	-9	33	3	-9
Tyr	-7	-7	-3	-4	7	-3	-5	-5	12	-4	-3	-6	-5	15	-7	-4	-5	3	24	-5
Val	2	-6	-3	-5	-11	-9	-5	-7	-6	9	5	-5	3	-2	-7	-3	1	-9	-5	13

TABLE 2.11 BLOSUM85 matrix derived from data in Table 2.8, scaled $\lambda=\ln(2)/2$. The matrix is for illustration only because of the limited data in Table 2.8.

	Ala	Arg	Asn	Asp	Cys	Gln	Glu	Gly	His	Ile	Leu	Lys	Met	Phe	Pro	Ser	Thr	Trp	Tyr	Val
Ala	8	-10	-6	-6	-11	-10	-7	-6	-10	-8	-14	-6	-9	-8	-6	-4	-2	-11	-11	-4
Arg	-10	8	-6	-10	-9	-5	-6	-4	-6	-11	-11	0	-7	-11	-9	-6	-5	-9	-11	-9
Asn	-6	-6	8	-2	-11	-9	-6	-6	-3	-6	-11	-6	-7	-9	-9	-1	-2	-11	-7	-8
Asp	-6	-10	-2	9	-10	-12	0	-4	-5	-10	-11	-5	-10	-10	-9	-4	-6	-10	-7	-8
Cys	-11	-9	-11	-10	10	-11	-11	-11	-8	-11	-12	-12	-10	-9	-10	-9	-6	-7	-7	-8
Gln	-10	-5	-9	-12	-11	8	-6	-12	-3	-13	-7	-3	-9	-11	-11	-8	-8	-11	-9	-13
Glu	-7	-6	-6	0	-11	-6	8	-4	-8	-12	-11	-3	-11	-11	-8	-8	-8	-11	-8	-7
Gly	-6	-4	-6	-4	-11	-12	-4	7	-9	-15	-15	-8	-11	-12	-11	-4	-8	-11	-12	-11
His	-10	-6	-3	-5	-8	-3	-8	-9	11	-10	-7	-8	-6	-6	-11	-7	-7	-6	0	-11
Ile	-8	-11	-6	-10	-11	-13	-12	-15	-10	7	-2	-12	-2	-2	-13	-7	-3	-11	-9	0
Leu	-14	-11	-11	-11	-12	-7	-11	-15	-7	-2	7	-12	-3	-3	-13	-8	-9	-7	-10	-5
Lys	-6	0	-6	-5	-12	-3	-3	-8	-8	-12	-12	7	-7	-13	-6	-6	-5	-11	-11	-10
Met	-9	-7	-7	-10	-10	-9	-11	-11	-6	-2	-3	-7	10	-6	-13	-8	-5	-9	-9	-3
Phe	-8	-11	-9	-10	-9	-11	-11	-12	-6	-2	-3	-13	-6	10	-11	-9	-9	-7	0	-9
Pro	-6	-9	-9	-9	-10	-11	-8	-11	-11	-13	-13	-6	-13	-11	8	-5	-6	-11	-10	-12
Ser	-4	-6	-1	-4	-9	-8	-8	-4	-7	-7	-8	-6	-8	-9	-5	8	-2	-11	-8	-11
Thr	-2	-5	-2	-6	-6	-8	-8	-8	-7	-3	-9	-5	-5	-9	-6	-2	8	-11	-9	-6
Trp	-11	-9	-11	-10	-7	-11	-11	-11	-6	-11	-7	-11	-9	-7	-11	-11	-11	10	-5	-11
Tyr	-11	-11	-7	-7	-7	-9	-8	-12	0	-9	-10	-11	-9	0	-10	-8	-9	-5	10	-8
Val	-4	-9	-8	-8	-8	-13	-7	-11	-11	0	-5	-10	-3	-9	-12	-11	-6	-11	-8	8

PAM200, ..., PAM250 (which is shown in Table 2.10). As expected, a mismatch between Lys and Arg has a positive score, so does that between Asp and Glu. In fact, a site with Arg in one sequence and Lys in another suggests as much sequence homology as a site with a Lys on both sequences (PAM250 score = 8 in both cases, Table 2.10). However, a site with an Arg in both sequences suggests a stronger homology (PAM250 score = 10). This is because Arg is rarer than Lys in this set of sequences (Table 2.9). If n is small, e.g., $n = 1$, then a PAM1 score for a Lys:Arg mismatch would be negative and that for a Lys:Lys match would be positive. In other words, with a short divergence time, a Lys:Lys match would suggest homology, but a Lys:Arg would not and this makes sense.

While we can derive a whole series of PAM matrices from the empirical matrix A in Table 2.8, we can obtain only one BLOSUM matrix from the data. This BLOSUM matrix may be called BLOSUM85 because the sequence pairs that generated the matrix A have sequence similarity close to 85%. This BLOSUM85 matrix will only be good for very closely related protein sequences. If we want to align highly diverged HIV-1 gag proteins, we have to obtain a different set of aligned sequences with a lower sequence similarity. The BLOSUM85 matrix derived from Table 2.8 is shown in Table 2.11.

We note that the score is 7 for a Lys:Lys pair, but 0 for a Lys:Arg pair. In other words, for low-divergence sequences, a Lys:Arg mismatch does not suggest homology, but a Lys:Lys pair does. If we use a set of highly diverged sequences, then the resulting BLOSUM matrix is expected to have a positive score for a Lys:Arg pair.

2.4 PAIRWISE ALIGNMENT WITH GAP PENALTY SPECIFIED BY THE AFFINE FUNCTION

There are two popularly used gap penalty schemes in sequence alignment, the constant gap penalty that we have already learned and the affine function gap penalty. The former does not distinguish between gap open and gap extension and the total gap cost of an alignment is $N \times G$, where N is the total gap length and G is penalty for one gap against a single nucleotide or amino acid. The alignment algorithm with this gap penalty scheme needs only one scoring matrix and one backtrack matrix. It is frequently used for illustrating the dynamic programming algorithms in bioinformatics textbooks. The affine function gap penalty distinguishes between gap open and gap extension, with greater penalty for gap open than for gap extension. The total gap penalty for an alignment is $N_{GO} \times GO + N_{GE} \times GE$, where N_{GO} and N_{GE} are the number of gap open and gap extension, respectively, and GO and GE are penalties for one gap open and one gap extension, respectively. The default GO and GE in BLAST (Altschul et al., 1990) are -5 and -2, respectively. The affine function gap penalty is used in essentially all practical computation where local or global sequence alignment is needed.

There are two formulations in the affine function gap penalty, in both literature and programming source codes. For an indel with a gap length N, one formulation specifies the gap penalty as equal to $GO + N \times GE$ (e.g., Gusfield, 1997; Pevzner, 2000). The BLAST suite of programs uses this formulation as well. The other formulation specifies the gap cost to be equal to $GO+(N-1)GE$ (e.g., Higgs and Attwood, 2005). The latter is theoretically more preferable than the former because it is reduced to constant gap penalty when $GO = GE$. It is the second formulation that I will use here in detailing the alignment with the affine function gap penalty.

The need for replacing constant gap penalty by affine function gap penalty may be illustrated by the two alignments in Figure 2.7C and D. The alignment in Figure 2.7C is generally considered by biologists as more likely than that in Figure 2.7D because indels are rare evolutionary events, with a single indel of length 2 more likely than two independent indels of length 1. Given the simple scoring scheme with constant penalty (match score = 2 and constant gap penalty of -2), the two alignments are equally good. However, if distinguish G_O from G_E, e.g., assign $G_O = -5$ and $G_E = -2$ (which is the BLAST default), then the alignment score will be 1 (=4*2–5–2) for the alignment in Figure 2.7C but -2 (=4*2–5–5) for the alignment in Figure 2.7D. With this new gap penalty scheme, the alignment in Figure 2.7C is better than that in Figure 2.7D. The rule of thumb is that $G_O > G_E$ and that the difference between G_O and G_E should increase with the frequency of long indels. The absolute values of G_O and G_E should be set in such a way that the alignment score between homologous sequences is positive. Setting $GO = 3*$(average mismatch score) appears to be a good compromise.

Pairwise alignment with the affine function gap penalty is complicated, and I will take a verbose approach instead of a condensed one to make sure that all details are covered to smooth your understanding. The cost of failing to understand is much greater than that of a few extra minutes of reading. I also separate the computation of the scoring matrices from that of the backtrack matrices although the matrices are computed simultaneously in all algorithmic implementations.

2.4.1 COMPUTING SCORING MATRICES

In contrast to dynamic programming with constant gap penalty where only one alignment scoring matrix is needed, alignment with affine function gap penalty needs to have three scoring matrices to keep alignment scores(Gotoh, 1982). The algorithm is based on the insight that there are three kinds of alignment blocks (Fig. 2.11A). Block G represents alignments with $x(i)$ aligned with $y(j)$, Block E represents those with $y(j)$ facing a gap character (a deletion) and Block F represents those with $x(i)$ facing a gap character (Fig. 2.11A). We need three matrices, designated by G, E, and F, respectively, to keep track of these three blocks. For clarity, I will also use an extra matrix, designated by V, to keep track of the maximum of $G(i,j)$, $E(i,j)$, and $F(i,j)$. These designations follow Gusfield (1997).

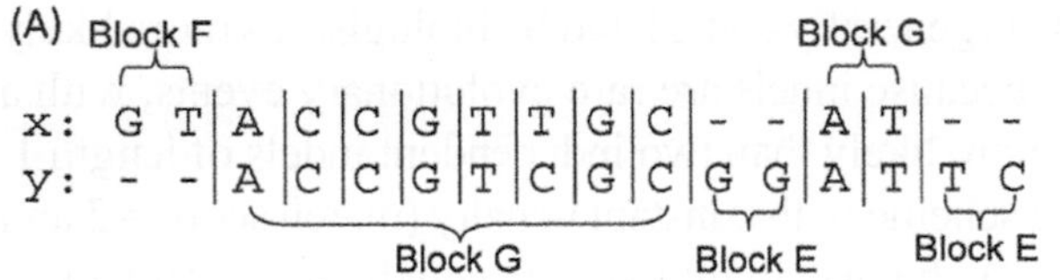

FIGURE 2.11 Three kinds of alignment blocks in dynamic programming with affine function gap penalty, together with a match/mismatch matrix (B), designated by S in the text.

Recall that, when we use constant gap penalty in pairwise alignment, we calculated UPLEFT, UP, and LEFT values and choose the maximum of the three to fill in the score matrix. We could have used matrices G, E, F, and V as well in that case, with matrix G storing all UPLEFT values, and E and F storing all UP and LEFT values and $V(i,j)$ storing the maximum of $G(i,j)$, $E(i,j)$, and $F(i,j)$. While we do not need G, E, and F matrices then, we do need them now with the affine function gap penalty.

To align two sequences x and y with lengths m and n, respectively, we designate x as the column sequence and y as the row sequence and set up the matrices with the following values (if leading gaps at beginning of the alignment are penalized). If leading gaps are not penalized, then set $V(i,0) = V(0,j) = 0$. The leading gaps are penalized in the numerical illustration below.

$$V(0,0) = 0$$
$$V(i,0) = -GO - (i-1)GE, \text{ for } 1 \leq i \leq m$$
$$V(0,j) = -GO - (j-1)GE, \text{ for } 1 \leq j \leq m \tag{2.10}$$

$$E(0,j) = 0, \text{ for } 0 \leq j \leq n$$
$$E(i,0) = -GO - (i-1)GE, \text{ for } 1 \leq i \leq m$$
$$F(i,0) = 0, \text{ for } 0 \leq i \leq m$$
$$F(0,j) = -GO - (j-1)GE, \text{ for } 1 \leq j \leq n \tag{2.11}$$
$$G(i,0) = 0, \text{ for } 0 \leq i \leq m$$
$$G(0,j) = 0, \text{ for } 0 \leq j \leq n$$

We will use a MM matrix designated by S (Fig. 2.11B), GO (gap open penalty) = 3 and GE (gap extension penalty) = 2. The general recurrences are

$$G(i,j) = V(i-1,j-1) + S(x_i, y_j)$$
$$E(i,j) = \max[E(i,j-1) - GE, V(i,j-1) - GO]$$
$$F(i,j) = \max[F(i-1,j) - GE, V(i-1,j) - GO] \tag{2.12}$$
$$V(i,j) = \max[G(i,j), E(i,j), F(i,j)]$$

In the spirit of recycling, we will reuse the two sequences used previously for illustrating the dynamic programming with constant gap penalty, with x ="ACGGCT" and y = "ACGT." The initialization values according to Eq. (2.10) and Eq. (2.11) are in the first row and first column of G, E, F, and V matrices in Table 2.12. Sequences x and y are also referred to as the column sequence and row sequence, respectively, as set up in the matrices shown in Tables 2.13.

We fill up the values of G, E, F, and V matrices according to Eq. (2.12) from left to right and from top to bottom, just as we have done previously with the constant gap penalty. The first value in the matrices are

TABLE 2.12 Alignment scoring matrices $G(i,j)$, $E(i,j)$, $F(i,j)$, and $V(i,j)$ with $GO = 3$, $GE = 2$ and the match-mismatch scores as shown in Figure 2.11B.

G matrix

	A	C	G	T
	0	0	0	0
A	2	-4	-6	-8
A	-4	4	-2	-4
C	-6	-2	6	0
G	-8	-4	3	5
G	-10	-6	-2	2
C	-12	-8	-4	3
T	-12	-8	-4	3

E matrix

	A	C	G	T
	0	0	0	0
A	-5	-1	-3	-5
A	-7	-4	1	-1
C	-9	-6	-2	3
G	-11	-8	-4	0
G	-13	-10	-6	-2
C	-15	-12	-8	-4
T	-13	-10	-6	-2

F matrix

	A	C	G	T
	0	0	0	0
A	-3	-5	-7	-9
A	-5	-7	-6	-8
C	-1	-4	-2	-4
G	-3	1	3	0
G	-5	-1	-2	2
C	-7	-3	1	0
T	-9	-5	-1	0

V matrix

	A	C	G	T
	0	-3	-5	-7	-9
A	-3	2	-1	-3	-1
A	-5	-1	4	1	3
C	-7	-3	1	6	5
G	-9	-5	-1	3	3
G	-11	-7	-3	1	2
C	-13	-9	-5	-1	3

$$G(1,1) = V(0,0) + S(A, A) = 0 + 2 = 2$$
$$E(1,1) = \max[E(1,0) - GE, V(1,0) - GO] = \max[-3-2, -3-3)] = -5$$
$$F(1,1) = \max[F(0,1) - GE, V(0,1) - GO] = \max[-3-2, -3-3)] = -5 \quad (2.13)$$
$$V(1,1) = \max[G(1,1), E(1,1), F(1,1)] = 2$$

What is nice with the dynamic programming is that once we know how to compute the first value, we know how to compute all the values because they are all computed exactly the same way. The complete scoring matrices G, E, and F for aligning the two sequences are shown in Tables 2.13, with the final optimal alignment score being 3 in $V(m,n)$ which is the maximum of $G(m,n)$, $E(m,n)$ and $F(m,n)$ in Table 2.12. Note that, because G matrix is for aligning sections containing no indels, its entries are always the alignment score $V(i-1, j-1)$ plus the MM score for the next nucleotide pair $x(i)$ and $y(j)$. Also note that each entry in the V matrix is the alignment score up to the corresponding nucleotide. For example, the number 4 in $V(2,2)$ (Table 2.12) is the alignment score for aligning sequences AC and AC, the number 2 in $V(5,4)$ is the alignment score for aligning ACGT and ACGGC, and the final number of 3 at the bottom right is the alignment score of aligning ACGT and ACGGCT (Table 2.12).

2.4.2   COMPUTING BACKTRACK MATRICES

We need backtrack matrices to obtain the actual sequence alignment. The use of affine function gap penalty demands three backtrack matrices, designated B_0, B_1, and B_2, in contrast to just one with constant gap penalty. Backtrack matrices are computed concurrently with the scoring matrices. It is only for clarity that I illustrate their computation separately below.

The three backtrack matrices are filled from left to right and from top to bottom, according to Eqs. (2.14)–(2.16). I have used values of 0, 1, and 2 for different states, but readers and teachers using the book are welcome to use arrows or whatever symbols to improve clarity.

$$B_0(i, j) = 0 \text{ when } \max[G(i, j), E(i, j), F(i, j)] = G(i, j)$$
$$B_0(i, j) = 1 \text{ when } \max[G(i, j), E(i, j), F(i, j)] = E(i, j) \quad (2.14)$$
$$B_0(i, j) = 2 \text{ when } \max[G(i, j), E(i, j), F(i, j)] = F(i, j)$$

$$B_1(i,j) = 1 \text{ when } E(i,j-1) - GE \leq V(i,j-1) - GO$$
$$B_1(i,j) = 2 \text{ when } E(i,j-1) - GE > V(i,j-1) - GO$$
$$(2.15)$$

$$B_2(i,j) = 1 \text{ when } F(i-1,j) - GE \leq V(i-1,j) - GO$$
$$B_2(i,j) = 2 \text{ when } F(i-1,j) - GE > V(i-1,j) - GO$$
$$(2.16)$$

Note that I used the $\leq$ sign for B_1, and B_2 matrices. This lumps two events (< and =) into one so that, if there are multiple equally optimal alignments, only one will be reported. The numerical illustration for the first two cells in each of the tree matrices are in Eq. (2.17). Note that the backtrack matrices here are indexed from 1, whereas the three scoring matrices are indexed from 0. The x and y sequences are also indexed from 1, e.g., $x(1) = $ 'A', and $y(1) = $ 'A'.

$$B_0(1,1) = 0 \text{ because } \max[G(1,1), E(1,1), F(1,1)] = G(1,1)$$
$$B_1(1,1) = 2 \text{ because } E(1,0) - GE > V(1,0) - GO$$
$$B_2(1,1) = 2 \text{ because } F(0,1) - GE > V(0,1) - GO$$
$$(2.17)$$

$$B_0(1,2) = 1 \text{ because } \max[G(1,2), E(1,2), F(1,2)] = E(1,2)$$
$$B_1(1,2) = 1 \text{ because } E(1,1) - GE < V(1,1) - GO$$
$$B_2(1,2) = 2 \text{ because } F(0,2) - GE > V(0,2) - GO$$
$$(2.18)$$

The complete backtrack matrices, shown in Table 2.13, are needed to obtain sequence alignment. However, they do not need extra memory space because scoring matrices are not needed for obtaining sequence alignment, the memory space for scoring matrices can be sequentially over-written by backtrack matrices.

TABLE 2.13   Three backtrack matrices (B_0, B_1 and B_2) for obtaining sequence alignment, with the match-mismatch matrix S specified in Figure 2.11B, GO (gap open penalty) = 3 and GE (gap extension penalty) = 2.

	B_0				B_1				B_2			
	A	C	G	T	A	C	G	T	A	C	G	T
A	0	1	1	1	2	1	2	2	2	2	2	2
C	2	0	1	1	2	1	1	2	1	1	1	1
G	2	2	0	1	2	1	1	1	2	1	1	1
G	2	2	0	0	2	1	1	1	2	2	1	1
C	2	0	2	0	2	1	1	1	2	2	2	1
T	2	2	2	0	2	1	1	1	2	2	2	2

2.4.3   OBTAIN SEQUENCE ALIGNMENT FROM BACKTRACK MATRICES

Many students get confused with applying the backtrack matrices to obtain the sequence alignment. The confusion mainly arises from the necessity of jumping from one backtrack matrix to another in recovering the alignment. The only case when you do not need to jump from one backtrack matrix to another is when the optimal alignment has no indel.

We start by checking the bottom-right value of matrix B_0, that is, $B_0(m,n)$. If it is 0, then we align $x(m)$ against $y(n)$, and move upleft to $B_0(m-1,n-1)$. If we continue to encounter 0 in $B_0(m-1,n-1)$, $B_0(m-2,n-2)$, etc., we will align $x(m-1)$ against $y(n-1)$, $x(m-2)$ against $y(n-2)$, ..., until $B_0(i,j) \neq 0$, or until we reach the left or top edge of the matrix.

If $B_0(i,j) = 1$, then we move to the corresponding cell in matrix B_1, that is, $B_1(i,j)$ which takes a value of either 1 or 2. If $B_1(i,j) = 2$, then we will (1) align a gap against $y(j)$ and (2) move left to the next cell, $B_1(i,j-1)$. As long as the next cell is 2 in B_1 matrix, we will continue to align a gap against nucleotide in y and move left until we encounter a 1 in B_1 matrix or when we reach the left edge of the matrix. Encountering a value of 1 in B_1 matrix means that we will (1) align a gap against $y(j)$, (2) move left to the next cell, and do the additional (3) jump back to the corresponding cell in B_0 matrix and decide what to do by checking the cell value in B_0.

If $B_0(i,j) = 2$, then we move to the corresponding cell in matrix B_2, that is, $B_2(i,j)$. If $B_2(i,j) = 2$, then we will (1) align a gap character against $x(i)$, and (2) move up the matrix to the next cell, that is, $B_2(i-1,j)$. We continue to align the gap character against nucleotide in x until we encounter a value of 1 in B_2, or until we reach the top edge of the matrix. A value of 1 in B_2 means that (1) we will align a gap against $x(i)$, (2) move upward to the next cell, and finally (3) jump back to the corresponding cell in B_0.

Take, for example, the backtrack matrices B_0, B_1, and B_2 shown in Tables 2.13. We note that $B_0(m,n) = B_0(6,4) = 0$, so we align $x(6)$, the last T in x, against $y(4)$, the last T in y (Step 1 in Fig. 2.12). We always move to the upleft cell after encountering a 0 in B_0, so this moves us from $B_0(6,4)$ to $B_0(5,3)$. Whenever we encounter a 2 in B_0, we move to the corresponding cell in matrix B_2 which is $B_2(5,3)$. $B_2(5,3) = 2$. A number 2 in B_2 always means that (1) we align a gap against the nucleotide in the column sequence, that is, against $x(5) = $ 'C' (Step 2 in Fig. 2.12), and (2) move upward to the next cell, $B_2(4,3)$ which is 1. A change of value from

2 to 1 in B_2 always means that (1) we align a gap against the nucleotide in the column sequence, that is, against $x(4)$ = 'G' (Step 3 in Fig. 2.12), and (2) move upward to the next cell, $B_2(3,3)$, and (3) jump back to the corresponding cell in B_0, i.e., $B_0(3,3)$. Because $B_0(3,3) = 0$, we align the two corresponding nucleotides (G:G, Step 4 in Figure 2.12) and move to $B_0(2,2)$. Because both $B_0(2,2)$ and $B_0(1,1)$ are zero, we align the corresponding nucleotides (Steps 5 and 6) to complete the alignment shown in Figure 2.12.

```
Seq x:  ACGGCT
Seq y:  ACG--T
Step    654321
```

FIGURE 2.12   Steps taken to align the two sequences using the backtrack matrices.

One simple way to check if our backtracking is correct is to compute the alignment score in Figure 2.12. There are four matches each getting 2 points, one gap open with penalty 3 and one gap extension with penalty 2. The alignment score is therefore $2*4 - 3 - 2 = 3$ which is the same as the value in $V(6,4)$ in Table 2.12.

2.5   MULTIPLE SEQUENCE ALIGNMENT

Dynamic programming algorithms for sequence alignment are slow and memory-hungry. Consequently, it is impractical to perform MSA by extending the dynamic programming approach from two dimension to multiple dimensions. An alternative is to use an approximate evaluation criterion termed the sum-of-pairs score (SPS) (Althaus et al., 2002; Gupta et al., 1995; Lipman et al., 1989; Reinert et al., 2000; Stoye et al., 1997). Each multiple alignment of N sequences implies $N(N-1)/2$ pairwise alignments. SPS is simply the summation of all pairwise alignment scores without penalizing shared gaps. Obtaining SPS from MSAs is easy. All we need is a scoring scheme, i.e., gap-open and gap-extension penalties plus a match/mismatch matrix. However, while applying the SPS criterion is conceptually simple, i.e., an MSA with the highest SPS is the best one, there has been no workable algorithms developed for practical sequence alignment, partly because of an inconsistency problem illustrated in the next section.

An alternative is to use a guide tree to reduce the multiple alignment problem to the pairwise alignment problem (Feng and Doolittle, 1987; Hogeweg and Hesper, 1984). All practical multiple alignment programs, e.g., Clustal series of programs (Higgins, 1994; Thompson et al., 1994), MAFFT (Katoh et al., 2005; Katoh and Toh, 2010) and MUSCLE (Edgar, 2004) take this approach. In short, we start from leaves of the tree and progress toward the root by aligning sequences represented by the two sister nodes. If the sister nodes are two tips on the tree, then it is the conventional pairwise alignment. If the sister nodes involve a tip and one internal node, then the internal node is represented by either a sequence profile or a reconstructed ancestral sequence (both covered in later sections of this chapter). So, we either align two sequences or align a sequence against a sequence profile (or against a reconstructed ancestral sequence). If the sister nodes are both internal nodes, then we will align either two profiles or two ancestral sequences, depending on whether the internal node is represented by either a sequence profile or an ancestral sequence. The pairwise alignment of sister nodes progresses to the root of the guide tree to complete the multiple alignment. This progressive multiple alignment represents a practical compromise between accuracy and speed. There are advantage and disadvantages of representing ancestral sequences by either a profile or an ancestral sequence. We will make a brief comparison later in this chapter.

This progressive multiple alignment creates a chicken-egg problem. To obtain a good alignment, one needs a good guide tree, but to have a good guide tree, one needs a good alignment. A guide tree is typically built from a matrix of pairwise alignment scores. Because pairwise alignment scores are similarity indices, they are sometimes converted to a distance matrix before constructing a guide tree. Such a guide tree is typically poor. One way to get a much better guide tree is to use the PhyPA method (Xia, 2016).

There is another chicken-egg problem associated with sequence alignment. We use a MM matrix, e.g., BLOSUM (Henikoff and Henikoff, 1992) to score sequence alignment. If we are to have a good alignment for highly diverged sequences, then we need a good MM matrix such as BLOSUM45. However, we cannot have a good BLOSUM45 if we do not have a set of diverged but well-aligned sequences. The BLOSUM approach alleviates this problem by excluding alignment segments with indels. In contrast, PAM matrices (Dayhoff et al., 1978) do not have this chicken-egg problem because they are all derived from a transition probability matrix based on very similar sequences whose alignment is not ambiguous.

2.5.1 PROFILE ALIGNMENT

Profile alignment aligns either one sequence (designated T) against a set of already aligned sequences in the form of a profile (designated S), or align two profiles S_1 and S_2. It is an essential technique for MSA. There are various approaches to profile alignment. The simplest is to get a consensus sequence from S (designated C_S) and align T and C_S by using the pairwise alignment method we learned in previous sections. Whenever we insert a gap in C_S, we insert a corresponding gap in all sequences in S. However, a profile is more informative than C_S.

Suppose we want to align sequence $T =$ "ACG" against the three aligned sequences in Figure 2.13A. The first step in profile alignment is to represent the three aligned sequences with a site-specific frequency profile (S). The set of three aligned sequences have five symbols (A, C, G, T, and the gap symbol "-") and can be represented by S shown in the first five rows in Figure 2.13B. The first column of S is a list of the five symbols, followed by five data columns corresponding to five aligned sites. Each data column corresponds to frequencies of symbols in an aligned site. The first data column represents the frequencies of symbols in the first aligned site, with the frequencies of A and G being 2/3 and 1/3, respectively. The second data column represents the frequencies of the second aligned site with the frequency C being 1 and the frequencies of other symbols being 0 and so on. Thus, a set of aligned sequences can always be represented by S in the form of an $N \times L$ matrix, where N is the number of symbols (five for nucleotide sequences and 21 for amino acid sequences) and L is the sequence length. It is important to note that any phylogenetic information among aligned sequences is lost in converting the set of aligned sequences to S.

The second step is to perform a special version of the dynamic programming to generate the scoring matrix and backtrack matrix. I will illustrate the profile alignment principle by using the constant gap penalty. With the length of T being 3 and the length of S being 5, there are only 15 cells to fill in. Because one needs to compute three values (DIAG, UP, and LEFT) for each cell, the total number of values to compute is 45, so manual calculation can only be done with very short sequences.

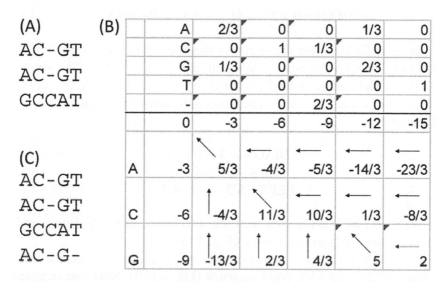

FIGURE 2.13 Dynamic programming to align a sequence T (="ACG") against three already aligned sequences in (A), with scoring and backtrack matrices in (B), and final alignment in (C). The first five rows in (B) is a sequence profile representing the three aligned sequences in (A). Christian Delamarche corrected a miscalculated value in the table.

The score matrix and the backtrack matrix (Fig. 2.13B) were obtained with a special scoring scheme. There are two kinds of matches, a match between two identical nucleotides, or a match between two gap symbols. The match score for the former and latter are designated M_{Nuc} and M_{Gap}, respectively, with corresponding values set to 2 and 1, respectively, in the example. There are also two kinds of mismatches, one involving a transitional difference and the other a transversional difference. They are designated as MM_s and MM_v, respectively, with corresponding values set to 1 and −1, respectively, in this example. We set the constant gap penalty with $G = -3$.

We now illustrate how the scoring matrix and backtrack matrix (Fig. 2.13B) are computed. For the first cell, the UP and LEFT values are simple:

$$UP = -3 + G = -3 - 3 = -6$$
$$LEFT = -3 + G = -3 - 3 = -6$$

For the DIAG value, we should keep in mind that the nucleotide A in the column sequence has a probability of 2/3 of an A-A match with $M_{Nuc} = 2$, and a probability of 1/3 of an A-G transition with $M_{Ms} = 1$. This leads to

$$\text{DIAG} = 0 + 2/3 \times M_{Nuc} + 1/3 \times MM_s = 5/3.$$

Because DIAG is the maximum of the three, it is used to fill the first cell, together with the associated upleft arrow (Fig. 2.13B). The second cell (to the right of the first cell) is simple because the profile at the second site contains C only. So, the computation is the same as in regular pairwise alignment:

$$\text{DIAG} = -3 - 1 = -4$$
$$\text{UP} = -6 - 3 = -9$$
$$\text{LEFT} = 5/3 - 3 = -4/3$$

Because LEFT is the largest of the three, the cell is filled with −4/3 together with a left-pointing arrow (Fig. 2.13B).

The cell likely to cause some confusion is the third, i.e., the one with a value of −5/3 and a left-pointing arrow (Fig. 2.13B). Note that an upleft arrow in that cell implies that A will (1) pair with C with a probability of 1/3, penalized by $MM_v = -1$, and (2) pair with "−" with a probability of 2/3, penalized by G = −3. Therefore,

$$\text{DIAG} = -6 - 2/3 \times 3 - 1/3 \times 1 = -25/3.$$

The calculation of UP is simply UP = −9 −3 = −12. A left-pointing arrow, however, implies a gap in the column sequence, so we have a gap with a probability of 2/3 of facing a gap in the row profile, with $M_{gap} = 1$ and a probability of 1/3 of facing a C, with G = −3. Therefore,

$$\text{LEFT} = -4/3 + 2/3 \times 1 - 1/3 \times 3 = -5/3.$$

Because LEFT is the largest of the three, the cell is filled with −5/3 and a left-pointing arrow. The rest of the cells are relatively straightforward. The alignment can again be obtained by tracing the backtrack matrix (Fig. 2.13B), which is shown in Figure 2.13C.

The profile alignment outlined above represents an extension of the pairwise alignment, with the row sequence replaced by a profile. One can also replace the column sequence by a profile to align two profiles instead of two sequences. This approach is used in Clustal and many other programs for MSA . The key skill for doing profile alignment is book-keeping. Anyone who is good at accounting should have no problem with profile alignment.

One might also argue that the profile alignment has a serious problem as follows. Sequence T may be phylogenetically more closely related to some sequences than others in S. However, the profile alignment approach does not take this into consideration. Unfortunately, alternative approaches by combining both phylogenetic reconstruction and MSA (Hein, 1990, 1994; Sankoff et al., 1973) are generally too computationally intensive to be practical. However, recent advances in Gibbs sampler, which in molecular biology is used mainly for de novo motif discovery and numerically illustrated in detail before (Xia, 2012b; 2018a, Chapter 4) has suggested alternative ways for pairwise sequence alignment (Zhu et al., 1998) and MSA conditional on a phylogenetic tree (Holmes and Bruno, 2001; Jensen and Hein, 2005).

2.5.2   REPLACING A SEQUENCE PROFILE BY A RECONSTRUCTED ANCESTRAL SEQUENCE

There is a major problem with representing ancestral nodes by sequence profiles. With increasing number of sequences, the identity of each site is gradually eroded. For example, the frequencies at each site become progressively more and more similar to the global frequencies when more and more divergent sequences are included. For this reason, representing ancestral node with a reconstructed sequences may have two advantages. First, it may alleviate the problem of information erosion. Second, aligning two sequences with ambiguous codes is simpler than aligning two profiles.

One advantage of a reconstructed ancestral sequence over a profile is illustrated in Figure 2.14 with a topology and a single nucleotide site shown. A sequence profile for the root node will have the site fully ambiguous because the leaves have exactly the same number of A, C, G, and T, whereas the site is C when reconstructed by the Fitch algorithm. The Fitch algorithm, together with Sankoff algorithm, will be illustrated in detail in the chapter on MP method for phylogenetic reconstruction.

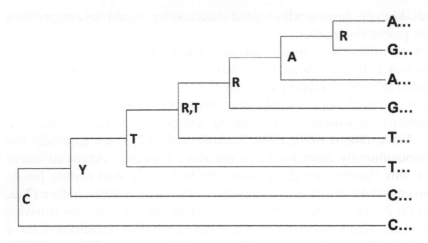

FIGURE 2.14   An 8-species topology with one nucleotide site shown. A profile for the root node would have equal nucleotide frequencies for the site (i.e., a fully ambiguous site), whereas a reconstructed sequence for the root node will have nucleotide C.

In summary, for MSA with a guide tree, we perform pairwise alignment between sister taxa from the leaves, reconstruct ancestral sequences for their parental nodes and traverse down the tree to the root to align the sequences for the sister nodes until all sequences have been aligned. When a gap is inserted in the sequence for the ancestral node, then sequences for all the descendent leaf nodes will receive the gap character as well.

2.5.3   MULTIPLE ALIGNMENT WITH A GUIDE TREE

Multiple alignment with a guide tree consists of three steps. The first is to perform all pairwise alignments by dynamic programming. With N sequences, there are $N(N-1)/2$ pairwise alignments, leading to a triangular matrix of alignment scores. The second step is to construct a guide tree by using the alignment score matrix as a sequence similarity matrix in conjunction with a clustering algorithm. Alternatively, one can convert the similarity matrix into a distance matrix and then use either UPGMA or neighbor-joining method (Saitou and Nei, 1987) to build a guide tree such as the one shown in Figure 2.15. The third step is to traverse the node to align sequences by pairwise alignment and profile alignment. Some multiple alignment programs, such as MAFFT (Katoh et al., 2005; Katoh and Toh, 2010) and MUSCLE (Edgar, 2004) take an iterative approach. That is, after obtaining the first multiple alignment, they will build a tree from this first multiple alignment and then use this tree (which is typically better than the original guide tree from pairwise alignment scores) to guide the multiple alignment again. This can be repeated a number of times until an index measuring the quality of multiple alignment does not show further improvement.

The multiple alignment starts from the most similar sequences. So, we move to internal node 11 and align Seq2 and Seq6 (Fig. 2.15). We then move to internal node 10 and align Seq5 against either an ancestral sequence for node 11 or a sequence profile representing aligned Seq2 and Seq6 using the method outlined in Figure 2.13. A profile or an ancestral sequence for node 10 is then created to represent the three aligned sequences (Seq2, Seq6, and Seq5). Moving to internal node 9, we found one of its two child nodes (internal node 12) having two child nodes with unaligned sequences (Seq3 and Seq4) which are then first aligned by using the dynamic programming method. A profile or an ancestral sequence for node 12 is then created to represent the aligned Seq3 and Seq4. This profile is then aligned against the profile representing the aligned Seq2, Seq6, and Seq5. The process continues until all sequences are aligned.

It is easy to see why we should start with the most similar sequences because any alignment error from pairwise alignment of child nodes will be propagated in subsequent alignment involving their parental nodes. Obviously, a wrong guide tree will bias the subsequent alignment which in turn will bias subsequent phylogenetic reconstruction based on the alignment. Unfortunately, a guide tree built from alignment scores is typically a very poor tree. For this reason, it is better to input a well-established tree, whenever available, as a guide tree for MSA. All frequently used multiple alignment programs allow users to input their own guild tree. My program DAMBE (Xia, 2013b) can build high-quality trees based on pairwise alignment with simultaneously estimated evolutionary distances ("simultaneous estimation" mean the distances are estimated using all pairs of sequences instead of just one pair) by using the PhyPA method (Xia, 2016). One can use the PhyPA function to build a tree and then input to an MSA program as a guide tree.

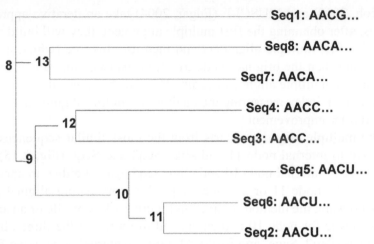

FIGURE 2.15   An example of a guide tree for multiple sequence alignment of eight sequences, called leaves or terminal nodes. The internal nodes are numbered from 8 to 13 (with terminal nodes, or leaves, numbered from 0 to 7).

2.6   THE INCONSISTENCY PROBLEM WITH PAIRWISE ALIGNMENT IN CONTRAST TO MULTIPLE ALIGNMENT

Pairwise alignment can be inconsistent (Fig. 2.16). Given the three amino acid sequences (*S1–S3*) in Figure 2.16a, we can get three pairwise alignments shown in Figure 2.16b with the scoring scheme defined by BLOSUM62, gap open equal to 20 and gap extension equal to 2. The residue W in *S1* at site 3 (designated by W_{13}, where the first subscript 1 indicates the 1st sequence (*S1*) and the second subscript 3 indicates the 3rd site in *S1*) is inferred to be homologous to W_{22} based on the pairwise alignment between *S1* and *S2*, and homologous to W_{33} based on the pairwise alignment between *S1* and *S3* (Fig. 2–16b). These two homologous site pairs (W_{13}/W_{22}, W_{13}/W_{33}) imply a homologous site pair W_{22}/W_{33} which, however, is not true in the pairwise alignment between *S2* and *S3* (Fig. 2.16b) where site W_{22} pairs with K_{32} instead of W_{33}. This inconsistency in site homology identification in pairwise alignment disappears in a multiple alignment (Fig. 2.16c) obtained with the same scoring scheme. When pairwise alignment is derived from the multiple alignment (Fig. 2.16d), then two inferred homologous pairs (W_{13}/W_{22}, W_{13}/W_{33}) imply a homologous site pair W_{22}/W_{33} which is observed in Figure 2.16d.

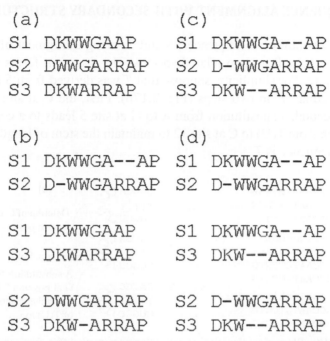

FIGURE 2.16 Identification of homologous sites in pairwise and multiple alignment, illustrating the problem of inconsistency in site homology identification associated with pairwise alignment. (a) Three amino acid sequences *S1* to *S3*; (b) three PSAs from the three sequences in (a), with scoring scheme of BLOSUM62, gap open equal to 20 and gap extension equal to 2; (c) MSA of three sequences in (a) with the same scoring scheme; (d) three PSAs derived from the MSA in (c).

For any particular pair of sequences *S1* and *S2*, other sequences may contribute both phylogenetic information and noise to the identification of homologous sites between *S1* and *S2*. With low sequence divergence, phylogenetic information contributed by other sequences overwhelms noise and reduces the problem of inconsistency in homologous site identification often seen in pairwise alignment. Thus, when a reliable multiple alignment can be obtained, one should use this multiple alignment for phylogenetic inference instead of pairwise alignment (Xia, 2016). However, when sequences are so diverged that additional sequences will contribute mostly noise instead of phylogenetic information, then building trees with only pairwise alignment might be more preferable (Xia, 2016).

2.7   SEQUENCE ALIGNMENT WITH SECONDARY STRUCTURE

Figure 2.17a shows two sequences, S and T, being a fragment of a fictitious rRNA gene from two related species. The fragment forms a stem-
loop structure. For simplicity, suppose that T was derived from S through
the intermediate T' in two steps (Fig. 2.17b). First, the C at site 11 was
deleted. Second, a substitution from A to G at site 5 leads to a correlated
substitution from T(U) to C at site 12 to maintain the stem of length 5. The
resulting sequence is T.

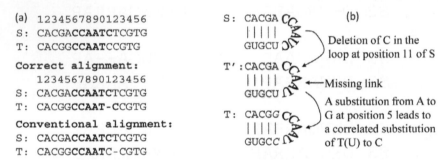

FIGURE 2.17 Illustration that the correct alignment may differ from the optimal
alignment. Nucleotide T becomes U in the secondary structure. (a) Two sequences (S and
T) with T derived from S via two steps shown in (b). The loop region is shown in **bold**.

The "Correct alignment" in Figure 2.17 captures the evolutionary
process shown in Figure 2.17b with two changes between S and T. There
is a deletion of nucleotide C in the loop region, as well as a substitution
from A in sequence S at site 5 to G in sequence T leading to a correlated
change of T to C at site 12 to maintain the base-pairing in the stem region.
The secondary structure information in Figure 2.17b suggests that the
first five and the last five nucleotides of S are respectively homologous
to the first five and the last five nucleotides of T. However, any currently
used alignment program based on linear sequence information, with any
sensible scoring scheme, would recover the "conventional alignment"
(Fig. 2.17a) that identified the gap at site 12. The two C's at site 11 in
the "conventional alignment" are nicely aligned but are not homologous
given the evolutionary steps generating T (Fig. 2.17b). It is easy to see
that the conventional alignment will have a greater alignment score than
the correct alignment and consequently is more "optimal." Thus, optimal

alignment (the alignment with the largest alignment score) may not necessarily be the correct alignment.

Aligning rRNA genes with the constraint of secondary structure has now been frequently used in practical research in molecular evolution and phylogenetics (Hickson et al., 2000; Kjer, 1995; Notredame et al., 1997; Xia, 2000; Xia et al., 2003a). However, one cannot always assume that rRNA secondary structure is stable over evolutionary time in different lineages. It is now well established that variation in rRNA secondary structure is strongly affected by the optimal growth temperature in prokaryotes (Galtier and Lobry, 1997; Hurst and Merchant, 2001; Nakashima et al., 2003; Wang and Hickcy, 2002; Wang et al., 2006). Two programs can automate sequence alignment guided by secondary structure: PROMALS3D (Pei et al., 2008) for protein sequences and PHASE (Gowri-Shankar and Rattray, 2007) for rRNA and tRNA sequences.

2.8 ALIGN NUCLEOTIDE SEQUENCES AGAINST AMINO ACID SEQUENCES

During the evolution of protein-coding genes, an entire codon or multiple codons may be deleted or inserted but it is much rarer to see an insertion or deletion (often abbreviated as indel) of one or two nucleotides because, such indel events lead to frameshifting mutations that almost always disrupt the original protein function and are strongly selected against. However, alignment of protein-coding nucleotide sequences often produces indels of one or two bases as alignment artifacts. The correctly aligned sequences should have complete codons, not one or two nucleotides, inserted or deleted.

One way to avoid the introduction of frameshifting indels as alignment artifacts is to align the protein-coding nucleotide sequences against aligned amino acid sequences, which was implemented in software DAMBE since 1999 (Xia, 2001; Xia and Xie, 2001). The approach obviously requires amino acid sequences which can be obtained by translating the protein-coding nucleotide sequences into amino acid sequences. This can be done automatically in DAMBE which implements all known genetic codes for translating protein-coding sequences from diverse organisms. Second, if you are working on nucleotide sequences deposited in GenBank, then typically you will find the corresponding translated amino acid sequences.

The alignment of protein-coding nucleotide sequences is typically done in three steps. First, the nucleotide sequences are translated into amino acid sequences. These amino acid sequences are then aligned and the nucleotide sequences are then aligned against the aligned amino acid sequences. This is illustrated in Figure 2.18A-D.

```
(A)  S1  ATG  CCG  GGA  CAA                (D)  S1  ATG  CCG  GGA  - - -  CAA
     S2  ATG  CCC  GGG  ATT  CAA                S2  ATG  CCC  GGG  ATT  CAA
                                                    ***  **   **         ***
(B)  S1  MPGQ
     S2  MPGIQ
                                           (E)  S1  ATG  CC-  GGG  A- -  CAA
(C)  S1  MPG-Q                                  S2  ATG  CCC  GGG  ATT  CAA
     S2  MPGIQ                                      ***  **   ***  *     ***
```

FIGURE 2.18   Aligning protein-coding nucleotide sequences against aligned amino acid sequences. (A) Two protein-coding sequences (*S1* and *S2*). (B) Amino acid sequences translated from *S1* and *S2* in (A). (C) Aligned amino acid sequences. (D) Mapping codon sequences against aligned amino acid sequences. (E) Conventional alignment.

This alignment (Fig. 2.18D) has 10 matches, 2 mismatches, and 1 gap of length 3. Recall that the main objective of sequence alignment is to identify homologous sites and it is important to note that different alignments may lead to different interpretations of sequence homology. With the alignment in Fig. 2.18D, sites 6 of the two sequences (G in *S1* and C in *S2*) are interpreted as a homologous site, so is site 9 (A in *S1* and G in *S2*). These interpretations are not established facts. They are only inferences of what might have happened.

Depending on the scoring scheme, a conventional nucleotide-based sequence alignment without using aligned amino acid sequences as a mapping reference, may well generate the alignment in Figure 2.18E, with 12 matches, 0 mismatch and two gaps of lengths 1 and 2, respectively.

Note three different interpretations of the homologous sites between alignments in Figure 2.18D (Alignment 1) and Figure 2.18E (Alignment 2). First, the nucleotide G at site 6 of *S1* is now interpreted to be homologous to the nucleotide G at site 7 of *S2*. Second, the nucleotide A at site 9 of *S1* is now interpreted as homologous to the nucleotide A at site 10 of *S2*. Which of the two alignments makes more sense? If Alignment 1 is correct but we used a nucleotide-based alignment method and end up with Alignment 2, then the estimation of the genetic distance between the two sequences will be biased. The genetic distance measures the evolutionary dissimilarity between two sequences, often estimated by ignoring the indel sites. It is often used as an index of sequence divergence time in molecular phylogenetics, when calibrated by fossils with known divergence time. In this particular case, if we perform site-wise deletion of indels, then *S1* and *S2* would appear more similar to each other in Alignment 2 than in Alignment 1. Biased estimation of the genetic distance often results in failure in molecular phylogenetic reconstruction.

Given that a protein-coding gene is unlikely to remain functional after two consecutive indel mutations as in Alignment 2, we may argue that Alignment 1 based on the alignment of amino acid sequences is better than Alignment 2. In addition to eliminating indels of length one or two as alignment artifacts, aligning protein-coding amino acid sequences against aligned amino acid sequences also has the benefit associated with the fact that amino acid sequences can be aligned more reliably. Aligning amino acid sequences are also faster than aligning the corresponding codon sequences because the amino acid sequences are only 1/3 as long as the corresponding codon sequences. The size of the MM matrix has little effect of the speed of alignment because computers take a memory address to retrieve a value in a matrix and this is the same for a 4×4 as for a 20×20 matrix.

However, there are also cases where a nucleotide-based alignment may be better. Now consider the two protein-coding sequences in Figure 2.19, with all three alternative alignments involving one indel of length 3 so none will introduce frameshifts. Which one makes more sense to you?

```
(A)      3    6    9    12   15      (C) Alignment 2
   S1  ATG  CCC  GTA  TAA             S1  ATG  CCC  GT-  --A  TAA
   S2  ATG  CCC  GTG  TTA  TAA        S2  ATG  CCC  GTG  TTA  TAA
                                          ***  ***  **        ***
(B) Alignment 1                      (D) Alignment 3
   S1  ATG  CCC  GTA  ---  TAA        S1  ATG  CCC  G--  -TA  TAA
   S2  ATG  CCC  GTG  TTA  TAA        S2  ATG  CCC  GTG  TTA  TAA
       ***  ***  **        ***            ***  ***  **        ***
```

FIGURE 2.19 A case in which aligning codon sequences against aligned amino acid sequences may not be as preferable as conventional alignment. (A) Two codon sequences with sites numbered. (B) Aligned codon sequences based on aligned amino acid sequences. (C–D) Two alternative equally good alignments from conventional pairwise alignment.

Alignment 1 (Fig. 2.19B) is the outcome of aligning nucleotide sequences against aligned amino acid sequences and the other two alignments (Fig. 2.19C,D) are from nucleotide-based alignments. The three alignments represent three alternative hypotheses, all involving a gap of length 3, but differ in the position of the gap. Alignment 1 has only 11 matches, whereas the other two alignments each have 12 matches. In this case, the two hypotheses represented by Alignments 2 and 3 are better than Alignment 1 based on the parsimony criterion. Alignment 1 implies a triplet indel and an A↔G substitution, whereas Alignments 2 and 3 each require only a triplet deletion. However, from Alignment 1, one can easily obtain Alignments 2 or 3 by automated postalignment adjustment (Xia, 2016).

KEYWORDS

- **dynamic programming**
- **affine function gap penalty**
- **match-mismatch matrix**
- **PAM**
- **BLOSUM**
- **guide tree**
- **pairwise alignment**
- **multiple alignment**

CHAPTER 3

Nucleotide Substitution Models and Evolutionary Distances

ABSTRACT

Nucleotide substitution models in molecular phylogenetics are Markov chain models characterized a rate matrix. Transition probabilities derived from the rate matrix are needed for computing likelihood in likelihood-based phylogenetic method and for deriving and computing evolutionary distances for distance-based phylogenetic methods. Substitution models are essential for dating speciation and gene duplication events. They enable us to trace history back to the very early forms of life, by reconstructing the genomic "books" erased and obliterated by billions of years of mutations. This chapter focuses on nucleotide-based substitution models, presenting three different ways of deriving transition probability matrices from various rate matrices. These three different ways should allow students of different mathematical background to understand substitution models and their uses in phylogenetics. Almost all frequently used substitution models are nested models with the simple one being a special case of the more general one. The likelihood ratio test, as well as the information-theoretic indices as an alternative approach for model selection, is numerically illustrated in choosing the substitution model that best describes the aligned sequences.

3.1 INTRODUCTION

This and the next five chapters belong to the core domain of molecular phylogenetics, including phylogeny-based comparative methods. Substitution models are the subject of this and the next chapter, which is followed by phylogenetic reconstruction methods. The objective is to trace evolutionary history as far back as possible so that we, in Aristotle's words, can all have the most advantageous view of things by viewing them from the very beginning.

It is often difficult to stretch our vision back to time immemorial. Substitutions occur over time and can overwrite each other at the same nucleotide or amino acid site. Such a process has been going on for millions or billions of years. When we compare two homologous nucleotide sequences and find differences in N sites, the actual number of substitutions (designated by M) could be much greater than N because multiple substitutions could have happened at the same site, overwriting each other (Fig. 3.1). How can we infer the unobservable M from the observable N?

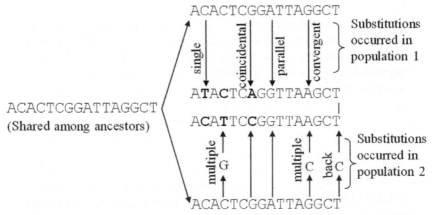

FIGURE 3.1 Illustration of nucleotide substitutions and the difficulty in correcting for multiple hits. The ancestor has diverged into northern and southern populations that have independently accumulated substitutions indicated by arrows. A total of 12 substitutions have happened but only three sites differ between the two extant sequences.

Substitution models aim to achieve two related objectives. The first is to correct for multiple hits. That is, to infer M (=12 in Fig. 3.1) from N (= 3 in Fig. 3.1). The second is to characterize substitution patterns among sites and in different evolutionary lineages. Many factors can modulate substitution rates of nucleotide sequences, such as transition bias (Xia et al., 1996) and rate heterogeneity among codons (Xia, 1998b), and of amino acid sequences, such as genetic codes and functional constraints (Xia and Li, 1998). To trace the evolutionary history back to time t_0, we need to know how nucleotide or amino acid sequences have come to their current states, i.e., how the sequences have changed during the interval from time t_0 to present.

If we understand substitution process well and can characterize the process by a substitution model, then it is possible to reconstruct ancestral protein-coding sequence based on substitution models, synthesize the reconstructed protein and explore its function and evolution (Chang et al., 2002a; Chang et al., 2002b; Ugalde et al., 2004). Given that substitution models are used widely in molecular phylogenetics, we need to develop an appreciation of the differences among different substitution models and to understand how to choose one substitution model over others in practical applications.

This chapter covers three related topics. The first is how to derive transition probabilities and evolutionary distances from an instantaneous rate matrix, which is the most fundamental aspect of substitution models. Transition probabilities are needed both for computing likelihood in likelihood-based method and for computing evolutionary distances in the distance-based method. Most of the chapter is taken up by my detailed illustration of three different approaches to do the derivation. The second is how far we can trace evolutionary history back in time if sequences do evolve according to a specified substitution model. The third is how to choose the best substitution models, i.e., likelihood ratio test (LRT) for nested models and information-theoretic indices, such as Akaike information criterion (AIC) and Bayesian information criterion (BIC), for nested or nonnested models.

There are three types of molecular sequences, i.e., nucleotide, AA, and codon sequences. Consequently, there are three corresponding types of substitution models. Many substitution models have been proposed for nucleotide, amino acid, and codon sequences. All substitution models used in molecular phylogenetics are Markov chain models characterized by (1) either a transition probability matrix (P) with discrete time or a rate matrix (Q) in continuous time where P can be derived from Q and vice versa and (2) equilibrium frequencies. Note that the phrase 'transition probability' in transition probability matrix means the probability of remaining in one state or changing from one state to another (e.g., nucleotide A to one of the other three nucleotides) in one unit time. The general form of a rate matrix for nucleotide sequences is, in the order of A, G, C, and T:

$$Q = \begin{bmatrix} A & - & a & b & c \\ G & g & - & d & e \\ C & h & i & - & f \\ T & j & k & l & - \end{bmatrix} \tag{3.1}$$

Frequently used nucleotide-based substitutions and their relationships are illustrated in Figure 3.2, with the JC69 model (Jukes and Cantor, 1969) being the simplest. The K80 model (Kimura, 1980) generalizes the JC69 model by allowing transitions and transversions to have different rates (α for transitions and β for transversions). F81/TN84 (Felsenstein, 1981; Tajima and Nei, 1984) generalizes JC69 by adding the frequency parameters. F84 (used in DNAML since 1984 Hasegawa and Kishino, 1989; Kishino and Hasegawa, 1989) and HKY85 (Hasegawa et al., 1985) may be viewed as extension from F81/TN84 with additional differential rates for transitions and transversions or from K80 by adding frequency parameters. TN93 (Tamura and Nei, 1993) extended F84/HKY85 by allowing C↔T and A↔G to have different rates, and GTR (Lanave et al., 1984; Tavaré, 1986) extended TN93 by allowing the four types of transversions to have different rates.

Many more substitution models and genetic distances have been proposed (Tamura and Kumar, 2002), with the number of all possible time-reversible models of nucleotide substitution being 203 (Huelsenbeck et al., 2004). In addition, there are more complicated models underlying the LogDet and the paralinear distances (Lake, 1994; Lockhart et al., 1994) that can presumably accommodate nonstationary substitution processes. Such models have not been implemented in a maximum likelihood framework until very recently (Jayaswal et al., 2005). Different substitution models often lead to different trees produced and constitute a major source of controversy in molecular phylogenetics (Rosenberg and Kumar, 2003; Xia, 2000; Xia et al., 2003a).

Transition probability matrix often referred to as the P matrix, specifies the probability of a nucleotide or amino acid changing into another one after time t. It is needed to calculate likelihood and to derive evolutionary distances. Thus, whether a substitution model can be implemented in a distance-based or maximum likelihood method essentially depends on whether the model's transition probabilities can be calculated. There are three ways to obtain transition probabilities from the Q matrix. These three ways will be explained and numerically illustrated in great detail in the next section. The derivation of variance for a single parameter or variance-covariance matrix for multiple parameters by the delta method is covered in Xia (2018a, Appendix).

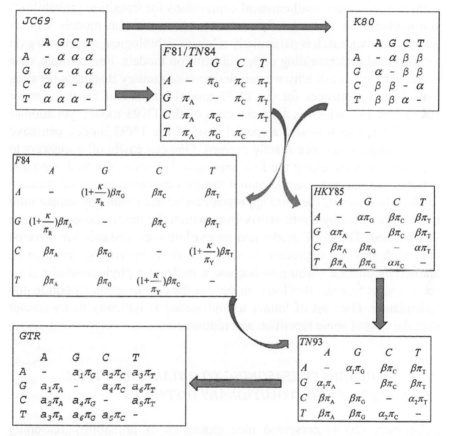

FIGURE 3.2 Relationship among commonly used substitution models for nucleotide sequences specified by their respective Q matrices. The diagonals of each matrix is constrained by the summation of each row is equal to 0.

3.2 THREE METHODS TO OBTAIN TRANSITION PROBABILITIES

Transition probabilities can be obtained by three approaches (Xia, 2018a) which will be covered in this section: (1) Probability reasoning, (2) solving differential equations involving rates, and (3) taking the matrix exponential of the rate matrix. The last two require some mathematical background, i.e., solving differential equations in the second and matrix algebra in the third. The first, in contrast, demands hardly any mathematical skill except for careful book-keeping and solving simultaneous equations, and can also yield nice and clean mathematical expressions for transition probabilities and evolutionary distances for a variety of substitution models. Consequently, this approach is particularly relevant to biological students to gain a conceptual understanding of the substitution models. For example, new researchers often ask why we can derive evolutionary distances between two aligned sequences for the TN93 model but cannot for the simpler HKY85 model, which is a special case of the TN93 model, yet another model, F84, which is also a special case of the TN93 model, can have its evolutionary distance readily derived. One can easily offer answers to such questions by taking the first approach. However, the first approach is not of general-purpose and cannot handle very complicated substitution models. In contrast, the third approach can be used with any substitution models specified by a rate matrix from which the matrix exponential can be obtained. The GTR model and its evolutionary distance are covered only with this last approach. In short, all these approaches need to be learned by anyone wishing to become a molecular phylogeneticist. This section aims to make this learning easy at the cost of some repetition and redundancy. The cost of failing to understand is typically much greater than the cost of some repetition and redundancy.

3.2.1   PROBABILITY REASONING TO OBTAIN TRANSITION PROBABILITIES AND EVOLUTIONARY DISTANCES

Felsenstein (2004) presented nice examples of probability reasoning to derive transition probabilities and evolutionary distances from rate matrices. This section presents the approach in a more systematic and accessible way following Xia (2017b).

3.2.1.1   JC69 MODEL

Consider nucleotide A in the JC69 model (Fig. 3.3a). Imagine that the nucleotide has a rate α of changing into any of the four nucleotides, i.e., including changing to itself (Fig. 3.3b). This is effectively the same specification as the JC69 model. After time t, the expected number of substitutions is $4at$ and the probability of no substitution is $p(x=0,\alpha,t) = e^{-4at}$ according to the Poisson distribution, and the probability of having at least one change is then $p(x \geq 1, \alpha, t) = 1 - e^{-4at}$ (Fig. 3.3c). Because nucleotide A can change into any one of the four nucleotides (including nucleotide A itself), each nucleotide gets $1/4$ of $p(x \geq 1, \alpha, t)$. We, therefore, have in Figure 3.3d

$$p_{ij}(t) = \frac{p(x \geq 1, \alpha, t)}{4} = \frac{1}{4} - \frac{1}{4}e^{-4at} \tag{3.2}$$

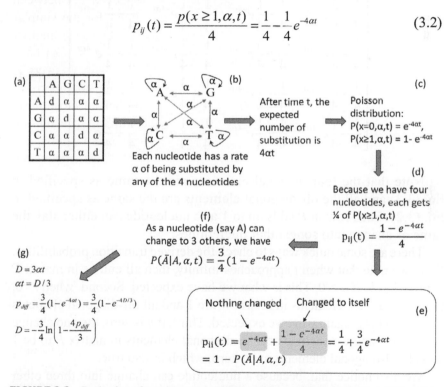

FIGURE 3.3 Derivation of transition probabilities and the evolutionary distance (D) based on the JC69 model. The d value in the diagonal of the rate matrix (a) is constrained by the row sum equal to 0, i.e., $d = -3a$. $P(j|i,t)$ means the probability of changing from the original nucleotide i to nucleotide j after time t, and is synonymous to $p_{ij}(t)$ or simply p_{ij} in this chapter.

The transition probability $p_{ii}(t)$ is the summation of two probabilities: the probability of no change (which is e^{-4at}) and the probability of changing to itself which is the same as specified in Eq. (3.2), as shown in Figure 3.3e, i.e.,

$$p_{ii}(t) = e^{-4\alpha t} + \frac{p(x \geq 1, \alpha, t)}{4} = \frac{1}{4} + \frac{3}{4}e^{-4\alpha t} \tag{3.3}$$

Thus, the transition probability matrix for the JC69 model is (in the order of A, G, C, T):

$$P_{JC69} = \begin{bmatrix} \frac{1}{4}+\frac{3}{4}e^{-4\alpha t} & \frac{1}{4}-\frac{1}{4}e^{-4\alpha t} & \frac{1}{4}-\frac{1}{4}e^{-4\alpha t} & \frac{1}{4}-\frac{1}{4}e^{-4\alpha t} \\ \frac{1}{4}-\frac{1}{4}e^{-4\alpha t} & \frac{1}{4}+\frac{3}{4}e^{-4\alpha t} & \frac{1}{4}-\frac{1}{4}e^{-4\alpha t} & \frac{1}{4}-\frac{1}{4}e^{-4\alpha t} \\ \frac{1}{4}-\frac{1}{4}e^{-4\alpha t} & \frac{1}{4}-\frac{1}{4}e^{-4\alpha t} & \frac{1}{4}+\frac{3}{4}e^{-4\alpha t} & \frac{1}{4}-\frac{1}{4}e^{-4\alpha t} \\ \frac{1}{4}-\frac{1}{4}e^{-4\alpha t} & \frac{1}{4}-\frac{1}{4}e^{-4\alpha t} & \frac{1}{4}-\frac{1}{4}e^{-4\alpha t} & \frac{1}{4}+\frac{3}{4}e^{-4\alpha t} \end{bmatrix} \tag{3.4}$$

Note that the four diagonal elements are the same as specified in Eq. (3.3) and all the off-diagonal elements are the same as specified in Eq. (3.2). Each row in P adds up to 1 as a nucleotide can either stay the same or change into some other nucleotides.

There are some quick ways to check the derived transition probabilities. First, we note that when t approaches infinity, then all entries in matrix P approaches ¼ if $\alpha > 0$. This is what we have expected. Second, when $t = 0$, then all diagonal elements in matrix P are 1 and all off-diagonal elements are zero. This is again what we expected. Third, if α is zero, then no change is possible, and we again expect all diagonal elements in matrix P to be 1 and all off-diagonal elements to be zero, which is also true.

We also notice that, because a nucleotide can change into three other nucleotides, the expected proportion of sites that are different between two aligned homologous sequences (p_{diff}) is $3*p_{ij}(t)$, i.e.,

$$p_{\text{diff}} = 3p_{ij}(t) = \frac{3}{4} - \frac{3}{4}e^{-4\alpha t} \tag{3.5}$$

Note that p_{diff} approaches ¾ when t is infinitely large, which implies a limit in correcting for multiple hits, i.e., correction is not possible with full substitution saturation. Eq. (3.5) offers another way of deriving $p_{ii}(t)$ in Eq. (3.3), i.e., $p_{ii}(t)$ is simply $1-p_{diff}$.

Eq. (3.5) allows us to derive the JC69 distance (D_{JC69}) because a distance is defined as μt where μ is the substitution rate which is equal to 3α in the JC69 model. This is the same as the distance that you have driven is the product of the speed (rate) and time. We can derive D_{JC69} (Fig. 3.3g) by substituting $\alpha t = D_{JC69}/3$ into Eq. (3.5) and obtain,

$$D_{JC69} = -\frac{3}{4}\ln\left(1-\frac{4p_{diff}}{3}\right) \tag{3.6}$$

where p_{diff} (the expected number of sites that are different between the two homologous sequences) can be approximated by the observed proportion of sites ($p_{diff.obs}$) differing between the two aligned sequences. Note that $p_{diff.obs}$ may differ from p_{diff} even when the underlying substitution model indeed follows JC69 because of (1) stochastic factors due to the limited aligned length of the two sequences and (2) distortion caused by suboptimal sequence alignment. Thus, although p_{diff} in Eq. (3.5) cannot be greater than 0.75, $p_{diff.obs}$ could, even when sequences evolve strictly according to the JC69 model. D_{JC69} is not defined when $p_{diff} \geq 0.75$ as there is no logarithm for 0 or negative values.

We can show that D_{JC69} in Eq. (3.6) is the maximum likelihood distance. For two aligned sequences of length N, designate the number of sites that differ between the two sequences as N_D and the number of sites identical between the two sites as ($N-N_D$). Now the likelihood function is:

$$L = \left(\frac{1}{4}\right)^N p_{ii}^{(N-N_D)}(1-p_{ii})^{N_D}$$

$$\ln L = N\ln\left(\frac{1}{4}\right) + (N-N_D)\ln(p_{ii}) + N_D\ln(1-p_{ii}) \tag{3.7}$$

$$= N\ln\left(\frac{1}{4}\right) + (N-N_D)\ln\left(\frac{1}{4}+\frac{3}{4}e^{-4D_{JC69}/3}\right) + N_D\ln\left(\frac{3}{4}-\frac{3}{4}e^{-4D_{JC69}/3}\right)$$

where the constant term $N*\ln(1/4)$ can be dropped in maximizing lnL to obtain the distance estimate but needs to be kept when performing likelihood ratio test for comparing different substitution models (e.g., JC69 against TN93). We take the derivative of lnL with respect to D_{JC69}, set the derivative to 0 and solve for D_{JC69}. The resulting D_{JC69} is exactly the same as that in Eq. (3.6). I used D instead of D_{JC69} in the equations below:

$$\frac{d \ln L}{dD} = -\frac{(N - N_D)e^{-4D/3}}{\frac{1}{4} + \frac{3}{4}e^{-4D/3}} + \frac{N_D e^{-4D/3}}{\frac{3}{4} - \frac{3}{4}e^{-4D/3}} = 0$$

$$D = -\frac{3}{4} \ln\left(\frac{3N - 4N_D}{3N}\right) = -\frac{3}{4} \ln\left(1 - \frac{4p_{\text{diff}}}{3}\right)$$

(3.8)

The variance of D_{JC69} (designated as V_{JC69}) is obtained as the negative reciprocal of the second derivative of lnL:

$$V_{JC69} = -\frac{1}{\dfrac{d^2 \ln L}{dD_{JC69}^2}} = \frac{p_{\text{diff}}(1 - p_{\text{diff}})}{L\left(1 - \dfrac{4p_{\text{diff}}}{3}\right)^2}$$

(3.9)

Note that V_{JC69} decreases with sequence length L as one would have expected. We illustrate the application of Eqs. (3.6) and (3.9) by using the aligned sequences in Figure 3.4 where $N = 24$, $N_D = 6$, and $p_{diff} = 6/24 = 0.25$. So $D_{JC69} = 0.3041$, and var(D_{JC69}) = 0.0176.

```
S1:  AAG  CCT  CGG  GGC  CCT  TAT  TTT  TTG
     ||   |    |||  |||  |        |||  |||  ||
S2:  AAT  CTC  CGG  GGC  CTC  TAT  TTT  TTT
```

FIGURE 3.4   Two homologous sequences for illustrating the computation of pairwise evolutionary distances.

The equilibrium frequencies of the π vector can be derived by setting $t = \infty$ in Eqs. (3.2)–(3.3) which leads to $p_{ii} = p_{ij} = \frac{1}{4}$. This implies that the equilibrium frequencies of the four nucleotides will be equal for the JC69 model. This is not surprising because the frequencies did not even appear in the rate matrix (Fig. 3.3a).

The JC 69 model is not realistic because nucleotides typically do not replace each other with equal probability. In particular, the ratio of transitional substitutions over transversional substitutions in almost all sequence comparisons is far greater than 1/2 expected under the JC69 model. This is often referred to as transition bias documented in both protein-coding and RNA genes. There are two factors contributing to the transition bias. First, the two purines are chemically similar to each other. Consequently, a purine is more likely to be misincorporated for another purine during DNA synthesis than for a pyrimidine. The same applies to the two pyrimidines. Second, transitions are more likely to be synonymous than transversions. In vertebrate mitochondrial genetic code, all transitions at 2-fold degenerate sites are synonymous, but all transversions at the 2-fold degenerate sites are nonsynonymous. Because nonsynonymous substitutions often disrupt protein function with deleterious effects, they are selected against and consequently have a low fixation probability. Xia et al. (1996) characterized the effect of these two factors on transition bias by

$$\frac{s_{obs}}{v_{obs}} = \frac{\mu_s}{\mu_v} \cdot \frac{P_s}{P_v} \tag{3.10}$$

where s_{obs} and v_{obs} are observed transitions and transversions from sequence comparisons between aligned mitochondrial genes, μ_s and μ_v are the mutation rate of transitions and transversions, respectively, and P_s and P_v are the fixation probability of a transitional mutation and a transversional mutation, respectively. Thus, transition bias can arise either from differential mutation pressure favoring transitions (i.e., a large μ_s/μ_v ratio) or from differential purifying selection against transversions, which would decrease P_v and consequently increase the P_s/P_v ratio. At 4-fold degenerate sites, both transitions and transversions are synonymous and may be assumed to be nearly neutral with $P_{s4} \approx P_{v4}$, where the subscript 4 denotes 4-fold degenerate sites. The s_{obs}/v_{obs} ratio at these 4-fold degenerate sites are about 2 after correcting for multiple hits, which leads to an estimate of μ_s/μ_v, assuming $P_{s4}/P_{v4} \approx 1$ at 4-fold sites:

$$\frac{s_{obs}}{v_{obs}} = \frac{\mu_s}{\mu_v} \cdot \frac{P_{s4}}{P_{v4}} \approx \frac{\mu_s}{\mu_v} \approx 2 \tag{3.11}$$

Similarly, if we assume that purifying selection acts roughly equally against nonsynonymous transitions and nonsynonymous transversions, then $P_{s0} \approx P_{v0}$ (where the subscript 0 denotes nondegenerate sites). The s_{obs}/v_{obs} ratio at these nondegenerate sites are also about 2, which provides an independent corroboration of $\mu_s/\mu_v \approx 2$.

At 2-fold degenerate sites, the s_{obs}/v_{obs} ratio is about 80 after correcting for multiple hits. This, together with the previous estimate of $\mu_s/\mu_v \approx 2$, provides an estimate of P_{s2}/P_{v2}:

$$\frac{s_{obs}}{v_{obs}} = \frac{\mu_s}{\mu_v} \frac{P_{s2}}{P_{v2}} \approx 2 \frac{P_{s2}}{P_{v2}} \approx 80; \frac{P_{s2}}{P_{v2}} \approx 40 \tag{3.12}$$

Because transitions are synonymous and transversions are nonsynonymous at 2-fold degenerate sites in animal mitochondrial genes, the ratio may be taken approximately as the ratio of fixation probability for synonymous mutations over fixation probability for nonsynonymous mutations. This P_{s2} / P_{v2} ratio can serve as a measure of the contribution of purifying selection to transition bias and is expected to increase with increasing intensity of purifying selection. Given the documented ubiquity of transition bias, the JC69 model is rarely used in practice.

3.2.1.2   K80 MODEL

The K80 model (Fig. 3.5a) generalizes the JC69 model to accommodate the transition bias by introduce one additional rate parameter. It has a transition substitution rate α and a transversion rate β (Fig. 3.5a). We will focus on nucleotide A and conceptualize the model with two events (Fig. 3.5b), in contrast to only one event in the JC69 model. The first event (e_1) occurs when nucleotide A changes into any of the four nucleotides (including to itself). In other words, the original A is replaced by a nucleotide randomly drawn from a nucleotide pool with equal nucleotide frequencies. This event occurs with a rate β. The second event (e_2) occurs when nucleotide A changes either to G or to itself, i.e., the original A is replaced by a nucleotide randomly drawn from a purine pool with an equal number of A and G. This e_2 occurs with a rate γ, thus, the transition rate α equals $\beta+\gamma$ according to this conceptualization. Note that whenever e_1 happens, the original nucleotide is replaced by any one of the four nucleotides with equal probability, no matter how many e_2 events has occurred before or after the occurrence of e_1. It might help to think of a long sequence with L sites being A at time 0. If these L sites each have experienced at least one e_2 event, then these sites will either be A or G with equal probability (i.e., 0.5), and we expect to have $L/2$ sites being A and the other $L/2$ sites being G. In contrast, if each of these L sites has experienced at least one e_1 event, then the site will be replaced by either A, C, G, or T with equal probability and we expect to observe A, C, G, and T in $L/4$ sites each. Any e_2 events occurring before or after the e_1 event does not change this expectation. This means that e_1 erases e_2 but not vice versa. The probability that an e_2 event happened is informative only when no e_1 event has happened.

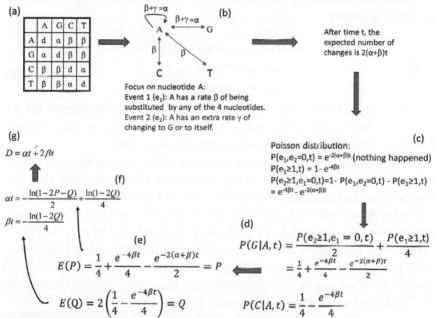

FIGURE 3.5 Derivation of transition probabilities and the evolutionary distance (D) based on the K80 model. The rate matrix (a) has the diagonal elements constrained by the row sum equal to 0, i.e., $d = -\alpha - 2\beta$. P and Q are the observed proportion of transitional and transversional changes between two aligned homologous sequences. Equating them to their respective expected values, E(P) and E(Q), leads to the solution of αt and βt shown, and the evolutionary distance D. $P(j|i,t)$ means the probability of changing from the original nucleotide i to nucleotide j after time t and is synonymous to $p_{ij}(t)$ or simply p_{ij} in this chapter.

After time t, the expected number of substitutions is $2(\alpha + \beta)t$, i.e., the nucleotide A has two ways of change with a rate of α (to A and to G) and another two ways of change with a rate β (to C and to T), so the probability of no change, according to Poisson distribution (Fig. 3.5c), is

$$p(e_1 = 0, e_2 = 0, t) = e^{-2(\alpha + \beta)t} \qquad (3.13)$$

Note that α is conceptualized as $(\beta+\gamma)$ in Figure 3.5, so $e^{-2(\alpha+\beta)t}$ in Eq. (3.13) is equivalent to $e^{-(4\beta+2\gamma)t}$. The probability that at least one e_1 event has occurred is

$$p(e_1 > 0, t) = 1 - e^{-4\beta t} \tag{3.14}$$

Thus, the probability that at least one e_2 has occurred but e_1 has not occurred is simply

$$\begin{aligned} p(e_2 > 0, e_1 = 0, t) &= 1 - p(e_1 = 0, e_2 = 0, t) - p(e_1 > 0, t) \\ &= 1 - e^{-2(\alpha+\beta)t} - (1 - e^{-4\beta t}) \\ &= e^{-4\beta t} - e^{-2(\alpha+\beta)t} \end{aligned} \tag{3.15}$$

These probabilities are also shown in Figure 3.5c. The reason for the condition that "e_1 has not occurred" is because e_1 event can erase e_2 event (see the discussion in the first paragraph of this section).

Now the probability of the starting nucleotide A changing to G during time t, designated as $p(G|A,t)$, is the summation of two probabilities. The first is 1/2 of the probability of $p(e_2>0,e_1=0,t)$ in Eq. (3.15) because the other 1/2 is for A to itself. The second is 1/4 of $p(e_1>0,t)$ in Eq. (3.14) because A→A, A→G, A→C and A→T each get 1/4, so only 1/4 of $p(e_1>0,t)$ is for A→G. The summation of these two probabilities (Fig. 3.5d) is $p(G|A,t)$. This probability is equal to $p(A|G,t)$, $p(C|T,t)$, and $p(T|C,t)$ in the K80 model. In other words, the summation of these two probabilities is the probability of a transition during time t (P_s). Thus,

$$\begin{aligned} P_s &= \frac{p(e_2 > 0, e_1 = 0, t)}{2} + \frac{p(e_1 > 0, t)}{4} \\ &= \frac{e^{-4\beta t} - e^{-2(\alpha+\beta)t}}{2} + \frac{1 - e^{-4\beta t}}{4} \\ &= \frac{1}{4} + \frac{e^{-4\beta t}}{4} - \frac{e^{-2(\alpha+\beta)t}}{2} = P(G|A,t) = P(A|G,t) = P(T|C,t) = P(C|T,t) \end{aligned} \tag{3.16}$$

Similarly, the probability of the starting A changing to C (or to T) is 1/4 of $p(e_1>0,t)$ in Eq. (3.14) because 1/4 is for A→A, 1/4 is for A→G and 1/4 is for A→T, so only 1/4 is for A→C (Fig. 3.5d). This probability is the probability for a transversional change during time t,

$$P_v = \frac{p(e_1 > 0, t)}{4} = \frac{1 - e^{-4\beta t}}{4} \tag{3.17}$$

As a quick check of the derived transition probabilities, we note that P_s and P_v are zero when $t = 0$ (or when $\alpha=0$ and $\beta=0$). This also implies that all diagonal elements in the transition probability matrix are equal to 1, and is what we have expected. When $t = \infty$ with $\alpha > 0$ and $\beta > 0$, all entries in matrix P approach $\frac{1}{4}$ (the equilibrium frequency of the K80 model). This is also what we expected.

For two aligned homologous sequences, P_s can be approximated by the proportion of sites differing by a transition (P), and $2P_v$ by the portion of sites differing by a transversion (Q, Fig. 3.5e). Note that the expected Q is equal to $2P_v$ because each nucleotide has two ways of having a transversional change. Therefore,

$$P = \frac{1}{4} + \frac{e^{-4\beta t}}{4} - \frac{e^{-2(\alpha+\beta)t}}{2} \tag{3.18}$$

$$Q = 2P_v = 2\left(\frac{1-e^{-4\beta t}}{4}\right) = \frac{1-e^{-4\beta t}}{2} \tag{3.19}$$

We can now first solve for βt from Eq. (3.19), and then substitute the solution for βt into Eq. (3.18) to solve for αt. This leads to

$$\alpha t = -\frac{\ln(1-2P-Q)}{2} + \frac{\ln(1-2Q)}{4}$$

$$\beta t = -\frac{\ln(1-2Q)}{4} \tag{3.20}$$

Recall that evolutionary distance is defined as μt, where μ is the substitution rate which is equal to $(\alpha + 2\beta)$ in the K80 model. Thus, the evolutionary distance based on the K80 model (D_{K80}) is $(\alpha + 2\beta)t$, which comes to

$$D_{K80} = \alpha t + 2\beta t = -\frac{\ln(1-2P-Q)}{2} - \frac{\ln(1-2Q)}{4} \tag{3.21}$$

where P and Q can be approximated by the observed proportion of sites differing by a transition or a transversion from two aligned sequences, designated as P_{obs} and Q_{obs}. Similar to what I have mentioned with reference to D_{JC69}, P and Q may differ from P_{obs} and Q_{obs} even if the K80 model is followed during the sequence evolution. This is because (1) limited aligned length of the two sequences may result in stochastic variation in P_{obs} and Q_{obs} and (2) the two observed proportions may be distorted by alignment errors. For example, for two homologous sequences that have diverged for an infinite length of time according to the K80 model, we would have expected P and Q to be 0.25 and 0.5, respectively. However, we may actually have $P_{obs} > 0.25$ or $Q_{obs} > 0.5$, which would render D_{K80} inapplicable. On the other hand, after sequence alignment and deletion of indels (because evolutionary distances are typically calculated without using sites with indels), P_{obs} and Q_{obs} may well be much smaller than the expected 0.25 and 0.5 leading to a severe underestimation of the true distance. It is also possible to have P_{obs} and Q_{obs} values that, when used to replace P and Q in Eq. (3.20), result in negative αt or βt values that make no biological sense. The same applies to D_{JC69} (in fact to any evolutionary distances based on a substitution model). Methods for handling such situations are discussed later in the section on the GTR model.

D_{K80} in Eq. (3.21) is also a maximum likelihood estimator of the distance based on the K80 model, just like the D_{JC69} distance in Eq. (3.6). To see this, it is simpler to reparameterize the K80 model by replacing αt and βt by D_{K80} and κ using the following relationship:

$$D_{K80} = \alpha t + 2\beta t$$
$$\kappa = \alpha t / \beta t \tag{3.22}$$

Solving these two equations gives us

$$\alpha t = \frac{D_{K80}\kappa}{\kappa + 2}$$
$$\beta t = \frac{D_{K80}}{\kappa + 2} \tag{3.23}$$

Substituting αt and βt into Eqs. (3.17) and (3.18) so that P and Q will be functions of D_{K80} and κ, and the likelihood function for deriving D_{K80} and κ is

$$L = \left(\frac{1}{4}\right)^N P^{N_s} Q^{N_v} (1 - P - Q)^{N - N_s - N_v}$$

$$\ln L = N \ln\left(\frac{1}{4}\right) + N_s \ln P + N_v \ln Q + (N - N_s - N_v)\ln(1 - P - Q) \tag{3.24}$$

where the constant term $N*\ln(1/4)$ can be dropped in maximizing lnL to obtain the distance estimate but need to be kept when performing likelihood ratio test for comparing different substitution models (e.g., K80 against TN93). Taking partial derivatives with respect to D_{K80} and κ, setting them to zero and solving the simultaneous equations, we have

$$D_{K80} = -\frac{\ln(1 - 2P_{obs} - Q_{obs})}{2} - \frac{\ln(1 - 2Q_{obs})}{4} \qquad (3.25)$$

$$\kappa = \frac{2\ln(1 - 2P_{obs} - Q_{obs})}{\ln(1 - 2Q_{obs})} - 1 \qquad (3.26)$$

where $P_{obs} = N_s/N$, and $Q_{obs} = N_v/N$. Using the two aligned sequences in Figure 3.4, we have $N = 24$ and $P_{obs} = 4/24$ and $Q_{obs} = 2/24$. These lead to $D_{K80} = 0.3151$, and $\kappa = 4.9126$. It may be relevant to add that, while D_{JC69} and D_{K80} are maximum likelihood estimates, distance formulae for F84 and TN93 models, obtained in the same way by equating the observed number of substitutions to expected number of substitutions, are generally not maximum likelihood estimates. This will become clear when we deal with these models.

We have previously derived the variance of D_{JC69} as the negative reciprocal of the second derivative of lnL with respect to D_{JC69}. This can be used only when the log-likelihood function is used to estimate a single parameter. When there are multiple parameters (e.g., D_{K80} and κ), we cannot use the same approach unless the parameters are not correlated. There are two related methods for deriving variances of parameters. The first is the delta method (Kimura and Ohta, 1972; Waddell and Steel, 1997a; Xia, 2007a, pp 256–262) covered in Xia (2018a, Appendix), and the second uses the Fisher information matrix to obtain both the variances of parameters and covariances between parameters. The method of Fisher information matrix is shown below.

To estimate variance involving multiple parameters, such as D_{K80} and κ, we first take the second-order partial derivatives of lnL with respective to D_{K80} and κ substituting the estimated D_{K80} and κ in Eqs. (3.25) and (3.26) into the second-order partial derivatives, arranging them into what is called a Fisher information matrix (M_{FI}) below, and computing the matrix inverse of M_{FI} (designated by M_{FI}^{-1}):

$$M_{FI} = \begin{bmatrix} -\dfrac{\partial^2 \ln L}{\partial \kappa^2} & -\dfrac{\partial^2 \ln L}{\partial \kappa \, \partial D_{K80}} \\ -\dfrac{\partial^2 \ln L}{\partial D_{K80} \partial \kappa} & -\dfrac{\partial^2 \ln L}{\partial D_{K80}^2} \end{bmatrix} \qquad (3.27)$$

The diagonal elements of M_{FI}^{-1} are the variances for κ and D_{K80} and the off-diagonal elements of M_{FI}^{-1} are covariances. The mathematical expression for the variance of κ is tedious but that for the variance of D_{K80} is simpler:

$$V(D_{K80}) = \frac{a^2 P + c^2 Q - (aP + cQ)^2}{N}, \text{ where}$$

$$a = \frac{1}{1 - 2P - Q}, b = \frac{1}{1 - 2Q}, c = \frac{a+b}{2}$$

(3.28)

With the aligned sequences in Figure 3.4, we have $N = 24$ and empirical $P = 4/24$ and $Q = 2/24$. These lead to $D_{K80} = 0.3151$ and $\kappa = 4.9126$. The M_{FI} and M_{FI}^{-1} are

$$M_{FI} = \begin{bmatrix} 0.047435 & -0.286795 \\ -0.286795 & 49.641105 \end{bmatrix}$$

$$M_{FI}^{-1} = \begin{bmatrix} 21.84451668 & 0.126204037 \\ 0.126204037 & 0.020873724 \end{bmatrix}$$

(3.29)

where the two parameters are in the order of κ and D_{K80}, i.e., the variance is 21.8445 for κ and 0.0209 for D_{K80}. The off-diagonal elements are covariances between the two parameters. Note that the variance (which measures uncertainty about the parameter value) for D_{K80} is larger than that for D_{JC69}. This is why we should always aim to find the simplest possible but sufficient model for our data because increasing the number of parameters in the model increases uncertainty. The last section in this chapter explains methods for model selection.

3.2.1.3   F84 AND HKY85 MODEL

The F84 and HKY85 model accommodate not only the differential substitution rates between transitions and transversions but also different equilibrium nucleotide frequencies in contrast to JC69 and K80 which assume equal equilibrium nucleotide frequencies. The same probabilistic reasoning used before can be applied to derive transition probabilities for the F84 and HKY85 models.

The rate matrix for the F84 model, in the order of A, G, C, and T, is

$$
Q_{F84} = \begin{vmatrix}
- & \beta\pi_G + \gamma\pi_G / \pi_R & \beta\pi_C & \beta\pi_T \\
\beta\pi_A + \gamma\pi_A / \pi_R & - & \beta\pi_C & \beta\pi_T \\
\beta\pi_A & \beta\pi_G & - & \beta\pi_T + \gamma\pi_T / \pi_Y \\
\beta\pi_A & \beta\pi_G & \beta\pi_C + \gamma\pi_C / \pi_Y & -
\end{vmatrix} \quad (3.30)
$$

where π_A, π_G, π_C, and π_T are equilibrium frequencies, π_R and π_Y are frequencies of purines and pyrimidines, and the diagonal elements are constrained by each row summing up to 0. Note that the Q_{F84} shown in Figure 3.2 is parameterized differently, with β and κ instead of β and γ. If you replace γ in Eq. (3.30) by $\kappa\beta$, then Q_{F84} becomes identical to that in Figure 3.2. It is easier to understand the F84 model by using Q_{F84} specified in Eq. (3.30) than that specified in Figure 3.2.

We may view the F84 model as featuring two events (e_1 and e_2). Suppose we start with a nucleotide A. Event e_1 occurs with rate β. When it occurs, the original A will be replaced by a nucleotide drawn randomly from a nucleotide pool in which the nucleotide frequencies are the same as the equilibrium frequencies. This means that the original A has a rate of $\beta\pi_A$, $\beta\pi_G$, $\beta\pi_C$, and $\beta\pi_T$ to change to A, G, C, and T, respectively, when e_1 occurs. This is different from the K80 model where, when e_1 occurs, the original A has a rate of 0.25 to change to any of the four nucleotides. Event e_2 has a rate of γ to occur, and will result in the original A being replaced by a purine drawn randomly from a purine pool with A and G frequencies specified as π_A / π_R and π_G / π_R. This means that the original A has a rate of $\gamma\pi_A / \pi_R$ and $\gamma\pi_G / \pi_R$ to change to A and G when e_2 occurs. This is illustrated in Figure 3-6a, where we use x to represent $\beta + \gamma / \pi_R$. Note that it is not a good idea to use α to represent $\beta + \gamma / \pi_R$ for two reasons. First, if we had started with a nucleotide C or T instead of A, then we would have $\beta + \gamma / \pi_Y$ instead of $\beta + \gamma / \pi_R$ which would force us to use α_1 and α_2 to distinguish between the two. A casual reader will then be misled to think that F84 has three rate parameters (i.e., β, α_1, and α_2) without knowing that α_1 and α_2 are used as different functions of the same rate parameter γ. Second, I have reserved α to represent $\beta + \gamma$ in Figure 3.6b which simplifies the derivation of transition probabilities illustrated in Figure 3.6.

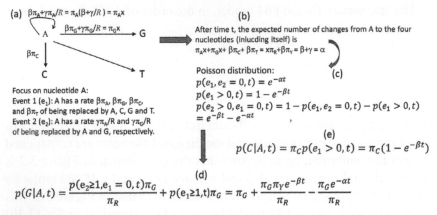

(a) $\beta\pi_A + \gamma\pi_A/R = \pi_A(\beta+\gamma/R) = \pi_A x$

$\beta\pi_G + \gamma\pi_G/R = \pi_G x$

A $\longrightarrow$ G

$\beta\pi_C \downarrow$

C $\longrightarrow$ T

Focus on nucleotide A:
Event 1 (e_1): A has a rate $\beta\pi_A$, $\beta\pi_G$, $\beta\pi_C$, and $\beta\pi_T$ of being replaced by A, C, G and T.
Event 2 (e_2): A has a rate $\gamma\pi_A/R$ and $\gamma\pi_G/R$ of being replaced by A and G, respectively.

(b)
After time t, the expected number of changes from A to the four nucleotides (inlucding itself) is
$\pi_A x + \pi_G x + \beta\pi_C + \beta\pi_T = x\pi_R + \beta\pi_Y = \beta+\gamma = \alpha$

Poisson distribution: (c)
$p(e_1, e_2 = 0, t) = e^{-\alpha t}$
$p(e_1 > 0, t) = 1 - e^{-\beta t}$
$p(e_2 > 0, e_1 = 0, t) = 1 - p(e_1, e_2 = 0, t) - p(e_1 > 0, t)$
$= e^{-\beta t} - e^{-\alpha t}$,

(e)
$p(C|A, t) = \pi_C p(e_1 > 0, t) = \pi_C(1 - e^{-\beta t})$

(d)
$p(G|A, t) = \dfrac{p(e_2 \geq 1, e_1 = 0, t)\pi_G}{\pi_R} + p(e_1 \geq 1, t)\pi_G = \pi_G + \dfrac{\pi_G \pi_Y e^{-\beta t}}{\pi_R} - \dfrac{\pi_G e^{-\alpha t}}{\pi_R}$

FIGURE 3.6 Derivation of transition probabilities based on the F84 model. π_A, π_G, π_C, π_T, and π_R, π_Y are equilibrium frequencies of A, C, G, T, purine (A+G) and pyrimidine (C+T), respectively. Event e_1 occurs at a rate of β and leads to the original A being replaced by any of the four nucleotides according to their equilibrium frequencies, and event e_2 occurs at a rate of γ and results in the original A being replaced by either A or G according to their frequencies in the purine pool, i.e., π_A / π_R, and π_G / π_R. I used x as a shorthand for $\beta + \gamma / \pi_R$. The rate γ does not appear in the final transition probabilities because it has been absorbed into α which equals $\beta + \gamma$ shown in (b). $P(j|i, t)$ means the probability of changing from the original nucleotide i to nucleotide j after time t and is synonymous to $p_{ij}(t)$ or simply p_{ij} in this chapter.

Note that whenever event e_1 happens, the original A is replaced by A, C, G, and T with probabilities π_A, π_G, π_C, and π_T, no matter how many e_2 events has occurred before or after the occurrence of e_1. This is similar to the scenario involving the K80 model, except that the K80 model assumes equal nucleotide frequencies. It might help to think of a long sequence with L sites being A at time 0. If these L sites each have experienced at least one e_2 event, then these sites will either be A or G with probabilities π_A and π_G, respectively, and we expect to have $\pi_A L$ sites being A and $\pi_G L$ sites being G. In contrast, if each of these L sites has experienced at least one e_1 event, then the site will be replaced by A, C, G, or T with probabilities π_A, π_G, π_C, and π_T, and we expect to observe A, C, G, and T in $\pi_A L$, $\pi_G L$, $\pi_C L$, and $\pi_T L$ sites, respectively. Any number of e_2 events occurring before or after the e_1 event does not change this expectation. This means that e_1 erases e_2 but not vice versa. The occurrence of an e_2 event is informative only when no e_1 event has happened.

After time t, the total flow of the original A to the four nucleotides (including itself, Fig. 3.6a,b) is

$$\pi_A x + \pi_G x + \beta \pi_C + \beta \pi_T = \pi_R x + \pi_Y \beta = \pi_R(\beta + \gamma / \pi_R) + \pi_Y \beta = \beta + \gamma = \alpha \quad (3.31)$$

so the probability that no substitution has happened during time t (Fig. 3.6c), according to Poisson distribution, is

$$p(e_1, e_2 = 0, t) = e^{-\alpha t} \quad (3.32)$$

The rate of A changing to A, G, C, and T through e_1 is $\beta \pi_A + \beta \pi_G + \beta \pi_C + \beta \pi_T = \beta$, so the probability that at least one e_1 has occurred during time t is

$$p(e_1 > 0, t) = 1 - e^{-\beta t} \quad (3.33)$$

The probability that e_2 has happened but e_1 has not is then

$$p(e_2 > 0, e_1 = 0, t) = 1 - p(e_1, e_2 = 0, t) - p(e_1 > 0, t) = e^{-\beta t} - e^{-\alpha t} \quad (3.34)$$

The reason for the condition that "e_1 has not occurred" is because e_1 event can erase e_2 event. With these it is easy to derive transition probability from A to G (Fig. 3.6d) as the summation of (1) a fraction of π_G of $p(e1>0,t)$, which is the probability of e_1 event that results in the original A being replaced by A, C, G, and T with probabilities π_A, π_G, π_C, and π_T, and (2) a fraction of π_G/π_R of $p(e_2>0,e_1=0,t)$, which is the probability that e_2 events not erased by $e1$. That is,

$$p(G \mid A, t) = p(e_1 > 0, t)\pi_G + \frac{p(e_2 > 0, e_1 = 0, t)\pi_G}{\pi_R} = \pi_G + \frac{\pi_G \pi_Y e^{-\beta t}}{\pi_R} - \frac{\pi_G e^{-\alpha t}}{\pi_R} \quad (3.35)$$

From now on, $p(j|i,t)$ will be written simply as p_{ij}, so $p(G|A,t)$ is p_{AG}. With the same reasoning, we can derive transition probabilities for other A↔G and C↔T substitutions. Note that the two rate parameters in the F84 model β and γ have been reparameterized into α $(=\beta + \gamma)$ and β in Eq. (3.35). The transition probability from the original A to C (a transversion, Fig. 3.6e) is simply

$$p_{AC} = \pi_C p(e_1 > 0, t) = \pi_C(1 - e^{-\beta t}) \quad (3.36)$$

For other transversions, e.g., p_{AT}, one just need to replace π_C by π_T. The complete transition probability matrix for the F84 model, in the order of A, G, C, and T, is

$$P_{F84} = \begin{vmatrix} \pi_A + \pi_A \pi_Y x_1 + \pi_G x_2 & \pi_G + \pi_G \pi_Y x_1 - \pi_G x_2 & \pi_C(1-e^{-\beta t}) & \pi_T(1-e^{-\beta t}) \\ \pi_A + \pi_A \pi_Y x_1 - \pi_A x_2 & \pi_G + \pi_G \pi_Y x_1 + \pi_A x_2 & \pi_C(1-e^{-\beta t}) & \pi_T(1-e^{-\beta t}) \\ \pi_A(1-e^{-\beta t}) & \pi_G(1-e^{-\beta t}) & \pi_C + \pi_C \pi_R x_3 + \pi_G x_4 & \pi_T + \pi_T \pi_R x_3 - \pi_T x_4 \\ \pi_A(1-e^{-\beta t}) & \pi_G(1-e^{-\beta t}) & \pi_C + \pi_C \pi_R x_3 - \pi_C x_4 & \pi_T + \pi_T \pi_R x_3 + \pi_C x_4 \end{vmatrix} \quad (3.37)$$

where

$$x_1 = \frac{e^{-\beta t}}{\pi_R}, x_2 = \frac{e^{-\alpha t}}{\pi_R}, x_3 = \frac{e^{-\beta t}}{\pi_Y}, x_4 = \frac{e^{-\alpha t}}{\pi_Y} \quad (3.38)$$

As a quick check of the transition probabilities, we first note that when $t = 0$ (or when $\alpha=0$ and $\beta=0$), then the diagonal elements are 1 and all off-diagonal elements are 0, which is what we expected. Second, when $t = \infty$ with $\alpha>0$ and $\beta>0$, then the transition probabilities will approach the equilibrium frequencies, which is also what we expected.

To obtain the distance for the F84 model (D_{F84}), recall that a distance is defined as μt where μ is the average substitution rate, i.e., substitution rates in Eq. (3.30) weighted by the equilibrium frequencies:

$$D_{F84} = 2\pi_A \pi_G (\beta t + \gamma t / \pi_R) + 2\pi_T \pi_C (\beta t + \gamma t / \pi_Y) + 2\pi_Y \pi_R \beta t \quad (3.39)$$

Now we need to obtain βt and γt in order to calculate D_{F84}. We can obtain αt and βt, and then obtain $\gamma t = \alpha t - \beta t$, remembering $\alpha = \beta + \gamma$ (Fig. 3.6b). The method we will use is the same as that for the K80 model, i.e., we obtain the expected transitions and transversions, designated E(S) and E(V), respectively, from transition probabilities and equate them to the observed S and V to solve for αt and βt. With the property of time reversibility, we have

$$\begin{aligned} E(S) &= 2\pi_A P_{AG} + 2\pi_C P_{CT} \\ E(V) &= 2\pi_A P_{AT} + 2\pi_A P_{AC} + 2\pi_G P_{GC} + 2\pi_G P_{GT} \end{aligned} \quad (3.40)$$

Equating E(S) and E(V) to the observed S and V, and solving these two equations with the two unknowns (αt and βt), we have

$$\alpha t = -\ln \left[1 - \frac{S}{2(\pi_C \pi_T / \pi_Y + \pi_A \pi_G / \pi_R)} - \frac{(\pi_C \pi_T \pi_R / \pi_Y + \pi_A \pi_G \pi_Y / \pi_R)V}{2(\pi_C \pi_T \pi_R + \pi_A \pi_G \pi_Y)} \right] \quad (3.41)$$

$$\beta t = -\ln\left(1 - \frac{V}{2\pi_R \pi_Y}\right) \tag{3.42}$$

Substituting βt and γt $(= \alpha t - \beta t)$ into Eq. (3.39) and after some algebraic manipulation, we have a more useful form of D_{F84}:

$$D_{F84} = 2\alpha t\left(\frac{\pi_C \pi_T}{\pi_Y} + \frac{\pi_A \pi_G}{\pi_R}\right) - 2\beta t\left(\frac{\pi_C \pi_T \pi_R}{\pi_Y} + \frac{\pi_A \pi_G \pi_Y}{\pi_R} - \pi_Y \pi_R\right) \tag{3.43}$$

To illustrate the calculation of D_{F84}, we may use the two aligned sequences in Figure 3.4 which gives us $\pi_A = 6/48$, $\pi_C = 12/48$, $\pi_G = 10/48$, $\pi_T = 20/48$, $S = 4/24$, $V = 2/24$, $\alpha t = 0.5778363341$, $\beta t = 0.2076393648$, and $D_{F84} = 0.3198867$. The variance of the D_{F84} can be obtained by either the delta method or the method using the Fisher information matrix.

A substitution model similar to the F84 model is the HKY85 model, with its rate matrix specified as:

$$Q_{HKY85} = \begin{matrix} A \\ G \\ C \\ T \end{matrix} \begin{bmatrix} - & (\beta+\gamma)\pi_G & \beta\pi_C & \beta\pi_T \\ (\beta+\gamma)\pi_A & - & \beta\pi_C & \beta\pi_T \\ \beta\pi_A & \beta\pi_G & - & (\beta+\gamma)\pi_T \\ \beta\pi_A & \beta\pi_G & (\beta+\gamma)\pi_C & - \end{bmatrix} \tag{3.44}$$

where $(\beta+\gamma)$ is often written as α and the diagonal elements are constrained by each row summing up to 0. The HKY85 model and the F84 model differ only in the specification of rates involving transitions. q_{AG} and q_{CT} for the HKY85 model are $\pi_G(\beta+\gamma)$ and $\pi_T(\beta+\gamma)$ as specified in Eq. (3.44), in contrast to $\pi_G(\beta+\gamma/\pi_R)$ and $\pi_T(\beta+\gamma/\pi_Y)$, respectively, in the F84 model specified in Eq. (3.30). By comparing these rates, it becomes obvious that the F84 model would be equivalent to the HKY85 model if $\pi_R = \pi_Y$.

We can obtain the transition probabilities for the HKY85 model in the same way as that for the F84 model. In short, we again start with nucleotide A and envision two events e_1 and e_2. Event e_1 occurs with rate β and results in the original A replaced by any of the four nucleotides with probabilities equal to their respective equilibrium frequencies. Event e_2 occurs with a rate γ and results in the original A being replaced by either A or G with the probabilities equal to their respective equilibrium frequencies. Fictionalized in this way, the expected number of substitutions after time t is $[\beta(\pi_A+\pi_G+\pi_C+\pi_T) + \gamma(\pi_A+\pi_G)]t = (\beta+\gamma\pi_R)t$. According to the Poisson distribution, the probability that no substitution has happened during time t is

$$p(e_1, e_2 = 0, t) = 1 - e^{-(\beta + \gamma \pi_R)} \tag{3.45}$$

The probability that at least one e_1 occurred after time t is

$$p(e_1 > 0, t) = 1 - e^{-\beta t} \tag{3.46}$$

The probability that e_2 has occurred but e_1 has not is

$$p(e_2 > 0, e_1 = 0, t) = 1 - p(e_1, e_2 = 0, t) - p(e_1 > 0, t) = e^{-\beta t} - e^{-(\beta + \gamma \pi_R)t} \tag{3.47}$$

The transition probability $p(G|A,t)$, abbreviated as p_{AG}, is

$$p_{AG} = \pi_G p(e_1 > 0, t) + \frac{\pi_G}{\pi_R} p(e_2 > 0, e_1 = 0, t) = \pi_G + \frac{\pi_G \pi_Y e^{-\beta t}}{\pi_R} - \frac{\pi_G e^{-(\beta + \pi_R \gamma)t}}{\pi_R} \tag{3.48}$$

In the same way, we can derive other transition probabilities which are shown below in the order of A, G, C, and T:

$$
P_{HKY} = \begin{bmatrix}
\pi_A + \pi_A x_1 + \pi_G x_2 & \pi_G + \pi_G x_1 - \pi_G x_2 & \pi_C(1 - e^{-\beta t}) & \pi_T(1 - e^{-\beta t}) \\
\pi_A + \pi_A x_1 - \pi_A x_2 & \pi_G + \pi_G x_1 + \pi_A x_2 & \pi_C(1 - e^{-\beta t}) & \pi_T(1 - e^{-\beta t}) \\
\pi_A(1 - e^{-\beta t}) & \pi_G(1 - e^{-\beta t}) & \pi_C + \pi_C x_3 + \pi_T x_4 & \pi_T + \pi_T x_3 - \pi_T x_4 \\
\pi_A(1 - e^{-\beta t}) & \pi_G(1 - e^{-\beta t}) & \pi_C + \pi_C x_3 - \pi_C x_4 & \pi_T + \pi_T x_3 + \pi_C x_4
\end{bmatrix} \tag{3.49}
$$

where

$$x_1 = \frac{\pi_Y e^{-\beta t}}{\pi_R}; x_2 = \frac{e^{-(\beta + \pi_R \gamma)t}}{\pi_R}; x_3 = \frac{\pi_R e^{-\beta t}}{\pi_Y}; x_4 = \frac{e^{-(\beta + \pi_Y \gamma)t}}{\pi_Y} \tag{3.50}$$

As a quick check of the transition probabilities, we first note that when $t = 0$ (or when $\alpha = 0$ and $\beta = 0$), then the diagonal elements are 1 and all off-diagonal elements are 0, which is what we expected. Second, when t approaches infinity with $\beta > 0$ and $\gamma > 0$, then the transition probabilities will approach the equilibrium frequencies, which is also what we expected.

We cannot derive the distance for the HKY85 model by following the same approach as that for the F84 model. Hasegawa et al. (1985) has tried this approach but were not successful because there is no explicit solution for βt and γt. However, if we treat the A↔G transition and C↔T transition separate, then we can solve for βt and γt (Rzhetsky and Nei, 1995). In other words, we obtain one set of βt and γt from observed A↔G transitions and transversions, and another set of βt and γt from observed C↔T transitions and transversions. βt in the two sets are the same as that in Eq. (3.41), but γt is different between the two sets of estimates. We can then take a weighted average of γt. Admittedly, this does sound mathematically clumsy and explains why HKY85, while commonly implemented in a likelihood approach or Bayesian inference, is almost never used in a distance-based phylogenetic analysis.

Here is the protocol to get βt and γt from HKY85. The expected numbers of A↔G and C↔T transitions, designated S_R and S_Y, respectively, and transversions are

$$
\begin{aligned}
E(S_R) &= 2\pi_A P_{AG} \\
E(S_Y) &= 2\pi_C P_{CT} \\
E(V) &= 2\pi_A P_{AT} + 2\pi_A P_{AC} + 2\pi_G P_{GC} + 2\pi_G P_{GT}
\end{aligned}
\tag{3.51}
$$

Setting $E(S_R)$ and $E(V)$ to the observed S_R and V and solve for βt and γt, we have

$$
\begin{aligned}
\beta t &= -\ln\left(1 - \frac{V}{2\pi_R \pi_Y}\right) \\
\gamma_R t &= \frac{1}{\pi_R}\ln\left(\frac{\pi_A \pi_G (2\pi_R \pi_Y - V)}{2\pi_A \pi_G \pi_R \pi_Y - S_R \pi_Y \pi_R^2 - \pi_A \pi_G \pi_Y V}\right)
\end{aligned}
\tag{3.52}
$$

where βt is the same as that in Eq. (3.42), and $\gamma_R t$ in Eq. (3.52) is γt estimated from observed S_R and V.

We now obtain another set of solutions for βt and γt by setting $E(S_Y)$ and $E(V)$ to their observed S_Y and V and solve for βt and γt, we have the same βt but a different γt:

$$
\gamma_Y t = \frac{1}{\pi_Y}\ln\left(\frac{\pi_C \pi_T (2\pi_R \pi_Y - V)}{2\pi_C \pi_T \pi_R \pi_Y - S_Y \pi_R \pi_Y^2 - \pi_C \pi_T \pi_R V}\right)
\tag{3.53}
$$

A weighted average of γt could be

$$
\gamma t = \pi_R \gamma_R t + \pi_Y \gamma_Y t
\tag{3.54}
$$

The distance for the HKY model

$$D_{\text{HKY85}} = \mu t = 2\pi_A\pi_G(\beta t + \gamma t) + 2\pi_T\pi_C(\beta t + \gamma t) + 2\pi_Y\pi_R\beta t \qquad (3.55)$$

To compute D_{HKY85} using the two aligned sequences in Figure 3.4, we have π_A=6/48, π_C=12/48, π_G=10/48, π_T=20/48, S_Y =4/24, S_R =0, V=2/24, βt = 0.2076393648, $\gamma_R t$ = –0.2223239164, $\gamma_Y t$ = 1.047432870, weighted γt = 0.624180608, D_{HKY85} = 0.308904. For comparison, the same two sequences yield D_{F84} = 0.319887. One may be curious about the $\gamma_R t$ value because one would have expected its minimum to be $-\beta t$ so that q_{AG} and q_{GA} in Eq. (3.44) will not be negative (because a negative evolutionary rate does not make biological sense)

In general, D_{HKY85} is slightly smaller than D_{F84}. I used the eight vertebrate COI sequences in the FASTA file VertCOI.fas that comes with DAMBE (Xia, 2013b) to compute both D_{HKY85} and D_{F84} (Fig. 3.7). The difference is minor, although D_{HKY85} is consistently but slightly smaller than D_{F84}.

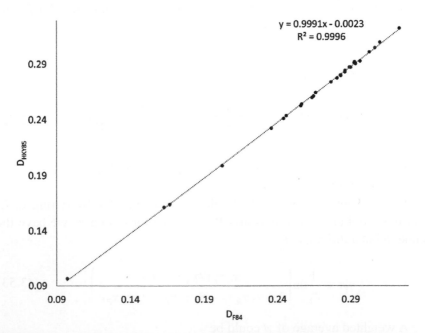

FIGURE 3.7   Evolutionary distances from the HKY85 and F84 models are nearly identical.

The HKY85 model itself may not carry much biological significance given the existence of the F84 model. However, the twists involved in computing the evolutionary distance, i.e., the separate estimation of $\gamma_{A \leftrightarrow G}$ and $\gamma_{C \leftrightarrow T}$, lead very naturally to a very useful TN93 model that we will cover next.

3.2.1.4 TN93 MODEL

We have come far, so far that we need hardly any extra effort to derive transition probabilities for the TN93 model. There are two equivalent specifications of the rate matrix for the TN93 model. The first, in the order of A, G, C, and T, is

$$
Q_{\text{TN93}} = \begin{bmatrix}
- & \beta \pi_G + \gamma_R \pi_G / \pi_R & \beta \pi_C & \beta \pi_T \\
\beta \pi_A + \gamma_R \pi_A / \pi_R & - & \beta \pi_C & \beta \pi_T \\
\beta \pi_A & \beta \pi_G & - & \beta \pi_T + \gamma_Y \pi_T / \pi_Y \\
\beta \pi_A & \beta \pi_G & \beta \pi_C + \gamma_Y \pi_C / \pi_Y & -
\end{bmatrix} \quad (3.56)
$$

where the diagonal elements are constrained by each row summing up to 0. The second specification, shown in Figure 3.2, simply replaces $(\beta + \gamma_R/\pi_R)$ by α_1 and $(\beta + \gamma_Y/\pi_Y)$ by α_2. We see that TN93 is reduced to F84 if $\gamma_R = \gamma_Y$, and to HKY85 if $\gamma_R / \pi_R = \gamma_Y / \pi_Y$.

The similarity between TN93 and F84 allows us to reuse Figure 3.6 for deriving transition probabilities for TN93. We only need to add a subscript R to γ and α in Figure 3.6 so that we have γ_R and α_R as rates for purine, keeping everything else the same and we instantly obtain the transition probabilities for transitional substitutions between purines and for transversional substitutions as shown in Figure 3.6. To get transition probabilities between pyrimidines, we can just replace the original nucleotide A in Figure 3.6 by nucleotide C or T and rename γ and α in Figure 3.6 to γ_Y and α_Y. Note that our $\alpha_R = \beta + \gamma_R$ and $\alpha_Y = \beta + \gamma_Y$, i.e., they are not new rate parameters.

The transition probability matrix for the TN93 model, in the order of A, G, C, and T, is

$$
P_{\text{TN93}} = \begin{bmatrix}
\pi_A + \pi_A \pi_Y x_1 + \pi_G x_2 & \pi_G + \pi_G \pi_Y x_1 - \pi_G x_2 & \pi_C(1-e^{-\beta t}) & \pi_T(1-e^{-\beta t}) \\
\pi_A + \pi_A \pi_Y x_1 - \pi_A x_2 & \pi_G + \pi_G \pi_Y x_1 + \pi_A x_2 & \pi_C(1-e^{-\beta t}) & \pi_T(1-e^{-\beta t}) \\
\pi_A(1-e^{-\beta t}) & \pi_G(1-e^{-\beta t}) & \pi_C + \pi_C \pi_R x_3 + \pi_T x_4 & \pi_T + \pi_T \pi_R x_3 - \pi_T x_4 \\
\pi_A(1-e^{-\beta t}) & \pi_G(1-e^{-\beta t}) & \pi_C + \pi_C \pi_R x_3 - \pi_C x_4 & \pi_T + \pi_T \pi_R x_3 + \pi_C x_4
\end{bmatrix} \quad (3.57)
$$

where x_1 and x_3 are the same as those in Eq. (3.38), but x_2 has α replaced by α_R and x_4 has α replaced by α_Y, i.e.,

$$x_1 = \frac{e^{-\beta t}}{\pi_R}, x_2 = \frac{e^{-\alpha_R t}}{\pi_R}, x_3 = \frac{e^{-\beta t}}{\pi_Y}, x_4 = \frac{e^{-\alpha_Y t}}{\pi_Y} \qquad (3.58)$$

To obtain the distance for the TN93 model (D_{TN93}), recall that a distance is defined as μt where μ is the average substitution rate, i.e., substitution rates in Eq. (3.56) weighted by the equilibrium frequencies, so

$$D_{TN93} = 2\pi_A \pi_G (\beta t + \gamma_R t / \pi_R) + 2\pi_T \pi_C (\beta t + \gamma_Y t / \pi_Y) + 2\pi_Y \pi_R \beta t \qquad (3.59)$$

Now we need to obtain $\alpha_R t$, $\alpha_Y t$, and βt from which we can calculate $\gamma_R t$ and $\gamma_Y t$. The method we will use is the same as that for the K80 and F84 models, i.e., we obtain the expected numbers of A↔G transitions, C↔T transitions and transversions, designated E(S_R), E(S_Y), and E(V), respectively, from transition probabilities and equate them to the observed S_R, S_Y, and V to solve for $\alpha_R t$, $\alpha_Y t$, and βt:

$$\begin{aligned}
E(S_R) &= 2\pi_A P_{AG} = S_R \\
E(S_Y) &= 2\pi_C P_{CT} = S_Y \\
E(V) &= 2\pi_A P_{AT} + 2\pi_A P_{AC} + 2\pi_G P_{GC} + 2\pi_G P_{GT} = V
\end{aligned} \qquad (3.60)$$

The resulting $\alpha_R t$, $\alpha_Y t$, and βt are

$$\alpha_R t = -\ln\left(1 - \frac{\pi_R S_R}{2\pi_A \pi_G} - \frac{V}{2\pi_R}\right) \qquad (3.61)$$

$$\alpha_Y t = -\ln\left(1 - \frac{\pi_Y S_Y}{2\pi_C \pi_T} - \frac{V}{2\pi_Y}\right) \qquad (3.62)$$

$$\beta t = -\ln\left(1 - \frac{V}{2\pi_R \pi_Y}\right) \qquad (3.63)$$

If one wishes to express D_{TN93} in S_R, S_Y, and V, then one may just substitute $\gamma_R t$, $\gamma_Y t$, and βt into Eq. (3.59), which yields

$$D_{TN93} = \frac{2\pi_A \pi_G}{\pi_R}(\alpha_R t - \pi_Y \beta t) + \frac{2\pi_C \pi_T}{\pi_Y}(\alpha_Y t - \pi_R \beta t) + 2\pi_R \pi_Y \beta t \qquad (3.64)$$

To illustrate the application of D_{TN93} with the two aligned sequences in Figure 3.4, we have $\pi_A = 6/48$, $\pi_C = 12/48$, $\pi_G = 10/48$, $\pi_T = 20/48$, $S_Y = 4/24$, $S_R = 0$, $V = 2/24$, $\alpha_R t = 0.13353$, $\alpha_y t = 0.90593$, $\beta t = 0.20764$, $\gamma_R t = \alpha_R t - \beta t = -0.07411$, $\gamma_y t = \alpha_y t - \beta t = 0.69829$, $D_{TN93} = 0.35299$. The variance of the D_{TN93} can be obtained by either the delta method or the method using Fisher information matrix. Note that $S_R = 0$ means no information for estimating $\alpha_R t$ properly.

In short, the approach of deriving transition probabilities by probability reasoning can go a long way if one can do good bookkeeping. In particular, the probability reasoning approach is very useful for conceptual understanding. However, the approach becomes increasingly difficult with more complicated substitution models, and we discuss alternatives in the following sections.

3.2.2 OBTAINING TRANSITION PROBABILITIES BY SOLVING DIFFERENTIAL EQUATIONS

To avoid too much redundancy, I will only illustrate this approach of deriving transition probabilities by solving (partial) differential equations with the JC69, K80, and TN93 models. One may use symbolic computation software such as MAPLE (http://www.maplesoft.com), which is a beautiful Canadian product, to solve equations. MAPLE essentially puts a capable mathematical assistant by your side.

3.2.2.1 JC69 MODEL

Suppose we start with a site occupied by a nucleotide A. Over time the site will change and we need to model the probability that it is still occupied by A after time t, designated as $P_{A(t)}$. The JC69 model has only one rate α. The rate of nucleotide A flowing away from A to the other nucleotides is $3\alpha P_{A(t)}$ and the rate flowing into A from the other three nucleotides is α, so we have

$$\frac{dP_{A(t)}}{dt} = -(3\alpha)P_{A(t)} + \alpha[P_{G(t)} + P_{C(t)} + P_{T(t)}] \tag{3.65}$$

One may add $[-\alpha P_{A(t)} + \alpha P_{A(t)}]$, which is 0, to Eq. (3.65) to facilitate its simplification to

$$\frac{dP_{A(t)}}{dt} = -4\alpha P_{A(t)} + \alpha \tag{3.66}$$

You can solve this equation by hand, but if you want to use MAPLE to solve the equation, just type in the following MAPLE statement:

dsolve({diff(PA(t),t)=–4*a*PA(t)+a,PA(0)=1},PA(t)),

where dsolve is for solving differential equations, the curly brackets enclose the differential equation and initial condition.

Solving the ordinary differential equation yields $P_{A(t)}$ which is the probability that the original nucleotide A will remain as A after time t and equals the diagonal elements of the transition probability matrix for the JC69 model:

$$P_{A(t)} = \frac{1}{4} + \frac{3}{4}e^{-4\alpha t} = P_{AA} = P_{GG} = P_{CC} = P_{TT} \tag{3.67}$$

The off-diagonal elements are all equal in the JC69 model. Because each row sums to 1, the three off-diagonal elements are simply

$$P_{ij} = \frac{1-P_{ii}}{3} = \frac{1}{4} - \frac{1}{4}e^{-4\alpha t} \tag{3.68}$$

To obtain the evolutionary distance between two aligned sequences, one simply equates $3p_{ij}$ to p_{diff} (the proportion of sites differing between the two sequences), solve for αt, and obtain the distance as $3\alpha t$. This leads to the previously derived distance in Eq. (3.6).

The equilibrium frequencies are reached when nucleotide frequencies do not change with time, e.g., when $dP_{A(t)}/dt = 0$, i.e., $-4\alpha P_{A(t)} + \alpha = 0$. This yields $P_{A(t)} = 1/4$.

This approach can be generalized as

$$\left[\frac{dP_{A(t)}}{dt} \quad \frac{dP_{G(t)}}{dt} \quad \frac{dP_{C(t)}}{dt} \quad \frac{dP_{T(t)}}{dt} \right] = P(t)Q$$

$$= \left[P_{A(t)} \quad P_{G(t)} \quad P_{C(t)} \quad P_{T(t)} \right] \begin{bmatrix} -a-b-c & a & b & c \\ g & -g-d-e & d & e \\ h & i & -h-i-f & f \\ j & k & l & -j-k-l \end{bmatrix} \tag{3.69}$$

where $P(t)$ is the frequencies of the four nucleotides at time t and Q is the rate matrix. One can obtain analytical solutions from the JC69 model all the way to the TN93 model.

3.2.2.2   K80 MODEL

The rate matrix of Kimura's two-parameter model is in Figure 3.2. Substituting it into Eq. (3.69) and solving the equations with the initial condition that $P_{A.0} = 1$ and $P_{C.0} = P_{G.0} = P_{T.0} = 0$ (i.e., we start with a nucleotide A) and the constrain of $P_A + P_G + P_C + P_T = 1$, we have

$$P_{A.t} = \frac{1}{4} + \frac{1}{4}e^{-4\beta t} + \frac{1}{2}e^{-2(\alpha+\beta)t} = P_{ii} \qquad (3.70)$$

$$P_{G.t} = \frac{1}{4} + \frac{1}{4}e^{-4\beta t} - \frac{1}{2}e^{-2(\alpha+\beta)t} = P_s \qquad (3.71)$$

$$P_{C.t} = P_{T.t} = \frac{1}{4} - \frac{1}{4}e^{-4\beta t} = P_v \qquad (3.72)$$

where P_s and P_v are the probability of observing a transition or a transversion, respectively, at a site, and are often approximated by the proportion of sites with a transition or a transversion difference.

One can obtain the results above by issuing the following statements in the MAPLE interface:

eq1:=diff(Pa(t),t)=−Pa(t)*(a+2*b)+Pg(t)*a+Pc(t)*b+Pt(t)*b;

eq2:=diff(Pg(t),t)=−Pg(t)*(a+2*b)+Pa(t)*a+Pc(t)*b+Pt(t)*b;

eq3:=diff(Pc(t),t)=−Pc(t)*(a+2*b)+Pa(t)*b+Pg(t)*b+Pt(t)*a;

eq4:=diff(Pt(t),t)=−Pt(t)*(a+2*b)+Pa(t)*b+Pg(t)*b+Pc(t)*a;

sols:=dsolve({eq1,eq2,eq3,eq4,Pa(0)=1,Pc(0)=0,Pg(0)=0,Pt(0)=0},
{Pa(t),Pg(t),Pc(t),Pt(t)});

The MAPLE statements above include specification of the four partial differential equations as eq1 to eq4, with the frequencies of nucleotides A, C, G, and T at time t specified as Pa(t), Pc(t), Pg(t), and Pt(t), respectively.

Rate parameters α and β are specified as a and b. We start with nucleotide A, so the initial conditions are Pa(0) = 1, and Pc(0)=0, Pg(0)=0, Pt(0)=0. Executing the statements generates Eqs. (3.70)–(3.72).

The other transition probabilities can be obtained in the same way. Once we have the transition probabilities, we can obtain the evolutionary distance between two aligned sequences by (1) equating the P_s to the proportion of sites differing by a transition (P) and $2P_v$ to the proportion of sites differing by a transversion (Q), (2) solve for αt and βt, and (3) obtain the distance as ($\alpha t + 2\beta t$). This yields the previously derived distance in Eq. (3.21).

3.2.2.3   TN93 MODEL

We will use the rate matrix specified in Figure 3.2 for the TN93 model. Substituting the Q matrix into Eq. (3.69) and solving the partial differential equations will generate transition probabilities. For example, we can use the following MAPLE statements to obtain transition probabilities p_{AA}, p_{AG}, p_{AC}, and p_{AT} by specifying the initial condition with a nucleotide A, i.e., $P_A(0) = 1, P_C(0) = 0, P_G(0) = 0, P_T(0) = 0$.

```
eq1 := diff(Pa(t),t) = Pa(t)*(–G*a1–C*b–T*b)+Pg(t)*A*a1+Pc(t)*A*b+Pt(t)*A*b;

eq2 := diff(Pg(t),t) = Pa(t)*G*a1+Pg(t)*(–A*a1–C*b–T*b)+Pc(t)*G*b+Pt(t)*G*b;

eq3 := diff(Pc(t),t) = Pa(t)*C*b+Pg(t)*C*b+Pc(t)*(–A*b–G*b–T*a2)+Pt(t)*C*a2;

eq4 := diff(Pt(t),t) = Pa(t)*T*b+Pg(t)*T*b+Pc(t)*T*a2+Pt(t)*(–A*b–G*b–C*a2);

sols:=dsolve({eq1,eq2,eq3,eq4,Pa(0)=1,Pc(0)=0,Pg(0)=0,Pt(0)=0},{Pa(t),Pg(t),Pc(t),Pt(t)});
```

The MAPLE statements above include specification of the four partial differential equations as eq1 to eq4, with the frequencies of nucleotides A, C, G, and T at time t specified as $Pa(t)$, $Pc(t)$, $Pg(t)$, and $Pt(t)$, respectively. Rate parameters α_R, α_Y, and β are specified as a1, a2, and b in the MAPLE statements. We start with nucleotide A, so the initial conditions are Pa(0) = 1, and Pc(0)=0, Pg(0)=0, Pt(0)=0. Executing the statements will generate $P_A(t)$, $P_G(t)$, $P_C(t)$, and $P_T(t)$, which are the probabilities that the initial A will remain A, or become G, C, or T. They are, after some algebraic manipulation,

$$P_A(t) = \frac{\pi_A \pi_R + \pi_A \pi_Y e^{-\beta t} + \pi_G e^{-(R\alpha_R + Y\beta)t}}{\pi_R} = p_{AA}$$

$$P_G(t) = \frac{\pi_G \pi_R + \pi_G \pi_Y e^{-\beta t} - \pi_G e^{-(R\alpha_R + Y\beta)t}}{\pi_R} = p_{AG}$$ (3.73)

$$P_C(t) = \pi_C \left(1 - e^{-\beta t}\right) = p_{AC}$$

$$P_T(t) = \pi_T \left(1 - e^{-\beta t}\right) = p_{AT}$$

Note that the rate parameter α_R appears only in the expression of p_{AA}, p_{GG}, p_{AG}, and p_{GA}, and the rate parameter α_Y appears only in p_{CC}, p_{TT}, p_{CT}, and p_{TC}. All other p_{ij} expressions not shown in Eq. (3.73) can be easily obtained in the same way by changing the initial conditions. Once we have the transition probabilities, the distance can be obtained as shown previously in Eq. (3.59)–(3.64).

3.2.3 OBTAIN TRANSITION PROBABILITIES FROM THE RATE MATRIX BY USING MATRIX EXPONENTIAL

The relationship between the transition probability matrix (P) and the rate matrix (Q) can be written as (Lanave et al., 1984)

$$P = e^{Qt}$$ (3.74)

This is a general approach, particularly useful when an analytical solution is not available or tedious to write out. We will first illustrate this method with JC69 and K80 in which simple analytical solutions for P are available but we will pretend not to have them. After gaining the familiarity with this approach, we will apply the method to derive P and evolutionary distance (D_{GTR}) for the GTR model for which we do not have an analytical solution for P. The basic skill we need is to obtain eigenvalues and eigenvectors from the rate matrix and the inverse of a matrix but there are many programs such as R, MAPLE, MatLab, etc., that can do it for us with one statement or two.

We will use the same set of sequence data throughout all these exercises. The two aligned sequences are 860 nt long, with site information shown in Table 3.1. By visual inspection of the values in Table 3.1, we see that A↔G transitions are the most frequent, followed by C↔T transitions, with the transversions least frequent. You will find D_{GTR} similar to D_{TN93} for these two sequences.

TABLE 3.1 Empirical substitution pattern between two aligned sequences ($S1$ and $S2$) of 860 nucleotides long. The first value in the first row, 100, means 100 sites have A in both sequences, the second value in the first row, 40, means 40 sites with A in $S1$ and G in $S2$ and so on.

	A	G	C	T
A	100	40	8	12
G	35	200	11	8
C	9	9	250	20
T	11	12	15	120
π	0.18314	0.299419	0.332558	0.184884

3.2.3.1 JC69 MODEL

Students often ask why JC69 has no rate to estimate. This is because (1) the evolutionary distance is defined as $D = \mu t$ where μ is the substitution rate equal to 3α in the case of JC69 model, i.e., $D = 3\alpha t$, and (2) we cannot estimate α and t separately, so that rate is scaled to 1. This means $3\alpha = 1$, so that t is measured by D, i.e., $D = 3\alpha t = 1*t = t$. Now $\alpha = 1/3$, which is why we say that the JC69 model has no rate parameter to estimate. The rate matrix Q for JC69 is made of all constants:

$$Q_{JC69} = \begin{bmatrix} -1 & 1/3 & 1/3 & 1/3 \\ 1/3 & -1 & 1/3 & 1/3 \\ 1/3 & 1/3 & -1 & 1/3 \\ 1/3 & 1/3 & 1/3 & -1 \end{bmatrix} \tag{3.75}$$

The sorted (in descending order) eigenvalues (λ) and eigenvectors (**U**) from Q_{JC69} are

$$\lambda = \begin{bmatrix} 0 \\ -4/3 \\ -4/3 \\ -4/3 \end{bmatrix}; U = \begin{bmatrix} 1 & -1 & -1 & -1 \\ 1 & 1 & 0 & 0 \\ 1 & 0 & 1 & 0 \\ 1 & 0 & 0 & 1 \end{bmatrix} \tag{3.76}$$

Now the transition probabilities for the JC69 model can be numerically calculated as

$$P = e^{QD}$$

$$= \begin{bmatrix} 1 & -1 & -1 & -1 \\ 1 & 1 & 0 & 0 \\ 1 & 0 & 1 & 0 \\ 1 & 0 & 0 & 1 \end{bmatrix} \begin{bmatrix} e^{0D} & 0 & 0 & 0 \\ 0 & e^{-4D/3} & 0 & 0 \\ 0 & 0 & e^{-4D/3} & 0 \\ 0 & 0 & 0 & e^{-4D/3} \end{bmatrix} \begin{bmatrix} 1/4 & 1/4 & 1/4 & 1/4 \\ -1/4 & 3/4 & -1/4 & -1/4 \\ -1/4 & -1/4 & 3/4 & -1/4 \\ -1/4 & -1/4 & -1/4 & 3/4 \end{bmatrix} \quad (3.77)$$

where the first matrix is U, the second diagonal matrix has diagonal elements being $e^{\lambda D}$, D is D_{JC69} that we wish to find, and the last matrix is the inverse of U, i.e., U^{-1}. I use D for D_{JC69} to save some typing. Eq. (3.77) simplifies the calculation of P (by matrix exponential) from Q for different D values. To obtain P for a different D, we only need to change the middle diagonal matrix. Note that, while P matrix changes with D between two aligned homologous sequences or with the branch length between two neighboring nodes on a tree, the rate matrix Q, with the assumption of homogeneity of rates over time, remains the same.

As we have mentioned several times in previous sections, the P matrix is needed to compute evolutionary distance (D) between two sequences (e.g., the two aligned sequences with data summarized in Table 3.1) or the log-likelihood in tree construction. We can obtain D in two ways, similar to what we have already learned in previous sections with analytical solutions of the P matrix. We will repeat these two ways as I found this repetition helpful to enhance understanding in students.

The first way is based on the fact that the P matrix represents our expected sequence divergence between two sequences with a given D, and we want to find a P matrix that ideally matches our observed sequence divergence. For the JC69 model, the observed sequence divergence is measured by the proportion of sites that differ between the two sequences (p_{diff}). From Table 3.1, $p_{diff} = 0.22093$. If we put $D = 0.22093$ into Eq. (3.77) then the resulting P matrix is

$$P_{D=0.22093} = \begin{bmatrix} 0.808636992 & 0.063787669 & 0.063787669 & 0.063787669 \\ 0.063787669 & 0.808636992 & 0.063787669 & 0.063787669 \\ 0.063787669 & 0.063787669 & 0.808636992 & 0.063787669 \\ 0.063787669 & 0.063787669 & 0.063787669 & 0.808636992 \end{bmatrix} \quad (3.78)$$

Note that the P matrix has only two distinct values, the diagonal value of 0.808636992 and the off-diagonal value of 0.063787669. The expected divergence from the P matrix given $D = 0.22093$, designated by $E(p_{diff})$ is the summation of the off-diagonal elements in the P matrix above divided by 4, i.e.,

$$E(p_{\text{diff}}) = \frac{\sum_{i=1}^{4}\sum_{j=1, j\neq i}^{4} p_{ij}}{4} = \frac{0.063787669 \times 12}{4} = 0.191363007 \qquad (3.79)$$

Alternatively, $E(p_{diff})$ is one minus the average of the four diagonal values. Apparently, $E(p_{diff})$ (=0.191363007) is smaller than the observed p_{diff} (=0.22093), so we need to try different D values larger than 0.22093 so as to find one that will result in $E(p_{diff})$ equal to the observed p_{diff}. There are efficient algorithms to automate this (Press et al., 1992) but suppose at this moment the god of mathematics happens to whisper $D = 0.2617147$ into our ears (otherwise we may have to guess various D values for a long time without using a computer). Replacing D in Eq. (3.77) with this holy value, we get a new P matrix with diagonal values being 0.779069767 and off-diagonal values being 0.073643411. With this new P matrix, $E(p_{diff}) = p_{diff} = 0.22093$, so we conclude that the best D is 0.2617147 for the JC69 model. For those who do not believe in the god of mathematics, consult the bible of numerical recipes (Press et al., 1992) and you will get the same answer.

The second way of estimating D is by the likelihood method, i.e., we want to find a D (and the associated P matrix) so that the following likelihood function is maximized:

$$\ln L = \sum_{i=1}^{4}\sum_{j=1}^{4} N_{ij} \ln(\pi_i p_{ij})$$
$$= N_{A,A} \ln(\pi_1 p_{1,1}) + N_{A,G} \ln(\pi_1 p_{1,2}) + \dots + N_{T,T} \ln(\pi_4 p_{4,4}) \qquad (3.80)$$

where N_{ij} is the number of sites where one sequence is occupied by nucleotide i and the other sequence by nucleotide j (e.g., $N_{AA} = 100$ in Table 3.1), π_i values are equilibrium frequencies, and p_{ij} values are entries in the P matrix (i.e., transition probabilities from nucleotide i to nucleotide j during D which measures time when the average rate is scaled to be 1). With the JC69 model, we could collapse the 16 terms in lnL into two terms because (1) all $\pi_i = 1/4$ and (2) there are only two distinct p_{ij} values with the four diagonal elements being the same to each other and the 12 off-diagonal elements being the same to each other. However, I choose to write them out in Eq. (3.80) because we eventually have to write out all individual terms with the GTR model.

What D value should we try first? As a distance corrected for multiple substitutions will always be greater than p_{diff}, the value of p_{diff} (=0.22093) can serve as the low bound for D. If we do set $D = 0.22093$, then the P matrix has already been shown in Eq. (3.78), so that lnL is

$$\ln L = 860 \ln(1/4) + 100 \ln(0.808637) + 40$$
$$\ln(0.0637877) + ... + 120 \ln(0.8086370) = -665.2286 \tag{3.81}$$

where 1/4 is the equilibrium frequencies for the JC69 model. The constant term 860*ln(1/4) can be omitted in finding D_{JC69} to maximize lnL.

We need to try various D values so as to find one that maximizes lnL. There are efficient numerical algorithms to do the guessing for us (Press et al., 1992), but again suppose at this moment the god of mathematics happens to whisper $D = 0.2617147$ into our ears. Replacing D in Eq. (3.77) with this holy value, we get a new P matrix with diagonal values being 0.779069767 and off-diagonal values being 0.073643411. This new P matrix leads to a larger lnL value of -1855.1007. In fact, this is the maximum lnL we can get (rounded to 4 decimal points), so we declare that D_{JC69} is 0.2617147, which is exactly the same by the first method. It is also the same as that from Eq. (3.6), which, as we have shown before, is a maximum likelihood estimate.

3.2.3.2 K80 MODEL

The K80 model has two rate parameters α and β and is often reparameter-ized by $\kappa = \alpha/\beta$ so that $\alpha = \kappa\beta$. Because we cannot separate rate from time and consequently time is measured by distance with the average rate scaled to one. This implies that $\alpha+2\beta =1$, so

$$\alpha+2\beta = \kappa\beta+2\beta = \beta(\kappa+2)=1$$
$$\beta = \frac{1}{\kappa+2} \tag{3.82}$$

Thus, the K80 model, although having two rates, ends up with only one rate ratio (κ) to be estimated. A given κ determines both β and α. For example, $\kappa = 2$ implies $\beta = 1/4$ and $\alpha = 1/2$ according to Eq. (3.82).

As transitions do appear to occur more frequently than transversions in Table 3.1, we will start with a guess of $\kappa = 2$. This leads to the rate matrix Q as follows

$$
Q = \begin{bmatrix}
A & -1 & 1/2 & 1/4 & 1/4 \\
G & 1/2 & -1 & 1/4 & 1/4 \\
C & 1/4 & 1/4 & -1 & 1/2 \\
T & 1/4 & 1/4 & 1/2 & -1
\end{bmatrix} \tag{3.83}
$$

We again obtain the sorted eigenvalues (λ) and eigenvectors ($\mathbf{U}$) and again arrange them in the following form as we have done before with Eq. (3.77). Note that eigenvectors are not unique, but the resulting P matrix will be the same.

$$
P = e^{QD} = \begin{bmatrix}
1 & -1 & 0 & -1 \\
1 & -1 & 0 & 1 \\
1 & 1 & -1 & 0 \\
1 & 1 & 1 & 0
\end{bmatrix}\begin{bmatrix}
e^{0D} & 0 & 0 & 0 \\
0 & e^{-1D} & 0 & 0 \\
0 & 0 & e^{-1.5D} & 0 \\
0 & 0 & 0 & e^{-1.5D}
\end{bmatrix}\begin{bmatrix}
1/4 & 1/4 & 1/4 & 1/4 \\
-1/4 & -1/4 & 1/4 & 1/4 \\
0 & 0 & -1/2 & 1/2 \\
-1/2 & 1/2 & 0 & 0
\end{bmatrix} \tag{3.84}
$$

where the first matrix is $\mathbf{U}$, the second diagonal matrix has diagonal elements being $e^{\lambda D}$, D is D_{K80} that we wish to find and the last matrix is the inverse of $\mathbf{U}$, i.e,. $\mathbf{U}^{-1}$. Now we have two parameters (D and κ) to estimate, in contrast to the JC69 model where we have only D to estimate.

Again, we have the same two methods for parameter estimation. The first is to find a pair of $\{D, \kappa\}$ that will maximize lnL defined in Eq. (3.80), and the second is to find a pair of $\{D, \kappa\}$ so that the observed proportion of sites with a transition (S) and the proportion of sites with a transversion (V) are the same as their expected values $E(S)$ and $E(V)$ derived from the P matrix:

$$
E(S) = \frac{p_{AG} + p_{GA} + p_{CT} + p_{TC}}{4} = \frac{4p_{AG}}{4};
$$

$$
E(V) = \frac{p_{AC} + p_{AT} + \dots + p_{TA}}{4} = \frac{8p_{AC}}{4} \tag{3.85}
$$

Note that the four p_{ij} values involving A$\leftrightarrow$G and C$\leftrightarrow$T are identical, so are the eight transversional p_{ij} values. Also, we have used S and V for the proportion of sites being transitions and transversions, respectively, instead of using P and Q as we did in previous sections. This is because we have already used P for the transition probability matrix and Q for rate matrix. The two methods lead to the same estimate for the JC69 and K80 models.

From Table 3.1, the observed S and V are

$$S = \frac{40+35+20+15}{860} = 0.127906977;$$

$$V = \frac{8+12+11+8+9+9+11+12}{860} = 0.093023256 \tag{3.86}$$

If we fix $\kappa = 2$, then no matter what D values we try, we cannot get E(S) and E(V) equal to the observed S and V. In fact, the closest we can get is when $D = 0.260446116$ (fixing $\kappa = 2$). The P matrix for this pair of $\{D = 0.260446116, \kappa = 2\}$ is

$$P_{\kappa=2, D=0.260446116} = \begin{bmatrix} 0.7809789 & 0.104374942 & 0.057323079 & 0.057323079 \\ 0.104374942 & 0.7809789 & 0.057323079 & 0.057323079 \\ 0.057323079 & 0.057323079 & 0.7809789 & 0.104374942 \\ 0.057323079 & 0.057323079 & 0.104374942 & 0.7809789 \end{bmatrix} \tag{3.87}$$

Note that there are only three distinct values in the P matrix above, with the four diagonal values being 0.7809789, the four transitions being 0.104374942 and eight transversions being 0.057323079. From this P matrix, E(S) = 0.104374942 (smaller than observed S) and E(V) = 0.114646158 (greater than the observed V). The difference between E(S) and S and between E(V) and V suggests that κ has to be larger than 2. So, we have to try different $\{D, \kappa\}$ combinations to find the optimal pair. Again, suppose the god of mathematics whispered $D = 0.265960816$ and $\kappa = 3.167999267$ into our ears or, alternatively, we have obtained the magic D and κ values by using the bible of numerical recipes (Press et al., 1992). This new κ value implies the following Q matrix:

$$Q = \begin{bmatrix} A & -1 & 0.613003041 & 0.193498479 & 0.193498479 \\ G & 0.613003041 & -1 & 0.193498479 & 0.193498479 \\ C & 0.193498479 & 0.193498479 & -1 & 0.613003041 \\ T & 0.193498479 & 0.193498479 & 0.613003041 & -1 \end{bmatrix} \tag{3.88}$$

This Q matrix gives us λ and $\mathbf{U}$ as

$$\lambda = \begin{bmatrix} 0 \\ -0.77399 \\ -1.613 \\ -1.613 \end{bmatrix} ; U = \begin{bmatrix} -0.5 & 0.5 & 0 & 0.70711 \\ -0.5 & 0.5 & 0 & -0.70711 \\ -0.5 & -0.5 & -0.70711 & 0 \\ -0.5 & -0.5 & 0.70711 & 0 \end{bmatrix} \quad (3.89)$$

With this set of λ and $\mathbf{U}$, if we try $D = 0.265960816$, then we will end up with the following P matrix:

$$P = \begin{bmatrix} 0.779069767 & 0.127906977 & 0.046511628 & 0.046511628 \\ 0.127906977 & 0.779069767 & 0.046511628 & 0.046511628 \\ 0.046511628 & 0.046511628 & 0.779069767 & 0.127906977 \\ 0.046511628 & 0.046511628 & 0.127906977 & 0.779069767 \end{bmatrix} \quad (3.90)$$

Now $E(S)$ and $E(V)$ as specified in Eq. (3.85) are 0.127906977 and 0.093023256, respectively. They are exactly the same as the observed S and V. So, we conclude that the combination of $D = 0.265960816$ and κ = 3.167999267 are the best estimates. To use the maximum likelihood approach, we will also find the same D and κ combination to yield the highest lnL (=−1831.1357). That is, $D = 0.265960816$ and $\kappa = 3.167999267$ are also maximum likelihood estimates.

There are two awkward situations one may occasionally encounter in deriving transition probabilities and estimating distances from an empirical substitution matrix. The first is that parameters such as κ in the K80 model may need to be negative for $E(S) = S$ and $E(V) = V$. A negative κ (which implies a negative evolutionary rate) makes no biological sense so computer programs such as DAMBE (Xia, 2013b) sometimes would constrain $\kappa \geq 0$. Unfortunately, users often are not aware that, among the estimated distances in a distance matrix, some distance may be subject to such constraints and some are not. The second awkward situation is when the distance formula is inapplicable, e.g., when $1-2P-Q \leq 0$ or $1-2Q \leq 0$ for the K80 model. Such cases are discussed in the next section with the GTR model. For this reason, simultaneously estimated (SE) distances (Tamura et al., 2004; Xia, 2009), which uses information from all pairwise comparisons, are much more robust and typically generate better distance estimates and better trees than independently estimated (IE) distances which use only information from two sequences. SE distances are covered in the chapter on distance-based phylogenetic methods.

3.2.3.3 GTR MODEL

We will illustrate two parameter-estimation approaches, by maximizing likelihood and by minimizing χ^2. After applying them to regular cases where a unique and biologically meaningful solution of parameters can be obtained, we will explore the approximate method for dealing with the two awkward cases we have mentioned before, one with negative rates and the other inapplicable cases.

The GTR model, as shown in Figure 3.2, has 6 rate parameters a_1-a_6. Because we cannot separate rate and time, the average rate is scaled to be 1 so that the time is measured by the distance and the six rate parameters are typically reparameterized as ratios over a_6 (the rate for G↔T) by the following:

$$2\pi_A\pi_G a_1 + 2\pi_A\pi_C a_2 + 2\pi_A\pi_T a_3 + 2\pi_C\pi_G a_4 + 2\pi_C\pi_T a_5 + 2\pi_G\pi_T a_6 = 1$$
$$\kappa_1 = a_1 / a_6, \kappa_2 = a_2 / a_6, \kappa_3 = a_3 / a_6, \kappa_4 = a_4 / a_6, \kappa_5 = a_5 / a_6 \tag{3.91}$$

where the first equation shows the scaling of the average rate to 1 and equations in the second line defines the five rate ratio parameters. We will use the empirical nucleotide frequencies in Table 3.1 as equilibrium frequencies π_i so we do not have too many parameters to estimate. Solving these six equations for a_i, we have

$$a_1 = \frac{\kappa_1}{2x}; a_2 = \frac{\kappa_2}{2x}; a_3 = \frac{\kappa_3}{2x}; a_4 = \frac{\kappa_4}{2x}; a_5 = \frac{\kappa_5}{2x}; a_6 = \frac{1}{2x} \tag{3.92}$$

where

$$x = \pi_A\pi_G\kappa_1 + \pi_A\pi_C\kappa_2 + \pi_A\pi_T\kappa_3 + \pi_C\pi_T\kappa_4 + \pi_G\pi_C\kappa_5 \tag{3.93}$$

This reparameterization is similar to what we have done with the K80 model where two rate parameters (α and β) are reparameterized to a single rate ratio parameter κ. Note that a_6 is not free if κ_1 to κ_5 are fixed.

Now we have six parameters to estimate (κ_1 to κ_5 and the distance D) if we use the empirical nucleotide frequencies for equilibrium nucleotide frequencies π_i. The computation is the same as before, i.e., we guess various parameter values to see which set of κ_i and D is the best by using either of the two criteria: (1) The observed transition probabilities matching the expected transition probabilities and (2) maximum likelihood. We will use both criteria simultaneously to evaluate and progressively improve the estimation of the six parameters.

3.2.3.3.1 Regular Cases

Regular cases in which κ_i and D have unique solutions are typically characterized by an empirical substitution matrix (Table 3.1) with diagonal values substantially greater than off-diagonal values. The observed transition probability matrix (P_{obs}) can be obtained by first averaging the two corresponding off-diagonal values in Table 3.1 (because time-reversibility implies that we cannot distinguish between A→G and G→A events and the two corresponding numbers should be averaged to generate a symmetrical matrix in columns 2–5 under C_{obs} in Table 3.2) and then divide each value in C_{obs} by their respective row sums. The resulting observed transition probabilities are shown under P_{obs} in Table 3.2.

We note that A↔G and C↔T transitions differ but the four transversions have roughly similar C_{obs} values in Table 3.2. As a first approximation, we will just use $\kappa_1 = 4$, $\kappa_2 = 1$, $\kappa_3 = 1$, $\kappa_4 = 1$, $\kappa_5 = 2$, and $D = 0.2$ as our initial guesses. These initial parameter values yield, according to Eqs. (3.91)–(3.92),

$$x = 0.5920065$$
$$a_1 = 3.378341, \; a_2 = 0.8445853; \; a_3 = 0.8445853;$$
$$a_4 = 0.8445853; \; a_5 = 1.689171; \; a_6 = 0.8445853$$

$$(3.94)$$

The rate matrix Q for GTR (Fig. 3.2) is determined by a_i and π_i, e.g., $Q_{AG} = a_1 * \pi_G = 1.0115383$ and the diagonal elements are constrained by the row sum equal to 0:

$$Q = \begin{array}{l} A \\ G \\ C \\ T \end{array} \begin{bmatrix} -1.4485621 & 1.0115383 & 0.2808737 & 0.1561501 \\ 0.6187079 & -1.0557317 & 0.2808737 & 0.1561501 \\ 0.154677 & 0.2528846 & -0.7198617 & 0.3123002 \\ 0.154677 & 0.2528846 & 0.5617475 & -0.969309 \end{bmatrix} \qquad (3.95)$$

With our initial $D = 0.2$, the Q matrix above leads to expected transition probability matrix P as

TABLE 3.2 Obtaining the empirical transition probability matrix from observed substitution data in Table 3.1. Each pair of corresponding off-diagonal values in Table 3.1 is first averaged to give values in columns 2–5 designated as C_{obs} (observed counts). These values are then divided by the "Sum" column to give the observed P matrix (P_{obs}) in the last four columns. The last columns represent expected counts (C_{exp}, see text) corresponding to C_{obs}.

	C_{obs}					P_{obs}				C_{exp}			
	A	G	C	T	Sum	A	G	C	T	A	G	C	T
A	100	37.5	8.5	11.5	157.5	0.634921	0.238095	0.053968	0.073016	100	37.5	8.5	11.5
G	37.5	200	10	10	257.5	0.145631	0.776699	0.038835	0.038835	37.5	200	10	10
C	8.5	10	250	17.5	286	0.02972	0.034965	0.874126	0.061189	8.5	10	250	17.5
T	11.5	10	17.5	120	159	0.072327	0.062893	0.110063	0.754717	11.5	10	17.5	120

$$P = \begin{bmatrix} A & 0.75935986 & 0.160218784 & 0.051686534 & 0.028734822 \\ G & 0.097997904 & 0.82158074 & 0.051686534 & 0.028734822 \\ C & 0.028463741 & 0.046535953 & 0.871009116 & 0.05399119 \\ T & 0.028463741 & 0.046535953 & 0.097116226 & 0.82788408 \end{bmatrix} \quad (3.96)$$

which differs much from P_{obs}, shown in Table 3.2. The lnL value, defined in Eq. (3.80), is -1796.492 and is not the maximum as a slight increase in D will generate a higher lnL value. If we do not change κ_i but optimize the D value, we will find lnL reaching its maximum of -1789.729 when $D = 0.269279$. But the resulting expected P matrix still does not match P_{obs} in Table 3.2, although somewhat closer than with $D = 0.2$. This means that our initial κ_i values are not good enough and need to be optimized as well.

We can proceed by trying various combination of the κ_i and D values to see which combination will give us the highest lnL. Efficient algorithms (Press et al., 1992) exist to find these κ_i and D values but suppose the god of mathematics has again whispered the following into our ears: $\kappa_1=5.2352836$, $\kappa_2=0.8195326$, $\kappa_3=2.4238604$, $\kappa_4=0.5354983$, $\kappa_5=1.8115580$, and $D=0.2785347$. These values would give the Q and P matrices as

$$Q = \begin{bmatrix} A & -1.7899718 & 1.2292351 & 0.2130239 & 0.3477128 \\ G & 0.7518622 & -1.0347866 & 0.1391862 & 0.1437382 \\ C & 0.1173121 & 0.1253162 & -0.5056578 & 0.2630294 \\ T & 0.3444325 & 0.2327835 & 0.4731222 & -1.0503382 \end{bmatrix} \quad (3.97)$$

$$P = \begin{bmatrix} A & 0.63492903 & 0.23810462 & 0.05395282 & 0.07301354 \\ G & 0.14563681 & 0.77668322 & 0.03883880 & 0.03884118 \\ C & 0.02971178 & 0.03496850 & 0.87410775 & 0.06121197 \\ T & 0.07232472 & 0.06290316 & 0.11010454 & 0.75466759 \end{bmatrix} \quad (3.98)$$

The P matrix, together with N_{ij} values in Table 3.1 and equilibrium frequencies, leads to $lnL = -1779.257$. If you try to use any other combination of κ_i and D values, the lnL will get smaller. Thus, the values whispered into our ears by the god of mathematics are the maximum likelihood estimates. The P matrix in Eq. (3.98), expected on the basis of D, π_i, and the Q matrix and hereafter referred to as P_{exp} is also nearly identical to P_{obs} in Table 3.2. P_{obs} and P_{exp} can be made more similar by increasing the precision of iteration.

We have not been explicit about the approach of matching the observed and the expected P matrix. With the substitution models from JC69 to TN93, we have analytical solutions for transition probabilities expressed as functions of D and substitution rates, so we simply equate the observed transition probabilities to their expected counterparts to obtain D and substitution rates. In the case of GTR, we do not have a handy analytical solution for the transition probabilities, so we aim to find a combination of D and κ_i values that will minimize the difference between P_{obs} and P_{exp}. One may note that if we multiply the values in P_{exp} in Eq. (3.98) by their corresponding row sum of counts (the "Sum" column in Table 3.2), we obtain the expected counts (C_{exp}) corresponding to observed counts (C_{obs}) in Table 3.2 (rounded to one decimal point). Thus, one may simply use C_{obs} and C_{exp} in Table 3.2 to computer χ^2 as an operational criterion for matching P_{obs} and P_{exp}, i.e.,

$$\chi^2 = \sum_{i=1}^{4}\sum_{j=i}^{4} \frac{(C_{obs.ij} - C_{exp.ij})^2}{C_{exp.ij}} \tag{3.99}$$

Note that Eq. (3.99) has 10 unique terms instead of 16 for the GTR model because the C_{obs} and C_{exp} are symmetrical due to the fact that we do not know the direction of nucleotide substitutions, e.g., we cannot distinguish between A→G and G→A and consequently averaged the off-diagonal counts (Table 3.2). For $i \neq j$, C_{obs}, and C_{exp} values in Table 3.2 would be multiplied by 2. Ideally, $\chi^2 = 0$, which means a perfect match between P_{obs} and P_{exp}. Thus, we have two similar ways to estimate D and κ_i. The likelihood method will find D and κ_i that maximize lnL defined in Eq. (3.80), and the χ^2 method will find D and κ_i that minimizes χ^2 defined in Eq. (3.99) both with constraints of $\kappa_i \geq 0$.

Note that parameter estimation by minimizing χ^2 in Eq. (3.99) is a special case of weighted least-squares method. The general form of weighted least-squares (WLS) is to minimize the residual sum of squares (RSS):

$$RSS = \sum \left[\frac{(o_i - e_i)^2}{w_i^m} \right] \tag{3.100}$$

where o_i and e_i are the observed and expected values, w_i is the weight typically equal to o_i or e_i, and m is an integer typically taking the value of 0, 1, or 2. If $m = 0$, Eq. (3.100) becomes an ordinary least-squares (OLS) method. If $m > 0$, then RSS represents weighted least-squares (WLS) method. If $m = 1$ and $w_i = e_i$, RSS in Eq. (3.100) becomes the same as χ^2 in Eq. (3.99). The Fitch-Margoliash method (Fitch and Margoliash, 1967) for reconstructing phylogenies from a distance matrix has $m = 2$ and $w_i = o_i$ (where o_i is the estimated evolutionary distance for species pair i and e_i is the patristic distance linking species pair i along the tree.)

In addition to the likelihood and the χ^2 methods, we can also obtain D and the Q matrix from P_{obs} in Table 3.2, as has been well illustrated by Felsenstein (Felsenstein, 2004, pp 208–209). Note that

$$P = e^{Qt} = e^{QD} \qquad (3.101)$$

where $t = D$ because the average rate is scaled to 1 so time is measured by distance. Thus, the matrix logarithm of P_{obs} in Table 3.2 gives us matrix QD

$$QD = \log(P_{obs}) = \begin{bmatrix} A & -0.49908268 & 0.2096211 & 0.03272184 & 0.09603549 \\ G & 0.34271386 & -0.28848954 & 0.03493475 & 0.0648886 \\ C & 0.05941871 & 0.03880131 & -0.14096078 & 0.13185534 \\ T & 0.09695011 & 0.04006713 & 0.07330419 & -0.29277942 \end{bmatrix} \qquad (3.102)$$

D can then be obtained as

$$D = -\sum_{i=1}^{4} QD_{i,i}\pi_i = 0.278789 \qquad (3.103)$$

The rate matrix Q can then be obtained as

$$Q = \frac{QD}{D} = \begin{bmatrix} A & -0.139138616 & 0.058439996 & 0.00912248 & 0.02677361 \\ G & 0.095544754 & -0.080427626 & 0.009739414 & 0.018090209 \\ C & 0.016565265 & 0.010817367 & -0.039298274 & 0.03675978 \\ T & 0.027028596 & 0.011170263 & 0.02043638 & -0.081623596 \end{bmatrix} \qquad (3.104)$$

which would lead to κ_i values similar to those from the maximum likelihood or χ^2 methods.

3.2.3.3.2 Two Awkward/Irregular Scenarios

The two awkward scenarios associated with independently estimated (IE) distances are (1) the best-fitting model has one or more negative substitution rates which make no biological sense, and (2) inapplicable cases (where distance formulae are not applicable). Two approaches have been used to handle them. The first is to constrain substitution rates to be nonnegative. The second is to use simultaneously estimated (SE) distances.

The first scenario with negative substitution rates may be simpler to illustrate with the K80 model than with the GTR model. Suppose we have empirical substitution pattern shown in Table 3.3 between two aligned highly diverged sequences with 211 aligned sites of which 40 sites differ by a transition, 104 sites by a transversion, and 67 sites are identical. So, the observed proportion of transitions (S) and transversions (V) are 0.18957346 and 0.492890995, respectively. From these, we can obtain a $D_{K80} = 2.091322$, a negative $\kappa = -0.033198953$ and the expected S and V, E(S), and E(V), will be exactly equal to S and V leading to $\chi^2 = 0$. The D_{K80} and κ values also result in the highest likelihood ($lnL = -581.551246$).

TABLE 3.3 Empirical substitution pattern between two aligned sequences illustrating parameter estimation when one or more substitution rates are negative.

	A	G	C	T
A	10	10	13	13
G	10	20	13	13
C	13	13	25	10
T	13	13	10	12

However, because a negative κ implies a negative substitution rate which makes no biological sense, we may want to constrain $\kappa \geq 0$. With such a constraint, we may not have a unique solution. You may imagine a likelihood surface as a hill with a single peak (with maximum lnL) which requires a negative κ to reach it. If we prevent ourselves from having a negative κ, then we are condemned to stay somewhere below the peak and there could a circle around the peak with every point on the circle having the same lnL. It would seem that we should sample this circle to get parameter values and then get an average of parameter values. However, in our particular case, a solution that reached convergence has an lnL equal to -581.551753 which, as will be shown later, is very close to that based on the GTR model allowing a negative κ. This new constrained solution has $\kappa = 0$, $\beta = 0.5$, and $D = 2.056021268$. Note that we tend to underestimate the distance whenever we force rates to be nonnegative.

The above treatment implies two models, one general model allowing negative κ and a constrained model forcing $\kappa = 0$ which eliminates one parameter to estimate. A likelihood ratio test between the constrained and nonconstrained models gives us $\chi^2 = 2*(-581.551753 + 581.551246)$ with one degree of freedom (DF) and the associated $p = 0.974596409$. Thus, there is no evidence that the constrained model with $\kappa = 0$ is worse than the model allowing a negative κ. We may also use AIC $(= -2lnL+2p)$, where p is number of parameters, for model selection. AIC is 1167.104 for the model with κ as a parameter, and 1165.102 for the model with $\kappa = 0$. The model with $\kappa = 0$ has a smaller AIC and is therefore favored.

We can also force $\kappa = 0$ and estimate D by minimizing χ^2 following Eq. (3.99) but this has the same problem as the maximum likelihood method. One of the converged solutions has the same $D = 2.056021268$ with resulting $E(S)$ and $E(V)$ equal to 0.190112531 and 0.491812852, respectively, which are slightly different from the observed S and V. We have three observed C_{obs} values, being 40, 104, and 67 for transitions, transversions, and identical sites, respectively, and three corresponding C_{exp} values, being 40.11374408 [$=E(S)*211$], 103.7725119 [$=E(V)*211$], and 67.11374407 $(= 211 - 40.11374408 - 103.7725119)$. The resulting χ^2 value is

$$\chi^2 = \frac{(40 - 40.11374408)^2}{40.11374408} + \frac{(104 - 103.7725119)^2}{103.7725119}$$
$$+ \frac{(67 - 67.11374407)^2}{67.11374407} = 0.001013994 \tag{3.105}$$

With such a small χ^2 value and one DF (one free parameter D), $p = 0.9746$.

If we fit the data in Table 3.3 to the GTR model allowing negative κ values, then we will get $\kappa_1 = -0.3016516$, $\kappa_2 = 1.0981328$, $\kappa_3 = 3.1294315$, $\kappa_4 = 0.3936567$, $\kappa_5 = -0.4275744$, and $D = 3.4131381$, with $lnL = -577.4771$. If we force $\kappa_i \geq 0$, then we will have multiple solutions with the same lnL, and all with the estimated distance smaller than that estimated by allowing negative κ_i. There has been no comprehensive evaluation of whether constraining κ_i leads to better phylogenetic resolution.

The second awkward scenario is when the distance cannot be estimated. The transition probability matrix from GTR (P_{exp}) is expected to have eigenvalues between 0 and 1 (Waddell and Steel, 1997b). However, P_{obs} could have negative eigenvalues, making it impossible to take a matrix logarithm of P_{obs}. Such inapplicable cases occur often with highly diverged sequences. For example, we cannot have D_{JC69} if p_{diff} in Eq. (3.6) is equal to or greater than 0.75. Distance calculation is typically more likely to become inapplicable for more complicated models. For example, the distance formula in Eq. (3.21) for the K80 model becomes inapplicable when P =0.2 and Q=0.5, but this is fine with the JC69 model because p_{diff} (=$P+Q$) is smaller than 0.75. For the GTR model, Felsenstein (Felsenstein, pp 209–210) included a fictitious data set (reproduced in Table 3.4) from which one cannot obtain D with the above method because P_{obs} has negative eigenvalues and therefore cannot have matrix logarithm. For such a data set, Felsenstein (2004, pp. 209–210) considers the correct distance as infinite and Waddell and Steel (1997b) suggest to set the distance for such inapplicable cases as twice as large as the maximum computable distance when computing evolutionary distances for a set of aligned sequences. The reason for doing this is that inapplicable cases often arise not because sequences have really diverged for an infinitely long period of time but because of random sampling effect. The data in Table 3.4 has a D_{K80} of only 0.799964455, which is not suggestive of an infinitely large distance.

TABLE 3.4 Observed substitutions between two sequences (C_{obs}) that would make the GTR distance inapplicable. P_{exp} is the expected transition probability matrix derived with D =1.404823107, κ_1 = 9862.39307, κ_2 = 485.5764748, κ_3 = 2484.380521, κ_4 = 459.8089364, and κ_5 = 469.2547688. C_{exp} is the expected substitutions based on P_{exp}.

	C_{obs}				P_{exp}				C_{exp}			
	A	G	C	T	A	G	C	T	A	G	C	T
A	32	40	8	20	0.358602	0.371038	0.080386	0.189974	35.9	37.1	8.0	19.0
G	40	40	8	12	0.371038	0.420328	0.079525	0.129109	37.1	42.0	8.0	12.9
C	8	8	76	8	0.080386	0.079525	0.760303	0.079786	8.0	8.0	76.0	8.0
T	20	12	8	60	0.189974	0.129109	0.079786	0.601132	19.0	12.9	8.0	60.1

With the likelihood method or the χ^2 method, we can constrain $\kappa_i \geq$ 0 and try to find D and κ_i that will maximize lnL or minimize χ^2. One of the points that has one of the largest lnL and the smallest χ^2 has D =1.404823107, κ_1 = 9862.39307, κ_2 = 485.5764748, κ_3 = 2484.380521, κ_4 = 459.8089364, and κ_5 = 469.2547688. These κ_i values do look extraordinarily large. However, the set of parameters does offer a good fit to the observed data (Table 3.4). With the resulting C_{exp} values shown in Table 3.4, the χ^2 value is

$$\chi^2 = \sum_{i=1}^{4} \sum_{j=i}^{4} \frac{(O-E)^2}{E} = \frac{(32-35.9)^2}{35.9} + \frac{(2\times40-2\times37.1)^2}{2\times37.1} + ...$$

$$+ \frac{(60-60.1)^2}{60.1} = 1.889137$$

(3.106)

The associated p value is 0.9296 given $\chi^2 = 1.889137$ and six degrees of freedom. Thus, the set of D and κ_i values offer a very good fit between the model and the data suggesting $D = 1.404823107$ as a statistically more reasonable alternative than an infinitely large distance or a distance twice as large as the largest applicable distance. The latter is odd to have a pairwise distance not depending on the two associated aligned sequences but on the most divergent pair of sequences with a definable distance.

An alternative approach that is better than constraining $\kappa_i \geq 0$ is to use simultaneously estimated (SE) distances which uses all sequence pairs for parameter estimation (Tamura et al., 2004; Xia, 2009) instead of using the independently estimated (IE) distances. SE distances eliminate or at least alleviate three serious problems with the IE approach for distance estimation: (1) inapplicable cases where the distance often cannot be computed for highly diverged sequences (Rzhetsky and Nei, 1994b; Tajima, 1993; Zharkikh, 1994), (2) internal inconsistency, with the substitution process between sequences A and B having κ_{AB} but that between sequences A and C having κ_{AC} (Felsenstein, 2004, p 200; Yang, 2006, pp 37–38), and (3) insufficient use of information because the computation of pairwise distances ignores information in other sequences that should also contain information about the divergence between the two compared sequences (Felsenstein, 2004, p 175; Yang, 2006, p 37). Both DAMBE (Xia, 2013b; Xia, 2017a) and MEGA (Kumar et al., 2016) implements SE distances. SE distances will be numerically illustrated in the chapter on distance-based phylogenetic methods.

All the models we have discussed above are time-reversible models. There are cases in which time-reversibility is violated. For example, vertebrate genomes are heavily methylated and, as a consequence, are associated with strong C→T substitutions. In contrast, most invertebrate genomes are little methylated and not associated with strong C→T substitutions. Thus, the balance between C and T is different between vertebrate and invertebrates. This violates the time-reversibility and cautions against analyzing vertebrate and invertebrate sequences in a single phylogenetic analysis with a single time-reversible model.

3.3 HOW FAR CAN WE TRACE BACK THE EVOLUTIONARY HISTORY?

Suppose we are dealing with extremely fast-evolving retroviruses whose per-generation transition probabilities are specified as

$$P = \begin{pmatrix} & A & G & C & T \\ A & 0.997 & 0.001 & 0.001 & 0.001 \\ G & 0.001 & 0.997 & 0.001 & 0.001 \\ C & 0.001 & 0.001 & 0.997 & 0.001 \\ T & 0.001 & 0.001 & 0.001 & 0.997 \end{pmatrix} \qquad (3.107)$$

Note that each row of a transition probability matrix sums up to 1, i.e., after one generation, a nucleotide either stays the same with a probability of 0.997 or changes into another nucleotide with a probability of 0.001. This is equivalent to the simplest JC69 model (Jukes and Cantor, 1969). Thus, if we start with a nucleotide A, which correspond to a frequency vector [1,0,0,0], then in two generations the frequency vector will become [0.994,0.002,0.002,0.002]. This means that the starting nucleotide A, after two generations, will remain the same with a probability of 0.994 and become nucleotide G, C, or T each with a probability of 0.002:

$$\begin{bmatrix} 1 & 0 & 0 & 0 \end{bmatrix} \begin{bmatrix} 0.997 & 0.001 & 0.001 & 0.001 \\ 0.001 & 0.997 & 0.001 & 0.001 \\ 0.001 & 0.001 & 0.997 & 0.001 \\ 0.001 & 0.001 & 0.001 & 0.997 \end{bmatrix} = \begin{bmatrix} 0.997 & 0.001 & 0.001 & 0.001 \end{bmatrix}$$

$$\begin{bmatrix} 0.997 & 0.001 & 0.001 & 0.001 \end{bmatrix} \begin{bmatrix} 0.997 & 0.001 & 0.001 & 0.001 \\ 0.001 & 0.997 & 0.001 & 0.001 \\ 0.001 & 0.001 & 0.997 & 0.001 \\ 0.001 & 0.001 & 0.001 & 0.997 \end{bmatrix} = \begin{bmatrix} 0.994 & 0.002 & 0.002 & 0.002 \end{bmatrix}$$

$$(3.108)$$

If we continue this multiplication for 3000 generations, the π vector will become [0.25,0.25,0.25,0.25], which means that all original historical information has been lost and we will have no information to infer what is the nucleotide to start with. In short, if a nucleotide has a probability of

0.001 to change into one of the three other nucleotides in each generation, then we cannot use the nucleotide sequences to reconstruct evolutionary history beyond 3000 generations because the sequences would have already reached full substitution saturation. Severe substitution saturation decreases the accuracy of phylogenetic reconstruction (Ritland and Clegg, 1990; Xia and Lemey, 2009; Xia et al., 2003b).

The human genomic mutation rate is ~2.5×10^{-8} (Nachman and Crowell, 2000). This allows us to trace evolutionary history back much further. Assuming that most mutations in human genome are neutral so that we can use this mutation rate as a proxy of substitution rate all the way back to the origin of life, we will find the starting frequency vector of [1,0,0,0] reaching [0.250,0.250,0.250,0.250] in fewer than 100,000,000 generations. If the average generation time from the beginning of life to human is one year, then the DNA sequences would be in full substitution saturation after 100,000,000 years and there is no way to trace evolutionary history beyond 100,000,000 years. It is likely that early organisms may have a generation time much shorter than one year (*Escherichia coli* replicate once every 20 minutes when nutrients are unlimited), so sequences may reach full substitution saturation much earlier than 100,000,000 years. Thus, one should be cautious in reporting molecular dating results back to billions of years. One may be able to reconstruct phylogenetic relationships among very ancient lineages because stabilizing selection can preserve coancestral information, such as functionally important amino acid residues at certain sites of a protein. If the amino acid residue is vital, then it will remain the same irrespective of time. However, such selection-preserved characters should not be used for dating.

3.4   SELECTING THE BEST-FITTING SUBSTITUTION MODEL

There are two approaches for model selection (Burnham and Anderson, 2002), one by the likelihood ratio test (LRT) for nested models and the other by information-theoretic indices. Nested models refer to one general and one special model with the latter being a special case of the former. For example, the JC69 model and the K80 model are nested because JC69 is a special case of K80. K80 is reduced to JC69 if transition rates and transversion rates are all equal. In the framework of LRT, the null hypothesis is that the special model fits the data just as well as the general model.

Rejecting the null hypothesis means that the special model performs significantly worse than the general model. One disadvantage of LRT, as in any other statistical significance test, is that we would be left with no decision when the null hypothesis is not rejected. However, the approach with information-theoretic indices, such as AIC or BIC, is not immune to this problem. Although we always choose a model with smaller AIC or BIC as if we always arrive at a decision unambiguously, our decision obviously would be weak if AIC or BIC values are similar between the two models.

We will use the aligned sequences in Figure 3.4 to illustrate the two model selection methods. The advantage of using sequences in Figure 3.4 is that different site patterns are easily counted. However, the aligned sequences are short (only 24 nt long). A very limited sample has two problems. First, it is expected to be subject to strong stochastic effect, and the resulting statistics may not be reliable. For example, LRTs assume that the sample is large enough for the resulting likelihood ratio chi-square to follow the χ^2 distribution. This assumption breaks down with small samples so we may get wrong p values. Second, small samples typically do not provide enough statistical power for discriminating between alternative hypotheses. For selecting substitution models, ideally, one should have aligned sequence lengths of a few hundred or longer. This requirement is not only for alleviating the two problems above but also to avoid the estimation based on no direct data. For example, TN93 allows A↔G and C↔T transitions to have different rates, so we need to estimate $\alpha_R t$ and $\alpha_Y t$. However, if we observe only C↔T transitions but no A↔G transitions, then our estimation of $\alpha_R t$ becomes weak. For GTR, we ideally should have data with not only observed A↔G and C↔T transitions but also the four distinct types of transversions. Missing some of them in observed data weakens parameter estimation. The short sequence alignment in Figure 3.4 highlights such problems.

3.4.1   LIKELIHOOD RATIO TEST

Recall that LRT is for significance test between two nested models, i.e., a general model and a special model which is a special case of the general model. The test statistic for LRT is the log-likelihood ratio chi-square defined as $2*(lnL_G - lnL_S)$, where lnL_G and lnL_S are the maximized log-likelihood of the general and the special models, respectively. It is sometimes abbreviated as $2\Delta lnL$. This statistic, if derived from a large amount of data, follows approximately the χ^2 distribution with the degree of freedom (DF) being the difference in the number of parameters between the two models (Wilks, 1938). That is, if the special and the general models have N_S and N_G parameters, respectively, then the DF is $(N_G - N_S)$, which is sometimes written as DF = Δp (difference in the number of parameters between the two models).

That a substitution model has N parameters is equivalent to saying the model has N unknowns that need to be estimated from the sequence data. A model can be expressed in different ways. For example, the P matrix for the JC69 model can be expressed either as functions of αt or as functions of D_{JC69} (=3 αt). Similarly, the P matrix of K80 can be expressed either as functions of αt and βt or as functions of D_{K80} (=$\alpha t + 2\beta t$) and κ (= α/β). In the same way, the P matrix for TN93 can be expressed as three rate parameters (Table 3.5) plus frequency parameters or as κ_R, κ_Y, and D_{TN93} plus frequency parameters. The P matrix of GTR can be expressed as functions of six rate parameters plus frequency parameters or as five rate ratio parameters (κ_1 to κ_5) and D_{GTR} plus frequency parameters. However, the number of parameters and lnL will remain the same no matter how we reparameterize the model.

Suppose we want to test whether K80 provides better fit to the aligned sequence pair in Figure 3.4 than JC69. For the JC69 model, lnL is specified in Eq. (3.7), which contains only one distance parameter (D_{JC69}). Maximum lnL_{JC69} is reached when D_{JC69} = 0.3041 and resulting lnL_{JC69} = −53.3588. Similarly, lnL for the K80 model is specified in Eq. (3.24) with a distance (D_{K80}) and a κ parameter. Maximum lnL_{K80} (= −51.9725) is reached with D_{K80} = 0.3151 and κ = 4.9126. So $2\Delta lnL$ = 2.7726 and DF = Δp =1. The p value, given $2\Delta lnL$ = 2.7726 and DF = 1, is 0.0959, which is not significant at 0.05 significance level.

It is relevant here to mention that all statistical significance tests confer two key pieces of information: (1) The effect size which is independent of sample size and (2) the p value that depends on sample size. The effect size is the deviation of observation from expectation based on the null hypothesis. For example, in a t-test between two group means ($\bar{x}_1$ and $\bar{x}_2$ with the null hypothesis of ($\bar{x}_1 = \bar{x}_2$), the observed difference (d_o) is ($\bar{x}_1 - \bar{x}_2$) and the expected difference (d_e) based on the null hypothesis is 0. So, the effect size is $d_o - d_e = d_o = (\bar{x}_1 - \bar{x}_2)$. This effect size does not change with sample size except for stochastic fluctuations. In contrast, the t statistic and the resulting p value depends on sample size. Similarly, in bivariate linear regression, the expected slope (b_e) under the null hypothesis of no linear relationship between the two variables is $b_e = 0$, so the effect size is the difference between the observed (fitted from the observed data) slope (b_o) and b_e, i.e., $b_o - b_e = b_o$. This effect size does not change with sample size. In contrast, in the t-test testing the significance of the slope, the t statistic and the associated p value depend on sample size.

In our LRT above contrasting K80 and JC69, the null hypothesis is that JC69 is just as good as K80. Under this null hypothesis, $\kappa = 1$ (which is assumed by the JC69 model). The observed κ is 4.9126 (estimated from the observed data). So, the effect size is $(4.9126 - 1)$, and the p value is 0.0959. If the aligned sequences are twice as long, everything else being equal, then we would still have $\kappa = 4.9126$ but $2\Delta lnL$ will become 5.5452 which is twice as large as before (the statistic increases linearly with sample size, everything else being equal), and the p value would then be 0.0185 (which would lead to rejection of the JC69 model at 0.05 significance level).

Table 3.5 lists parameters, their estimated values, and lnL for JC69, K80, TN93, and GTR so that we can contrast any of the two nested hypotheses. For example, applying LRT to JC69 and TN93, we will have $2\Delta lnL$ equal to 11.8320 with 5 degrees of freedom (TN93 has three rate parameters and three frequency parameters in contrast to JC69 with only one parameter, Table 3.5), p equals 0.0372 and we reject JC69 and conclude that TN93 is a better model for the aligned sequences in Figure 3.4. Similarly, contrasting between GTR and JC69 leads to $2\Delta lnL = 26.6832161$, DF = 8, $p = 0.0008$.

TABLE 3.5 Parameter values and lnL for JC69, K80, TN93, and GTR models. The equilibrium frequencies for A, G, C, and T are 0.1250, 0.2083, 0.2500, and 0.41667, respectively, and are needed for TN93 and GTR (i.e., three additional parameters as the four frequencies need to sum up to 1). AIC and BIC values for each model are also listed.

Model	Parameter[1]	Value	*lnL*	AIC	BIC
JC69	D	0.3041	−53.3588	108.718	109.896
K80	D	0.3151	−51.9725	107.945	110.301
	κ	4.9126			
TN93	$\alpha_R t$[2]	0.13354	−47.4428	106.886	113.954
	$\alpha_Y t$[2]	0.88225			
	βt[2]	0.20765			

TABLE 3.5   *(Continued)*

Model	Parameter[1]	Value	*lnL*	AIC	BIC
GTR	$a_{A \leftrightarrow G}^{[3]}$	0	−40.0172	98.034	108.637
	$a_{A \leftrightarrow C}^{[3]}$	0			
	$a_{A \leftrightarrow T}^{[3]}$	0			
	$a_{G \leftrightarrow C}^{[3]}$	−0.0612			
	$a_{C \leftrightarrow T}^{[3]}$	0.4515			
	$a_{G \leftrightarrow T}^{[3]}$	0.2464			

[1] D: evolutionary distance.

[2] Defined in Eq. (3.61)–(3.63). The three rate parameters in TN93 can be reparameterized to κ_R, κ_Y, and D_{TN93}.

[3] These six rate parameters can be reparameterized into 5 rate ratio parameters and D_{GTR}.

The accuracy and validity of LRT has often been questioned (Pinheiro and Bates, 2000, pp 82–93), mainly with the concern of whether the statistic $2\Delta lnL$ follows the χ^2 distribution. Unfortunately, there has not yet been a simple alternative for biologists. However, one can take some comfort from the observation that if one simulates sequence evolution according to a specific substitution model, the specific substitution model used to simulate the sequences is almost always identified by LRT as the best model.

3.4.2   INFORMATION-THEORETIC INDICES

Several information-theoretic indices have been formulated for model selection. The Akaike information criterion or AIC (Akaike, 1973, 1974) is defined as

$$AIC = -2\ln L + 2p \tag{3.109}$$

where p is the number of parameters. The smaller the AIC value, the better the model. The AIC values for JC69, K80, TN93, and GTR (Table 3.5) shows that AIC favors the more complicated model with GTR having the smallest AIC value (Table 3.5).

Bayesian information criterion or BIC (Schwarz, 1978) is defined as

$$BIC = -2\ln L + p\ln(n) \qquad (3.110)$$

where n is the sample size (or sequence length in our case). AIC and BIC differ only in the second term, with BIC penalizes parameter-rich models more than AIC. GTR is again the best model because it has the smallest BIC value (Table 3.5) but JC69 is better than K80 which is, in turn, better than TN93.

3.5 EMPIRICAL SUBSTITUTION MATRIX

We have already observed a few empirical substitution matrices, such as BLOSUM and Dayhoff matrices, in the chapter on sequence alignment. Sometimes a direct inspection of an empirical substitution matrix can often give us a good idea of what substitution model is appropriate for the sequences. There are two ways to obtain an empirical substitution matrix. One is by compiling all pairwise substitutions. The other is to make tree-guided comparisons in three steps: (1) construct a tree, (2) reconstruct ancestral sequences at internal nodes, and (3) compile substitution data between neighboring nodes along the tree. The sequence data we use for illustration are in the sample sequence file VertCOI.fas that comes with the software DAMBE (Xia, 2013b; Xia, 2017a). The file contains eight aligned mitochondrial *COI* gene sequences from eight vertebrate species with an aligned sequence length of 1512 bases and no gaps.

3.5.1 TWO WAYS OF COMPILING EMPIRICAL SUBSTITUTION MATRICES

3.5.1.1 ALL PAIRWISE SEQUENCE COMPARISONS

With N aligned sequences, there are $N*(N-1)/2$ pairwise comparisons. Table 3.6a shows an empirical substitution matrix from all 28 pairwise comparisons for the eight vertebrate mitochondrial COI sequences. I will highlight three patterns easily visible from the empirical substitution matrix, compiled from all 28 pairwise sequence comparisons. First, nucleotide frequencies are not equal, with G much fewer than others. This would exclude JC69 and K80 which assume equal nucleotide frequencies at equilibrium. Second, the A↔G transition occurred at a slower rate than

C↔T transitions. Note that G is relatively rare, so we do expect A↔G transition to be less frequent than C↔T transitions. However, the observed difference in the number of A↔G and C↔T transitions is more than what can be explained by the difference in nucleotide frequencies. This would exclude F84 and HKY85. Third, the four transversions occurred at very different rates with far more observed A↔C than G↔T. These lead us to choose GTR as the only appropriate substitution model for the set of sequences.

TABLE 3.6 Empirical substitution patterns from all pairwise comparisons (a) and tree-guided comparisons (b).

(a)	A	G	C	T	(b)	A	G	C	T
A	8919					5118			
G	1417	5930				248	2955		
C	2299	457	8992			336	53	5355	
T	1322	301	3438	9261		176	36	587	4792

3.5.1.2   TREE-GUIDED SEQUENCE COMPARISON

Compiling all pairwise substitutions has one disadvantage. Suppose we have N aligned sequences with $N-1$ sequence being very similar but one sequence being highly divergent. The substitutions occurred during the divergence of this deviant sequence will be counted $(N-1)$ times because this sequence will be pairwise compared with the other $(N-1)$ sequences. To alleviate this problem, we can perform a tree-guided compilation.

An unrooted tree for N aligned sequences has $(N-2)$ internal nodes which represent hypothesized ancestral organisms. We can use the empirical Bayes method (Yang, 2006, pp. 119–124) to reconstruct ancestral sequences for these internal nodes. For the eight vertebrate species with their tree in Figure 3.8, there are six internal nodes and 13 (= 2N–3, where N is the number of sequences) branches. Our comparison will be between neighboring nodes only, e.g., *Homo sapiens* against reconstructed internal node 12, *Pan troglodytes* against internal node 12, node 12 against node 11, and so on. The resulting compilation from 13 sequence comparisons between neighboring nodes, generated from DAMBE (Xia, 2013b; Xia, 2017a), is shown in Table 3.6b. In this particular case, the substitution pattern is similar to that from all pairwise comparison in Table 3.6a, i.e., the off-diagonal elements are nearly proportional between the two matrices. This is because there is no sequence that is extraordinarily diverged from the rest (Fig. 3.8).

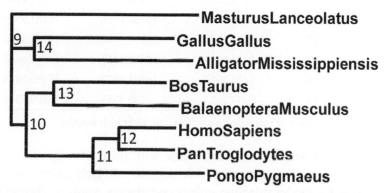

FIGURE 3.8 Phylogenetic tree for the eight vertebrate mitochondrial *COI* sequences in sample file VertCOI.fas file that comes with DAMBE (Xia, 2013b; Xia, 2017a).

3.5.1.3 DOES EMPIRICAL SUBSTITUTION MATRIX TELL US THE SUITABLE SUBSTITUTION MODEL?

We inferred, from visual inspection of the empirical substitution matrix in Table 3.6, that GTR is appropriate for fitting our aligned vertebrate mitochondrial *COI* sequences. To confirm our choice of GTR, we may apply the two model selection methods covered in the previous section, i.e., information-theoretic indices and likelihood ratio test. We have already applied them to a toy example before, and here is a more realistic application. The main part of the computation is to obtain the log-likelihood (lnL) given the tree, the substitution model, and the aligned sequences. This part of the calculation is detailed in a later chapter on maximum likelihood phylogenetic method and the pruning algorithm. Here we will simply run the program DAMBE to get the output in Table 3.7 by assuming the topology in Figure 3.8 and no rate heterogeneity over sites (which you can change).

TABLE 3.7 Information-theoretic indices for choosing substitution models, based on aligned vertebrate mitochondrial *COI* sequences in the sample file VertCOI.fas that comes with DAMBE (Xia, 2013b; Xia, 2017a). number of parameters (N_p) and log-likelihood (*lnL*) for each model are also shown. Output from DAMBE.

Model	$N_p^{(1)}$	*lnL*	AIC	BIC
GTR	21	−7947.2233	15936.4466	16048.1916
TN93	18	−8066.0868	16168.1736	16263.9550
HKY85	17	−8079.1840	16192.3680	16282.8282
F84	17	−8093.1009	16220.2018	16310.6620
K80	14	−8176.7961	16381.5922	16456.0888
JC69	13	−8357.2894	16740.5788	16809.7543

[1] N_p is the sum of number of rate ratio parameters and 13 branch lengths.

For a set of nested models, *lnL* value will always increase with an increasing number of parameters (Table 3.7), so *lnL* itself cannot be used as a criterion for model selection unless one always wants to choose the most parameter-rich model. Both AIC and BIC include a penalty for the increasing number of parameters, as shown in Eq. (3.109) and Eq. (3.110). Results in Table 3.7 show that GTR has the smallest AIC and BIC values, i.e., it is the most suitable model for the alignment COI sequences. This is consistent with our visual inspection of the empirical substitution model.

With the *lnL* values in Table 3.7, we can also perform likelihood ratio tests between nested models, with likelihood ratio chi-square being $2\Delta lnL$ and the DF being the difference in the number of parameters (N_p in Table 3.7). Take GTR and JC69 for example, *lnL* is −7947.2233 for GTR and −8357.2894 for JC69, so likelihood ratio chi-square is $2\Delta lnL = 820.1323$ and DF = 8. The null hypothesis tested states that GTR and JC69 are equally suitable for the aligned sequences, and is strongly rejected ($p = 0.00000$).

Table 3.8 displays results from all pairwise LRTs and shows that GTR is significantly better than all the alternative models, which is consistent with the model choice by our visual inspection of the empirical substitution matrix in Table 3.6 and the result from the information-theoretic indices. While a chosen substitution model from such model selection protocols is generally expected to perform best in molecular phylogenetic reconstruction, in reality it is not so simple, especially when one also include substitution models with rate heterogeneity over site modeled by gamma distribution, typically designated by adding "+Γ" to the model, such as TN93+Γ or GTR+Γ. Such models often perform poorly with highly diverged sequences. One way to show this is to take aligned protein-coding sequences from a set of vertebrate species with well-corroborated phylogenetic relationships (i.e., the true tree is effectively known). One can then use only the third codon positions for tree reconstruction, which is equivalent to highly diverged sequences. GTR+Γ is often the best model based on the model selection criteria, but maximum likelihood methods using such a GTR+Γ model (e.g., PhyML) often cannot recover the "true" tree as frequently as a distance-based method (e.g., FastME) with simultaneously estimated distances.

TABLE 3.8 Likelihood ratio tests for two nested models, with log-likelihood of the general and the special models ($lnL_{General}$ and $lnL_{Special}$, respectively), as well as the likelihood-ratio chi-square (X^2), degree of freedom (DF), and p value (for testing the null hypothesis that the general and the special models are equally good). Output from DAMBE.

Comparison	$lnL_{General}$	$lnL_{Special}$	X^2	DF	P
GTR..JC69	−7947.2233	−8357.2894	820.1323	8	0.00000
TN93..JC69	−8066.0868	−8357.2894	582.4053	5	0.00000
HKY85..JC69	−8079.184	−8357.2894	556.2108	4	0.00000
F84..JC69	−8093.1009	−8357.2894	528.3771	4	0.00000
K80..JC69	−8176.7961	−8357.2894	360.9867	1	0.00000
GTR..K80	−7947.2233	−8176.7961	459.1456	7	0.00000
TN93..K80	−8066.0868	−8176.7961	221.4186	4	0.00000
HKY85..K80	−8079.184	−8176.7961	195.2241	3	0.00000
F84..K80	−8093.1009	−8176.7961	167.3904	3	0.00000
GTR..HKY85	−7947.2233	−8079.184	263.9215	4	0.00000
TN93..HKY85	−8066.0868	−8079.184	26.1945	1	0.00000
GTR..F84	−7947.2233	−8093.1009	291.7552	4	0.00000
TN93..F84	−8066.0868	−8093.1009	54.0282	1	0.00000
GTR..TN93	−7947.2233	−8066.0868	237.7270	3	0.00000

3.5.2 PARTITION CODON SEQUENCES INTO 3RD CODON SITES AND 1ST AND 2ND CODON SITES

Substitutions are often synonymous at third codon sites (CS3) but tend to be nonsynonymous at first and second codon sites (CS12). Empirical data suggest that substitution pattern at CS3 conform to neutral evolution better than at CS12 (Xia, 2009). We, therefore, need different substitution models for CS3 and for CS12. Because *COI* is a protein-coding gene, we will use the *COI* sequences in the previous section to illustrate the partition of the codon sequences into the two categories of codon sites.

The empirical substitution patterns for CS12 and for CS3 (Table 3.9), compiled with the tree-guided method using the same tree in Figure 3.8, differ from each other and from those in Table 3.6. The most striking difference between CS12 and CS3 is the dramatic rarity in nucleotide G and T in CS3. This is because the coding strand of *COI* is located on the AC-rich light strand (Xia, 2005). CS3 and CS12 also have one striking similarity, that is, the off-diagonal values are quite predictable from nucleotide frequencies. In CS12 (Table 3.9a), there are more $C \leftrightarrow T$ transitions than $A \leftrightarrow G$ transitions ($N_{C \leftrightarrow T} = 115$ vs $N_{A \leftrightarrow G} = 68$) but that is largely attributable to more frequent C and T than A and G at CS12. $(\pi_C \pi_T)/(\pi_A \pi_G)$ ≈ 1.555 (where π_i is frequency of nucleotide i) which is almost exactly the ratio of $N_{C \leftrightarrow T}/N_{A \leftrightarrow G}$. Similarly, for CS3, the difference in $N_{C \leftrightarrow T}$ and $N_{A \leftrightarrow G}$ is also largely attributable to the differences in nucleotide frequencies. In short, for both CS12 and CS3, we see little advantage of TN93 model, which allows the $C \leftrightarrow T$ and $A \leftrightarrow G$ transitions to have different rates, over F84 and HKY85 which assume the same transitional substitution rate.

TABLE 3.9 Empirical substitution patterns compiled from tree-guided sequence comparisons separately for first and second codon sites (a) and third codon sites (b), referred to as CS12 and CS3, respectively, in the text.

(a)	A	G	C	T	(b)	A	G	C	T
A	2856					2378			
G	68	2835				226	37		
C	40	18	3135			396	12	2475	
T	18	16	115	4003		107	1	695	225

The observed number of transversions do seem to differ dramatically, especially in CS3 with $N_{A \leftrightarrow C} = 396$ and $N_{G \leftrightarrow T} = 1$ (Table 3.9b). However,

$(\pi_A\pi_C)/(\pi_G\pi_T) \approx 634$, so we actually expected even greater differences between $N_{A\leftrightarrow C}$ and $N_{G\leftrightarrow T}$. In short, the differences in the number of the four transversions, while not quite predictable from nucleotide frequencies, do not differ strongly to argue for GTR.

We may again subject CS12 and CS3 to quantitative model selection. Rather than presenting results equivalent to Table 3.7 and Table 3.8, I will just say that BIC is the smallest for F84 with CS3 data and for HKY85 with CS12 data. However, alternative models more complicated than F84 and HKY85 have very similar AIC and BIC values (Fig. 3.9). Model selection by AIC and BIC is often aided by a plot of AIC and BIC versus the number of parameters. The rule of thumb is to choose a model at the point of a sharp bend after which the curve becomes largely horizontal. For CS12 with BIC criterion (Fig. 3.9a), one may choose either the 2-parameter K80 model or 5-parameter HKU or F84 model. For CS3 with BIC criterion, one would choose the 5-parameter F84 or HKY85 model.

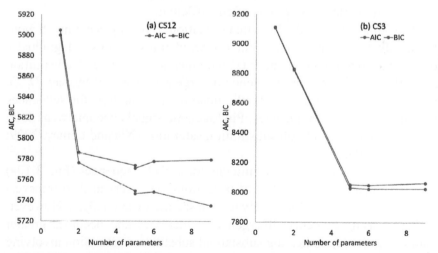

FIGURE 3.9 AIC and BIC change with the number of parameters of substitution models. See Table 3.7 for the number of parameters associated with each model.

One may ask why K80 is almost acceptable for CS12 but definitely not for CS3? The reason is obvious with data shown in Table 3.9. The nucleotide frequencies are almost equal for CS12 but dramatically different for CS3. As K80 assumes equal nucleotide frequencies at equilibrium, it is clearly wrong for CS3 but not so for CS12. The site partition example also shows that, given N sets of data each resulting from a simple substitution process, mixing them together will often demand a much more complicated model. For our *COI* data, the conclusion from the previous section that the sequence evolution conforms better to GTR when all codon sites are combined is an artifact of mixing the CS12 and CS3.

3.6   VISUALIZING SUBSTITUTION SATURATION

As we have learned before, a starting nucleotide, say A, will have a decreasing probability of remaining as A as time goes by. Eventually, the probability will approach the equilibrium frequency at which point all historical information is lost. This is the point when full substitution saturation has occurred. There are quantitative methods for testing substitution saturation (Xia et al., 2003b). However, for nucleotide sequences, graphic visualization of transitions and transversions versus an evolutionary distance (e.g., D_{F84} based on the F84 model), sometimes called a substitution saturation plot or SS plot is often sufficient.

The rationale of an SS plot is that transitions typically occur much more frequently than transversions but observed transversions (v) gradually outnumbers observed transitions (s) with increasing degree of substitution saturation (i.e., increasing sequence divergence measured by, say, D_{F84}), reaching a ratio of $v/s = 2$ at full substitution saturation for sequences of equal nucleotide frequencies. Phylogenetic signals become weak long before sequences reach full substitution saturation (Xia and Lemey, 2009; Xia et al., 2003b).

An SS plot for the aligned mitochondrial *COI* sequences (Fig. 3.10a) shows a much greater number of transitions (s) observed than transversional substitutions (v) for closely related species (a small D_{F84}). However, with increasing sequence divergence, v increases and becomes greater than s (Fig. 3.10a), indicating substantial substitution saturation involving more divergence sequences. In contrast, an SS plot based on CS12 (Fig. 3.10b) suggest little substitution saturation, as we would have expected.

3.7   BEYOND TIME REVERSIBLE MODELS

All substitution models we have learned, from the simplest JC69 to the most complicated GTR, are time-reversible models. While some of them, e.g., F84, HKY85, TN93, GTR, allow mutation bias to generate different nucleotide frequencies, they do assume that such mutation bias operates homogeneously among all lineages so that nucleotide frequencies remain similar among all phylogenetic lineages. This assumption is a mathematical convenience but does not reflect reality. There are many cases where this assumption is violated. Here we briefly mention four of them.

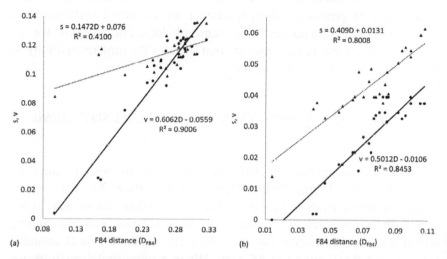

FIGURE 3.10   A substitution saturation plot, with proportions of transitions (s) and transversions on the Y-axis and an evolutionary distance based on the F84 model on the X-axis. (a) with all three codon sites included. (b) with only codon sites 1 and 2.

3.7.1   DNA METHYLATION

CpG-specific DNA methylation causes the methylated C to mutate to T through spontaneous deamination, leading to CpG deficiency documented in a large number of genomes covering a wide taxonomic distribution (Bestor and Coxon, 1993; Rideout *et al.*, 1990; Sved and Bird, 1990). Such CpG-specific methylation is observed not only in invertebrates, but also in prokaryotes (Cardon *et al.*, 1994; Josse *et al.*, 1961; Karlin and Burge, 1995; Karlin and Mrazek, 1996; Nussinov, 1984). For example, *Mycoplasma pulmonis* has several CpG-specific DNA methyltransferase genes encoded in its genome which exhibits extreme CpG deficiency and GC%. However, when CpG-specific methyltransferase genes were lost in some *Mycoplasma* lineages, such as *M. genitalium* and *M. pneumoniae*,

CpG dinucleotide frequencies as well as GC%, began to increase (Xia, 2003). This process of increasing CpG dinucleotide and GC% represents a nonstationary process violating the time reversibility of the substitution models used in nearly all model-based phylogenetic analyses.

While CpG-specific DNA methylation is prevalent in vertebrates with a strong signature of CpG deficiency, there is little such methylation in invertebrate genomes. Thus, whenever we include invertebrate and vertebrate genes or genomes in the same phylogenetic analysis, we are dealing with a nonstationary process that violates the time reversibility of commonly used substitution models.

3.7.2   GENOMIC STRAND ASYMMETRY AND GENES SWITCHING STRANDS

Genomic strand asymmetry has been observed in both prokaryotic genomes (Lobry, 1996a, 1996b; Marin and Xia, 2008; Xia, 2012a) and vertebrate mitochondrial genomes (Carullo and Xia, 2008; Xia, 2005, 2008). In prokaryotes, the leading strand is GT-rich and the lagging strand is AC-rich. In vertebrate mitochondrial genomes, the H-strand is GT-rich and the L-strand is AC-rich. When a gene switches from one strand to another, it is immediately thrown into a nonstationary process that violates the time-reversibility assumption of commonly used substitution models. The strand-switching is associated with two easily detectable evolutionary consequences. First, a gene switching from a GT-rich H-strand to an AC-rich L-strand will experience a reduction in G and T frequencies and an increase in A and C frequencies. Second, the gene will exhibit accelerated evolution with long branches associated with it (Xia, 2012c). Figure 3.11 shows four such strand-switching events involving a tRNA gene. The strand switching resulted in dramatically increased evolutionary rate (Fig. 3.11) as well as a rapid change in nucleotide composition (not shown).

The identification of strand-switching events is typically through an examination of gene synteny. If all phylogenetic relatives exhibit gene synteny shown in Figure 3.11e except for one which exhibits gene synteny shown in Figure 3.11f, then we may infer that gene 3 has switched strand. In phylogenetic reconstruction, one should pay special attention to genes that have switched their strand during evolution.

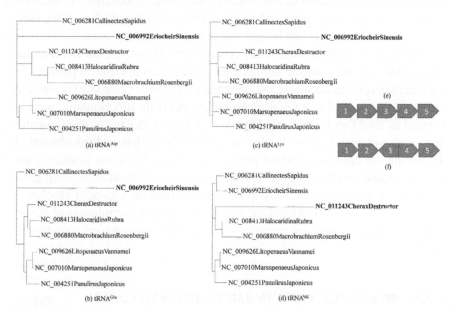

FIGURE 3.11   Trees constructed from four tRNA genes (a, b, c, and d), with the topology constrained by the *COXI* gene. Each tree has one lineage (**bolded**) where the tRNA gene has switched strand, which is associated with a dramatically increased evolutionary rate (Xia, 2012c). (e) and (f) illustrate the identification of strand-switching events, with arrows pointing in the 5' to '3 direction.

3.7.3   GC-RICH AND GC-POOR ISOCHORES IN VERTEBRATE GENOMES

Warm-blooded vertebrate genomes are structured into GC-rich and GC-poor isochores (Bernardi, 1985, 1989, 1993, 2000; Bernardi et al., 1988; Bernardi et al., 1985). A gene switching from a GC-rich isochore to a GC-poor isochore is expected to lose G and C and gain A and T, and vice versa. Before reaching the location-specific equilibrium frequencies, the gene is in a nonstationary process violating the time-reversibility of substitution models. The process is the most visible through pseudogenes which, if from a GC-rich isochore to a GC-poor isochore, would accumulate AT-biased mutations.

We may misunderstand spontaneous mutation spectrum without taking into consideration of the isochore structure. Spontaneous mutation spectrum is generally assumed to be AT-biased after studies (Gojobori et al., 1982; *Li* et al., 1984) that compared mutations accumulated on pseudogenes with their functional counterpart. However, such a general conclusion may miss subtle nuances in nucleotide substitution patterns in mammalian species because a pseudogene may also accumulate GC-biased mutation if it landed in a GC-rich isochore and if its functional counter is located in an AT-rich isochore. However, GC-rich isochores are typically gene-rich and pseudogenes landed in such isochores have a high chance of disrupting the function of some genes. In contrast, GC-poor isochores are gene-poor and can typically receive pseudogenes without disrupting gene functions. For this reason, most pseudogenes land on GC-poor isochores and tend to accumulate AT-biased mutation. Thus, accumulation of A and T in pseudogenes does not necessarily mean that spontaneous mutation is AT-biased.

3.7.4   *NONSTATIONARITY IN AMINO ACID AND CODON SUBSTITUTIONS*

Amino acid substitution can also occur in a nonstationary manner. One example involves the evolution of the mammalian gastric pathogen, *Helicobacter pylori*. Two mechanisms of acid-resistance have postulated to enable the pathogen to colonize the acidic environment of mammalian stomach (Xia, 2018a, Chapter 17; Xia and Palidwor, 2005): (1) A urease gene that converts urea to ammonia to neutralize the influx of proton and to facilitate the extrusion of proton, and (2) an increase in membrane protein isoelectric point to alleviate the influx of proton into cytoplasm. The high activity of arginase channels amino acid Arg to the production of urea and many membrane proteins have acquired Lys leading to an increased protein isoelectric point and positive charge. Thus, relative to its phylogenetic relative *H. hepaticus,* both Arg and Lys frequencies have changed in a large number of proteins in *H. pylori.*

Codon usage and substitution patterns are shaped by mutation and tRNA-mediated selection. We already mentioned how changing mutation bias can lead to nonstationarity. Here we show a case where changing tRNA availability also leads to nonstationarity. An evolutionary change in tRNA composition or relative abundance is expected to alter codon adaptation. This is not controversial theoretically, but empirically difficult to demonstrate. However, recent studies (Xia, 2012c; Xia, 2018a, Chapter 9; Xia et al., 2007) have documented that changes in tRNA^{Met} genes (where Met is the amino acid carried by the tRNA) in animal mitochondrial DNA (mtDNA) are associated with changes in Met codon usage.

In MtDNA of most animal species, Met is coded by AUA and AUG codons. In some animal species, e.g., vertebrates, these two codons are translated by a single tRNA$^{Met/CAU}$ species (where CAU is the anticodon in the 5' to 3' orientation) with a modified C (i.e., f^{5}C) at the first anticodon position (Grosjean et al., 2010) to allow C/A pairing. In other animal species, e.g., tunicates, an additional tRNA$^{Met/UAU}$ gene is present in the mtDNA. One would expect that, when tRNA$^{Met/UAU}$ is absent, AUA should be a less favorable codon for Met than when an additional tRNA$^{Met/UAU}$ is present. This is indeed the case. In tunicate and bivalve species where an additional tRNA$^{Met/UAU}$ is encoded in mtDNA, AUA codon is used relatively more frequently than in species without a tRNA$^{Met/UAU}$ gene. Thus, just the addition of a single tRNA gene could put protein-coding genes into a nonstationary process.

3.7.5 STATIONARITY AND TIME-REVERSIBILITY IN MARKOV CHAINS

Stationarity is defined as all substitution rates being constant over time, that is, they do not change over time. For this reason, stationarity is synonymous to time-homogeneity, both referring to a constant rate over time. The formal definition is

$$p\left(i_{t+1}|j_t\right) = p(i_t \mid j_{t-1}) = c \tag{3.111}$$

where i and j stand for different nucleotides or amino acids, c is a constant, and p is the probability of transition from nucleotide j to nucleotide i.

One can probably find many substitution processes where stationarity does not hold. For example, a bacterial intracellular pathogen is often AT-rich relative to its free-living sister species (Xia and Palidwor, 2005), suggesting that GC→AT substitution rates have changed during the evolution of intracellular parasitism. We cannot measure the substitution rates over millions of years to ascertain if they are constant. However, if we find a large clade of species all have very similar nucleotide or amino acid frequencies, then we may assume that substitution rates are roughly constant during the evolution of this clade of species and that the nucleotide or amino acid frequencies have reached a stationary distribution defined below:

$$\pi_{t+1} = \pi_t P \tag{3.112}$$

where π_t is a vector of frequencies (e.g., the nucleotide frequencies or amino acid frequencies) known as equilibrium frequencies and P is the transition probability matrix. All the substitution models covered in this chapter, including JC69, K80, F84, HKY85, TN93, and GTR, assume their π vectors to have reached a stationary distribution so that substitutions of nucleotide i by nucleotide j is exactly balanced by substitutions of nucleotide j by nucleotide i. This balance of forward and backward substitutions is known as time-reversible defined as:

$$\pi_i q_{ij} = \pi_j q_{ij} \ or \ \pi_i p(t)_{ij} = \pi_j p(t)_{ji} \tag{3.113}$$

where q_{ij} and p_{ij} are the elements in the rate matrix Q and transition probability matrix P, respectively.

Stationarity does not guarantee time-reversibility. Suppose we have

$$P = \begin{bmatrix} 0 & 1 \\ 1 & 0 \end{bmatrix} \tag{3.114}$$

If we now have a frequency vector $[x_1, x_2]$ at time 0. Multiplying the vector by P gives us $[x_2, x_1]$ at time 1. Multiplying $[x_2, x_1]$ by P again returns us back to $[x_1, x_2]$, the frequency vector at time 0. Such a Markov chain is known as periodic with period $k = 2$. Similarly, suppose we have

$$P = \begin{bmatrix} 0 & 1 & 0 & 0 \\ 0 & 0 & 1 & 0 \\ 0 & 0 & 0 & 1 \\ 1 & 0 & 0 & 0 \end{bmatrix} \tag{3.115}$$

If we now have a frequency vector $[x_1, x_2, x_3, x_4]$ at time 0. Multiplying the vector against P four times will return us a frequency vector identical to that at time 0. Such a Markov chain is periodic with period $k = 4$. Apparently, periodic Markov chains will not reach equilibrium frequencies and will not be time-reversible, although elements in P are all constants. Only aperiodic Markov chains can reach equilibrium frequencies. All our substitution models belong to aperiodic Markov chains.

KEYWORDS

- **substitution model**
- **substitution saturation**
- **transition probability**
- **Markov chain**
- **evolutionary distances**

CHAPTER 4

Protein and Codon Substitution Models and Their Evolutionary Distances

ABSTRACT

Substitution models based on amino acid or codon sequences are conceptually the same as nucleotide-based models, except that the matrices are larger, being 20 × 20 for amino acid sequences and 61 × 61 for the standard genetic code with 61 sense codons. Observed substitutions between two sense codons depend on codon frequencies, the physiochemical similarity between the two encoded amino acids, and the number of nucleotide site differences between the two codons (which could differ at 1, 2, or all 3 sites). Similarly, observed substitutions between two amino acids depend on amino acid frequencies and amino acid dissimilarities. Transition probabilities and evolutionary distance for amino acid sequences are derived from empirical substitution matrices, together with scenarios in which evolutionary distance cannot be obtained. Codon-based substitution models are then presented with a critical evaluation to highlight their deficiencies. Codon-based LBP93 distance is then derived, its problems highlighted, and several improvements are presented.

4.1 TRANSITION PROBABILITY AND EVOLUTIONARY DISTANCE FROM AMINO ACID SUBSTITUTION MODEL

Which amino acids are more likely to replace each other? This question has been addressed in two approaches reviewed in Xia (Xia, 2018a, Chapter 13). The first is based on the neutral theory of molecular evolution (Kimura, 1977, 1983; Miyata and Yasunaga, 1980) and the even earlier realization that most amino acid replacements tend to involve similar amino acids (Kimura, 1968; King and Jukes, 1969). Thus, a good measure of amino acid dissimilarity should serve as a good predictor of amino acid replacement frequencies. The second is the empirical approach, i.e., one simply compiles a large number of closely related amino acid sequences and count the actual number of observed amino acid replacement. This approach has generated Dayhoff matrices, BLOSUM matrices, and many others.

4.1.1 THREE FACTORS AFFECTING AMINO ACID REPLACEMENT

The three key factors affecting the empirical counts of amino acid replacement are amino acid dissimilarity (D_{ij}), amino acid frequency (P_i), and site differences between two codon families (D_{CF}). This last one requires some explanation. Asp (encoded by GAY) and Glu (encoded by GAR) codon families can change into each other through a single nucleotide substitution, whereas Glu and Phe codon families require three nucleotide substitutions to change into each other. This site difference between codon families is measured approximated by the minimum number of site differences between two most similar codons, one from each codon family, and designated D_{CF}. D_{CF} equals 1 between Asp and Glu codon families, and 3 between Phe and Glu codon families. Obviously, two amino acids with a small D_{CF} are more likely to replace each other than two with a large D_{CF}, everything else being equal. Table 4.1 is a partial list of these variables, together with a column headed "N_{JTT}" which is the observed frequency of pairwise replacement inferred from amino acid sequence alignment (Jones et al., 1992).

There are two major approaches for measuring amino acid dissimilarity. The first is based on physiochemical properties of the amino acids, such as volume, polarity, and the chemical composition of the side chain. This approach generated Grantham's (Grantham, 1974), Miyata's (Miyata et al., 1979) distances, and several others, and will be generally referred to as D_{ij} here. Grantham's distance combines the volume, polarity, and side chain composition, and Miyata's distance incorporates only volume and polarity. Hydropathy index (HI, Kyte and Doolittle, 1982) which is a good proxy for polarity and molecular weight (MW) for each amino acid (a good proxy for volume) were listed in Table 2.7 in Chapter 2 together with amino acid usage in *Escherichia coli* and *Saccharomyces cerevisiae*.

TABLE 4.1   Observed frequencies of amino acid replacement (N_{JTT}) compiled by Jones et al. (Jones et al., 1992), together with Miyata's distance (Miyata et al., 1979) and minimum codon family distance (D_{CF}, defined as the number of site differences between two most similar codons, one from each codon family). P_i is the frequency of amino acid i.

AA1	AA2	Miyata	D_{CF}	P_iP_j	N_{JTT}
Arg	Ala	2.9152	2	0.003934	426
Asn	Ala	1.7729	2	0.003295	333
Asn	Arg	2.0357	2	0.002309	185
Asp	Ala	2.3613	1	0.003858	596
Asp	Arg	2.3352	2	0.002703	80
Asp	Asn	0.6498	1	0.002264	2134
...	...	...	...	...	...
Val	Trp	2.5036	2	0.000916	44
Val	Tyr	1.5137	2	0.002111	63

Frequently used amino acids are expected to be more frequently observed in amino acid substitutions.

Another amino acid dissimilarity, based not on physiochemical properties of amino acid, but on structural compatibility, has also been proposed (Xia and Xie, 2002). Different protein structural elements such as α-helix, β-sheet, etc., exhibit their unique amino acid compositions because some amino acids are incompatible with certain structures. For example, amino acids Ala and Glu are good α-helix formers, whereas Pro is not as it introduces a sharp bend in the polypeptide chain. Similarly, Ile and Val are good β-sheet formers, whereas Glu and Pro are not. Thus, structurally compatible amino acids tend to be neighbors, so a distance derived in this way (Xia and Xie, 2002) may be termed structural compatibility distance. It is highly significantly and negatively correlated with the frequency of amino acid substitutions.

We expect the observed replacement frequencies to decrease with D_{ij}, which has been confirmed in numerous occasions involving diverse array of organisms (Grantham, 1974; Miyata et al., 1979; Palidwor et al., 2010; Xia, 1998b; Xia and Li, 1998; Xia and Xie, 2002; Yampolsky and Stoltzfus, 2005). Paradoxically, Miyata's distance typically predicts amino acid replacement frequencies better than Grantham's distance which include the additional variable of chemical composition of the side chain. This is presumably because this additional variable is somewhat messy and difficult to reduce to a clean number as volume and polarity.

N_{JTT} in Table 4.1 is known to be negatively correlated with Grantham's or Miyata's distance. Correlation between $\ln(N_{JTT})$ and Miyata's distance is -0.5832 with $P < 0.0001$ (Xia, 2018a), reflecting strong purifying selection against amino acid replacement involving very different amino acids. Such a strongly negative correlation suggests that any mechanical model aims to explain amino acid replacement or nonsynonymous codon substitutions should include amino acid dissimilarity measures. That is, the substitution rate should be a function of amino acid dissimilarity, as well as amino acid frequencies. However, there is one confounding factor that distorts the effect of amino acid dissimilarity on the frequency of amino acid replacement. Proteins have functionally important domains and unimportant domains. Amino acid dissimilarity can predict well the frequency of amino acid replacement involving functionally important amino acid sites, but the prediction does not work as well for functionally unimportant amino acid sites. Thus, to incorporate amino acid dissimilarity into an amino acid substitution model (or a codon-based substitution model), one needs to first assess site-specific functional importance in a multiple sequence alignment. In general, a low-variability site tend to be more functionally constrained than a high-variability site.

Surprisingly, in contrast to the relationship between $\ln(N_{JTT})$ and amino acid dissimilarities, the correlation is much higher between $\ln(N_{JTT})$ and D_{CF} being 0.7620 (Fig. 4.1). Such a high correlation is expected for homologous sequences that have experienced few multiple substitutions. The correlation will decrease as sequences evolve toward full substitution saturation. A significant relationship also exist between $\ln(N_{ij})$ and P_iP_j in Table 4.1 which is understandable because frequently used amino acids will be more likely involved in amino acid replacement. The three factors in Table 4.1 jointly accounts for 85.9% of the total variation in $\ln(N_{JTT})$. However, one should keep in mind that D_{CF} and amino acid dissimilarity are not independent of each other. The arrangement of codons in the genetic code is such that codons differing by one site typically code for more similar amino acids than codons differing by three sites (Xia, 1998b). This contributes to a positive correlation between D_{CF} and amino acid dissimilarity. Thus, the negative correlation between $\ln(N_{JTT})$ and D_{CF} is confounded by the relationship between $\ln(N_{JTT})$ and amino acid dissimilarity.

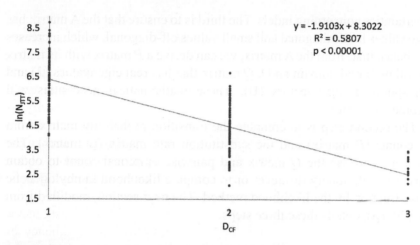

FIGURE 4.1   Amino acid replacement frequencies depend on by D_{CF} defined as the minimum number of site differences between two most similar codons, one from each codon family. Note that N_{JTT} has been log-transformed in the Y-axis.

The dependence of $\ln(N_{ij})$ on D_{CF} and amino acid dissimilarity changes with substitution saturation. For highly diverged sequences, each codon would have already experienced multiple substitutions, and $\ln(N_{ij})$ will no longer be dependent on D_{CF}. $\ln(N_{ij})$ remains highly dependent on amino acid dissimilarity because amino acid replacement becomes mainly constrained by functional conservation. In fact one can use this as a criterion to test substitution saturation at the nucleotide level. If $\ln(N_{ij})$ no long correlates with D_{CF}, then it is a good sign that phylogenetic signals at the nucleotide level is largely lost, and one should use amino acid sequences for phylogenetic reconstruction.

While molecular phylogeneticists may eventually find a good mechanistic model for codon or amino acid substitutions, at present model-based phylogenetic reconstruction for amino acid sequences relies mainly on empirical substitution matrix. The general procedure of obtaining evolutionary distances from protein sequences is of three steps. First, obtain empirical substitution counts between closely related sibling species. For example, if one wants to compute evolutionary distances for a protein among primates, then one would compile protein pairs from closely related primate sibling species, perform pairwise alignment and obtain a 20×20 matrix of empirical substitution counts. There are three reasons for choosing closely related species. The first is to minimize the need for correction for multiple substitutions at the same site. The second is to avoid uncertainties concerning indels. The third is to ensure that the A matrix has large values in the diagonal and small values off-diagonal, which increases the chance that, from the A matrix, we can derive a P matrix with its matrix logarithm in real domain and a Q matrix that has real eigenvalues (λ) and corresponding eigenvectors ($\mathbf{U}$). These mathematical necessities will become clear later.

The second step is to compute the transition probability matrix from the counts (P matrix) and the substitution rate matrix (Q matrix). The last step is to use the Q matrix and pairwise empirical count to obtain pairwise evolutionary distances or to compute likelihood in phylogenetic reconstruction by the likelihood method. The next section, modified from Xia (2018a), details these three steps.

4.1.2   DERIVING P AND Q MATRICES FOR COMPUTING EVOLUTIONARY DISTANCES

One may compute an evolutionary distance between two aligned amino acid sequences by using the equivalent of the JC69 model, i.e., assuming equal amino acid frequencies and the same rate of change between any two amino acids. However, such an evolutionary distance, although simple to compute, is of little practical use. An informative phylogenetic analysis with protein sequences typically involve the use of a pre-compiled matrix (e.g., JTT, BLOSUM, Dayhoff, etc.) or a home-made matrix to derive an empirical rate matrix (Q), and then use this Q matrix to compute either the distance between two species or branch lengths between two nodes in a tree. This section shows the process of using an empirical substitution matrix to compute evolutionary distances.

Table 4.2 is a compilation of 60 non-redundant pairwise comparison from 120 closely related HA (Hemagglutinin, <1% divergence) sequences from Influenza A viruses, i.e., Seq1 vs Seq2, Seq3 vs Seq4, etc. There are 1928 sites at which both sequences are Ala, one site with one sequence being Arg and the other being Asn, and so on (Table 4.2). Because sequences are very similar, we have large values in the diagonal and small values off-diagonal. As we cannot distinguish between substitutions such as Asn→Arg and Arg→Asn, the two corresponding off-diagonal elements are averaged. This resulting symmetrical matrix is often referred as the A matrix. We also designate N_i as the sum of row i in matrix A, $N = \Sigma N_i$ (i =Ala, Arg, ..., Val). Amino acid frequencies (π_i) are shown in the last row of Table 4.2, $\pi_i = N_i/N$, which we assume to be close to equilibrium frequencies.

Many elements in the A matrix are zero. This is an artefact of the limited sequence comparisons between HA sequences of low divergence. Ideally we should increase the number of comparisons to reduce the number of zero values in the matrix. I intentionally use this A matrix containing many zeroes to highlight a problem later about limited compilation.

HA sequences in the influenza A viruses, just as proteins in HIV-1, are not as functionally conserved as those proteins encoded in nuclear genomes used to compile empirical amino acid substitution matrices such as BLOSUM or JTT (Fig. 4.2). This implies that amino acid dissimilarity indices will not predict the frequency of amino acid replacement in the HA protein as well as in JTT, which is true (Fig. 4.2). The weaker relationship for the HA data (Fig. 4.2c) relative to that for the JTT data (Fig. 4.2a) is not due to smaller sample size in the HA data.

I should insert a caution here against using an empirical substitution matrix and assuming that it fits all amino acid substitution rates. While amino acid substitution frequencies tend to decrease with increasing amino acid dissimilarity (Fig. 4.2), this is not always true. For some proteins on the surface of parasites that can elicit immune response in the host, natural selection often favors more drastic changes that will help the parasite to evade host's immune system. This highlights the problem of using JTT, BLOSUM, Dayhoff, or any other precompiled matrix for phylogenetic analysis of your particular protein sequences. The substitution pattern may be quite different in your sequences than what is captured in any of the precompiled matrices.

The empirical P matrix is obtained by dividing every A_{ij} by N_i (Table 4.3). Note that P satisfies time-reversibility, i.e., $\pi_i P_{ij} = \pi_j P_{ji}$. Such a P matrix derived from empirical substitution data is sometimes subscripted as P_{obs} or P_{emp} to distinguish it from a mathematically derived P matrix based on an explicit substitution model. I will use P or P_{obs} interchangeably when there is no confusion.

Note that

$$P = e^{Qt} = e^{QD}$$
$$QD = \log(P)$$

(4.1)

where $t = D$ because the average substitution rate is scaled to 1 so time is measured by distance. Note that the empirical P matrix is from all pairwise

TABLE 4.2 Empirical substitution matrix A from HA (hemagglutinin) protein sequences of closely related Influenza A viruses. Because we cannot distinguish between substitutions such as Ala→Arg and Arg→Ala, the two corresponding off-diagonal values have been averaged. Amino acid frequencies (in %) shown at the last row are assumed to be equilibrium frequencies (π_j). Frequent replacements.

	Ala	Arg	Asn	Asp	Cys	Gln	Glu	Gly	His	Ile	Leu	Lys	Met	Phe	Pro	Ser	Thr	Trp	Tyr	Val
Ala	1928	0	0	0.5	0	0	0	0	0	0	0	0	0	0	0	1.5	18.5	0	0	3
Arg	0	1065	0.5	0	0	1	0	0	0	0	0	11	0.5	0	0	1.5	0	0	0	0
Asn	0	0.5	2591	9.5	0	0	0	0	0.5	0	0	1.5	0	0	0	21.5	1.5	0	0	0
Asp	0.5	0	9.5	1497	0	0	3.5	0	0	0	0	0	0	0	0	0	0	0	0	0
Cys	0	0	0	0	900	0	0	0	0	0	0	0	0	0	0	0	0	0	0	0
Gln	0	1	0	0	0	932	0	0	3	0	0	6	0	0	0	0	0	0	0	0
Glu	0	0	0	3.5	0	0	2028	1.5	0	0	0	20.5	0	0	0	0	0	0	0	0.5
Gly	0	0	0	0	0	0	1.5	2393	0	0	0	0	0	0	0	0	0	0	0	0
His	0	0	0.5	0	0	3	0	0	896	0	0	0	0	0	0	0	0	0	1	0
Ile	0	0	0	0	0	0	0	0	0	2093	1.5	0	2	0	0	0	11	0	0	14.5
Leu	0	0	0	0	0	0	0	0	0	1.5	2754	0	1.5	0.5	1	0.5	0	0	0	1.5
Lys	0	11	1.5	0	0	6	20.5	0	0	0	0	2481	0	0	0	0	0	0	0	0
Met	0	0.5	0	0	0	0	0	0	0	2	1.5	0	419	0	0	0	0.5	0	0	0
Phe	0	0	0	0	0	0	0	0	0	0	0.5	0	0	1139	0	0	0	0	0	0.5
Pro	0	0	0	0	0	0	0	0	0	0	1	0	0	0	1133	7.5	0	0	0	0
Ser	1.5	1.5	21.5	0	0	0	0	0	0	0	0.5	0	0	0	7.5	2611	10	0	0	0
Thr	18.5	0	1.5	0	0	0	0	0	0	11	0	0	0.5	0	0	10	2344	0	0	0
Trp	0	0	0	0	0	0	0	0	0	0	0	0	0	0	0	0	0	600	0	0
Tyr	0	0	0	0	0	0	0	0	1	0	0	0	0	0	0	0	0	0	1619	0
Val	3	0	0	0	0	0	0.5	0	0	14.5	1.5	0	0	0.5	0	0	0	0	0	2193
π_i	5.75	3.18	7.74	4.45	2.65	2.78	6.05	7.06	2.65	6.25	8.13	7.43	1.25	3.36	3.36	7.82	7.03	1.77	4.77	6.52

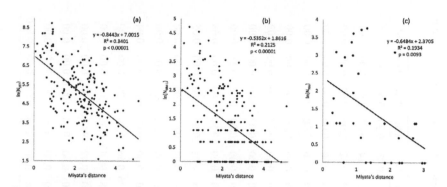

FIGURE 4.2 Miyata's distance can predict amino acid replacement better for the JTT matrix (a) than for the HIV-1 proteins (b) or Influenza HA proteins in Table 4.2. (a) and (b) are from Xia (2018a, Chapter 13).

comparisons between closely related HA proteins, so D represents the "average" distance among all sequence pairs. Given Eq. (4.1), the matrix logarithm of P in Table 4.3 gives us a QD matrix (Table 4.4). Note that not all empirical P matrices have a matrix logarithm in real domain, but large diagonal values relative to off-diagonal values increase the chance of the P matrix having a matrix logarithm. This is one of the reasons that we compile Matrix A from closely related species.

In contrast to a P matrix of which each row sums up to 1, a Q matrix has each row sums up to 0. The diagonal of a Q matrix represents the rate of each amino acid changing into other amino acids. Thus, the summation of diagonal values multiplied by the frequency of the corresponding amino acid represents the total change which is the evolutionary distance (D):

$$D = -\sum_{l=1}^{20} QD_{i,i}\pi_l = 0.00954 \qquad (4.2)$$

The small D is expected because the maximum percentage divergence of sequence pairs I used is 1%, with many sequence pairs with percentage divergence of only 0.1767%. If we had only two aligned sequences and if the A matrix in Table 4.2 were in fact obtained from the pairwise comparison between these two aligned sequences, then D above would be the evolutionary distance between the two sequences, and there would be no need to compute a Q matrix for obtaining distance. However, in molecular phylogenetics we typically have N sequences with $N \gg 2$. We will have $N(N-1)/2$ pairwise distances, and we want to have the same Q matrix to

TABLE 4.3 Empirical P matrix (P_{obs}) derived from A matrix in Table 4.2 (rounded to three decimal points). P_{obs} satisfies time-reversibility with $\pi_i P_{ij} = \pi_j P_{ji}$. All values multiplied by 100 to increase the number of significant digits shown.

	Ala	Arg	Asn	Asp	Cys	Gln	Glu	Gly	His	Ile	Leu	Lys	Met	Phe	Pro	Ser	Thr	Trp	Tyr	Val
Ala	98.80	0.00	0.00	0.03	0.00	0.00	0.00	0.00	0.00	0.00	0.00	0.00	0.00	0.00	0.00	0.08	0.95	0.00	0.00	0.15
Arg	0.00	98.66	0.05	0.00	0.00	0.09	0.00	0.00	0.00	0.00	0.00	1.02	0.05	0.00	0.00	0.14	0.00	0.00	0.00	0.00
Asn	0.00	0.02	98.67	0.36	0.00	0.00	0.00	0.00	0.02	0.00	0.00	0.06	0.00	0.00	0.00	0.82	0.06	0.00	0.00	0.00
Asp	0.03	0.00	0.63	99.11	0.00	0.00	0.23	0.00	0.00	0.00	0.00	0.00	0.00	0.00	0.00	0.00	0.00	0.00	0.00	0.00
Cys	0.00	0.00	0.00	0.00	100.0	0.00	0.00	0.00	0.00	0.00	0.00	0.00	0.00	0.00	0.00	0.00	0.00	0.00	0.00	0.00
Gln	0.00	0.11	0.00	0.00	0.00	98.94	0.00	0.00	0.32	0.00	0.00	0.64	0.00	0.00	0.00	0.00	0.00	0.00	0.00	0.00
Glu	0.00	0.00	0.00	0.17	0.00	0.00	98.73	0.07	0.00	0.00	0.00	1.00	0.00	0.00	0.00	0.00	0.00	0.00	0.00	0.02
Gly	0.00	0.00	0.00	0.00	0.00	0.00	0.06	99.94	0.00	0.00	0.00	0.00	0.00	0.00	0.00	0.00	0.00	0.00	0.00	0.00
His	0.00	0.00	0.06	0.00	0.00	0.33	0.00	0.00	99.50	0.00	0.00	0.00	0.00	0.00	0.00	0.00	0.00	0.00	0.11	0.00
Ile	0.00	0.00	0.00	0.00	0.00	0.00	0.00	0.00	0.00	98.63	0.07	0.00	0.09	0.00	0.00	0.00	0.52	0.00	0.00	0.68
Leu	0.00	0.00	0.00	0.00	0.00	0.00	0.00	0.00	0.00	0.05	99.76	0.00	0.05	0.02	0.04	0.02	0.00	0.00	0.00	0.05
Lys	0.00	0.44	0.06	0.00	0.00	0.24	0.81	0.00	0.00	0.00	0.00	98.45	0.00	0.00	0.00	0.00	0.00	0.00	0.00	0.00
Met	0.00	0.12	0.00	0.00	0.00	0.00	0.00	0.00	0.00	0.47	0.35	0.00	98.94	0.00	0.00	0.00	0.12	0.00	0.00	0.00
Phe	0.00	0.00	0.00	0.00	0.00	0.00	0.00	0.00	0.00	0.00	0.04	0.00	0.00	99.91	0.00	0.00	0.00	0.00	0.04	0.00
Pro	0.00	0.00	0.00	0.00	0.00	0.00	0.00	0.00	0.00	0.00	0.09	0.00	0.00	0.00	99.26	0.66	0.00	0.00	0.00	0.00
Ser	0.06	0.06	0.81	0.00	0.00	0.00	0.00	0.00	0.00	0.00	0.02	0.00	0.00	0.00	0.28	98.40	0.38	0.00	0.00	0.00
Thr	0.78	0.00	0.06	0.00	0.00	0.00	0.00	0.00	0.00	0.46	0.00	0.00	0.02	0.00	0.00	0.42	98.26	0.00	0.00	0.00
Trp	0.00	0.00	0.00	0.00	0.00	0.00	0.00	0.00	0.00	0.00	0.00	0.00	0.00	0.00	0.00	0.00	0.00	100.0	0.00	0.00
Tyr	0.00	0.00	0.00	0.00	0.00	0.00	0.00	0.00	0.06	0.00	0.00	0.00	0.00	0.00	0.00	0.00	0.00	0.00	99.94	0.00
Val	0.14	0.00	0.00	0.00	0.00	0.00	0.02	0.00	0.00	0.66	0.07	0.00	0.00	0.02	0.00	0.00	0.00	0.00	0.00	99.10

TABLE 4.4 QD matrix (multiplied by 100 to ease display) resulting from the matrix logarithm of P_{obs} in Table 4.3.

	Ala	Arg	Asn	Asp	Cys	Gln	Glu	Gly	His	Ile	Leu	Lys	Met	Phe	Pro	Ser	Thr	Trp	Tyr	Val
Ala	-1.22	0.00	0.00	0.03	0.00	0.00	0.00	0.00	0.00	0.00	0.00	0.00	0.00	0.00	0.00	0.08	0.96	0.00	0.00	0.16
Arg	0.00	-1.35	0.05	0.00	0.00	0.09	0.00	0.00	0.00	0.00	0.00	1.03	0.05	0.00	0.00	0.14	0.00	0.00	0.00	0.00
Asn	0.00	0.02	-1.35	0.37	0.00	0.00	0.00	0.00	0.02	0.00	0.00	0.06	0.00	0.00	0.00	0.83	0.06	0.00	0.00	0.00
Asp	0.03	0.00	0.64	-0.90	0.00	0.00	0.23	0.00	0.00	0.00	0.00	0.00	0.00	0.00	0.00	0.00	0.00	0.00	0.00	0.00
Cys	0.00	0.00	0.00	0.00	0.00	0.00	0.00	0.00	0.00	0.00	0.00	0.00	0.00	0.00	0.00	0.00	0.00	0.00	0.00	0.00
Gln	0.00	0.11	0.00	0.00	0.00	-1.07	0.00	0.00	0.32	0.00	0.00	0.64	0.00	0.00	0.00	0.00	0.00	0.00	0.00	0.00
Glu	0.00	0.00	0.00	0.17	0.00	0.00	-1.28	0.07	0.00	0.00	0.00	1.01	0.00	0.00	0.00	0.00	0.00	0.00	0.00	0.02
Gly	0.00	0.00	0.00	0.00	0.00	0.00	0.06	-0.06	0.00	0.00	0.00	0.00	0.00	0.00	0.00	0.00	0.00	0.00	0.00	0.00
His	0.00	0.00	0.06	0.00	0.00	0.34	0.00	0.00	-0.50	0.00	0.00	0.00	0.00	0.00	0.00	0.00	0.00	0.00	0.11	0.00
Ile	0.00	0.00	0.00	0.00	0.00	0.00	0.00	0.00	0.00	-1.38	0.07	0.00	0.10	0.00	0.00	0.00	0.53	0.00	0.00	0.69
Leu	0.00	0.00	0.00	0.00	0.00	0.00	0.00	0.00	0.00	0.05	-0.24	0.00	0.05	0.02	0.04	0.02	0.00	0.00	0.00	0.05
Lys	0.00	0.44	0.06	0.00	0.00	0.24	0.83	0.00	0.00	0.00	0.00	-1.57	0.00	0.00	0.00	0.00	0.00	0.00	0.00	0.00
Met	0.00	0.12	0.00	0.00	0.00	0.00	0.00	0.00	0.00	0.48	0.36	0.00	-1.07	0.00	0.00	0.00	0.12	0.00	0.00	0.00
Phe	0.00	0.00	0.00	0.00	0.00	0.00	0.00	0.00	0.00	0.00	0.04	0.00	0.00	-0.09	0.00	0.00	0.00	0.00	0.00	0.04
Pro	0.00	0.00	0.00	0.00	0.00	0.00	0.00	0.00	0.00	0.00	0.09	0.00	0.00	0.00	-0.75	0.66	0.00	0.00	0.00	0.00
Ser	0.06	0.06	0.82	0.00	0.00	0.00	0.00	0.00	0.00	0.00	0.02	0.00	0.00	0.00	0.29	-1.62	0.38	0.00	0.00	0.00
Thr	0.79	0.00	0.06	0.00	0.00	0.00	0.00	0.00	0.00	0.47	0.00	0.00	0.02	0.00	0.00	0.43	-1.76	0.00	0.00	0.00
Trp	0.00	0.00	0.00	0.00	0.00	0.00	0.00	0.00	0.00	0.00	0.00	0.00	0.00	0.00	0.00	0.00	0.00	0.00	0.00	0.00
Tyr	0.00	0.00	0.00	0.00	0.00	0.00	0.00	0.00	0.06	0.00	0.00	0.00	0.00	0.00	0.00	0.00	0.00	0.00	-0.06	0.00
Val	0.14	0.00	0.00	0.00	0.00	0.00	0.02	0.00	0.00	0.66	0.07	0.00	0.00	0.02	0.00	0.00	0.00	0.00	0.00	-0.91

compute all these distances, assuming that the evolutionary process has remained the same so that the Q matrix is applicable to all sequences. Therefore we need to derive the Q matrix as

$$Q = \frac{QD}{D} \qquad (4.3)$$

which is shown in Table 4.5. Note that the A matrix derived from two highly diverged homologous sequences may not have matrix logarithm in real domain, so we will not have matrix QD in Eq. (4.1) and consequently will not be able to calculate D according to Eq. (4.2). However, with an A matrix derived from closely related sequence pairs, we are almost guaranteed to obtain the Q matrix in Eq. (4.3). With this Q matrix, we can compute D for any pairs of homologous sequences.

You might be wondering why we need a Q matrix to compute D. This will become clear soon but, in short, a Q matrix and a distance D will allow us to obtain a P matrix and we can then check if the D fits the data well. If not, we will just replace D with another value and check until we find a D with the best fit. The P matrix is obtained by taking matrix exponential specified in Eq. (4.1), which needs eigenvalues and eigenvectors from the Q matrix. Because our A matrix is derived from closely related species with diagonal values much greater than the off-diagonal values, a Q matrix derived from such an A matrix is almost guaranteed to have real eigenvalues (λ) and corresponding eigenvectors (**U**). The 20 eigenvalues from the Q matrix in Table 4.5, sorted in ascending order, are -2.86995, -2.75689, -2.46387, -1.81284, -1.49779, -1.32248, -1.19482, -1.09364, -0.80343, -0.71024, -0.45099, -0.35980, -0.25654, -0.15149, -0.09002, -0.05503, -0.04275, 0.00000, 0.00000, 0.00000, with the associated eigenvector **U** in Table 4.6. To replicate these eigenvalues and eigenvectors, one needs to start from the data in Table 4.2 instead of Tables 4.3 or 4.4 because values in these last two tables have been rounded and consequently not precise.

Now the P matrix for a given distance D (designated P_D) is

$$P_D = U\Lambda U^{-1} \qquad (4.4)$$

where Λ is a diagonal matrix with values being $e^{D\lambda_1}$, $e^{D\lambda_2}$, ..., $e^{D\lambda_{20}}$, **U** the eigenvectors in Table 4.6, and **U**$^{-1}$ the matrix inverse of **U**. Values in P_D are probabilities and should range between 0 and 1. However, limited data compilation with many 0 values in the A matrix (Table 4.2), coupled with

TABLE 4.5 Instantaneous rate matrix (Q), computed according to Eq. (4.3), rounded to save space.

	Ala	Arg	Asn	Asp	Cys	Gln	Glu	Gly	His	Ile	Leu	Lys	Met	Phe	Pro	Ser	Thr	Trp	Tyr	Val
Ala	-1.27	0.00	0.00	0.03	0.00	0.00	0.00	0.00	0.00	0.00	0.00	0.00	0.00	0.00	0.00	0.08	1.00	0.00	0.00	0.16
Arg	0.00	-1.42	0.05	0.00	0.00	0.10	0.00	0.00	0.00	0.00	0.00	1.08	0.05	0.00	0.00	0.15	0.00	0.00	0.00	0.00
Asn	0.00	0.02	-1.41	0.38	0.00	0.00	0.00	0.00	0.02	0.00	0.00	0.06	0.00	0.00	0.00	0.87	0.06	0.00	0.00	0.00
Asp	0.03	0.00	0.66	-0.94	0.00	0.00	0.24	0.00	0.00	0.00	0.00	0.00	0.00	0.00	0.00	0.00	0.00	0.00	0.00	0.00
Cys	0.00	0.00	0.00	0.00	0.00	0.00	0.00	0.00	0.00	0.00	0.00	0.00	0.00	0.00	0.00	0.00	0.00	0.00	0.00	0.00
Gln	0.00	0.11	0.00	0.00	0.00	-1.12	0.00	0.00	0.34	0.00	0.00	0.67	0.00	0.00	0.00	0.00	0.00	0.00	0.00	0.00
Glu	0.00	0.00	0.00	0.18	0.00	0.00	-1.34	0.08	0.00	0.00	0.00	1.06	0.00	0.00	0.00	0.00	0.00	0.00	0.00	0.03
Gly	0.00	0.00	0.00	0.00	0.00	0.00	0.07	-0.07	0.00	0.00	0.00	0.00	0.00	0.00	0.00	0.00	0.00	0.00	0.00	0.00
His	0.00	0.00	0.06	0.00	0.00	0.35	0.00	0.00	-0.52	0.00	0.00	0.00	0.00	0.00	0.00	0.00	0.00	0.00	0.12	0.00
Ile	0.00	0.00	0.00	0.00	0.00	0.00	0.00	0.00	0.00	-1.44	0.07	0.00	0.10	0.00	0.00	0.00	0.55	0.00	0.00	0.72
Leu	0.00	0.00	0.00	0.00	0.00	0.00	0.00	0.00	0.00	0.06	-0.25	0.00	0.06	0.02	0.04	0.02	0.00	0.00	0.00	0.06
Lys	0.00	0.46	0.06	0.00	0.00	0.25	0.86	0.00	0.00	0.00	0.00	-1.64	0.00	0.00	0.00	0.00	0.00	0.00	0.00	0.00
Met	0.00	0.12	0.00	0.00	0.00	0.00	0.00	0.00	0.00	0.50	0.37	0.00	-1.12	0.00	0.00	0.00	0.12	0.00	0.00	0.00
Phe	0.00	0.00	0.00	0.00	0.00	0.00	0.00	0.00	0.00	0.00	0.05	0.00	0.00	-0.09	0.00	0.00	0.00	0.00	0.00	0.05
Pro	0.00	0.00	0.00	0.00	0.00	0.00	0.00	0.00	0.00	0.00	0.09	0.00	0.00	0.00	-0.78	0.69	0.00	0.00	0.00	0.00
Ser	0.06	0.06	0.86	0.00	0.00	0.00	0.00	0.00	0.00	0.00	0.02	0.00	0.00	0.00	0.30	-1.69	0.40	0.00	0.00	0.00
Thr	0.82	0.00	0.06	0.00	0.00	0.00	0.00	0.00	0.00	0.49	0.00	0.00	0.02	0.00	0.00	0.44	-1.84	0.00	0.00	0.00
Trp	0.00	0.00	0.00	0.00	0.00	0.00	0.00	0.00	0.00	0.00	0.00	0.00	0.00	0.00	0.00	0.00	0.00	0.00	0.00	0.00
Tyr	0.00	0.00	0.00	0.00	0.00	0.00	0.00	0.00	0.06	0.00	0.00	0.00	0.00	0.00	0.00	0.00	0.00	0.00	-0.06	0.00
Val	0.14	0.00	0.00	0.00	0.00	0.02	0.02	0.00	0.00	0.69	0.07	0.00	0.00	0.02	0.00	0.00	0.00	0.00	0.00	-0.95

TABLE 4.6 Eigenvectors (U) from the instantaneous rate matrix (Q), corresponding to the 20 eigenvalues sorted in ascending order, multiplied by 10 and rounded to save space.

Ala	Arg	Asn	Asp	Cys	Gln	Glu	Gly	His	Ile	Leu	Lys	Met	Phe	Pro	Ser	Thr	Trp	Tyr	Val
0.32	0.15	0.25	0.34	-0.15	0.14	0.19	0.25	0.59	0.08	0.02	0.19	0.21	0.14	-0.11	0.08	-0.13	-0.24	0	0
-0.08	0.25	-0.05	-0.04	-0.65	-0.08	-0.24	-0.26	0.03	0.13	-0.16	0.03	-0.08	-0.19	-0.08	-0.04	0.02	-0.13	0	0
-0.29	0.06	0.58	0.14	0.24	-0.27	-0.45	-0.23	-0.08	-0.38	0.13	-0.40	0.25	-0.09	-0.21	0.03	-0.09	-0.32	0	0
0.07	-0.06	-0.14	-0.08	-0.31	0.42	0.36	0.15	-0.12	-0.62	-0.05	-0.24	0.12	-0.12	-0.12	-0.01	-0.03	-0.18	0	0
0.00	0.00	0.00	0.00	0.00	0.00	0.00	0.00	0.00	0.00	0.00	0.00	0.00	0.00	0.00	0.00	0.00	0.00	1	0
-0.03	0.11	-0.03	0.01	0.25	0.63	-0.26	-0.05	0.02	0.07	0.18	0.11	-0.11	-0.20	-0.06	-0.02	0.07	-0.11	0	0
-0.12	0.47	-0.10	0.03	0.49	-0.34	0.42	0.33	-0.01	0.00	-0.41	0.04	-0.13	-0.35	-0.13	-0.12	0.04	-0.25	0	0
0.00	-0.01	0.00	0.00	-0.03	0.02	-0.03	-0.02	0.00	0.00	0.08	-0.01	0.05	0.31	0.39	-0.89	0.15	-0.29	0	0
0.01	-0.02	0.00	-0.01	-0.09	-0.26	0.15	0.04	-0.02	-0.09	0.68	0.15	-0.10	-0.15	-0.03	0.02	0.16	-0.11	0	0
0.29	0.14	0.24	-0.69	0.08	-0.01	0.00	-0.16	-0.25	-0.04	-0.08	0.37	0.06	0.22	-0.06	0.11	-0.16	-0.26	0	0
0.00	0.00	0.00	-0.02	-0.01	-0.02	-0.08	0.25	0.15	-0.10	0.03	-0.35	-0.81	0.44	0.10	0.19	-0.25	-0.34	0	0
0.20	-0.76	0.18	-0.01	0.00	-0.12	-0.03	0.04	0.04	0.18	-0.41	0.11	-0.20	-0.48	-0.18	-0.11	0.07	-0.31	0	0
-0.01	-0.01	-0.01	0.11	0.06	0.03	0.18	-0.63	-0.02	0.00	-0.02	0.03	-0.05	0.04	-0.01	0.02	-0.03	-0.05	0	0
0.00	0.00	0.00	-0.01	0.00	0.00	0.00	-0.01	0.01	0.01	0.01	-0.02	0.09	-0.23	0.78	0.17	-0.18	-0.14	0	0
-0.07	0.00	0.11	-0.01	-0.11	0.18	0.29	0.15	-0.25	0.60	0.16	-0.27	0.09	0.03	-0.08	0.03	-0.06	-0.14	0	0
0.49	0.01	-0.60	0.02	0.25	-0.32	-0.39	-0.19	0.00	0.15	0.17	-0.33	0.26	0.01	-0.20	0.06	-0.12	-0.32	0	0
-0.64	-0.26	-0.30	-0.32	0.05	0.00	0.06	0.00	0.43	0.09	0.04	0.16	0.22	0.16	-0.14	0.09	-0.15	-0.29	0	0
0.00	0.00	0.00	0.00	0.00	0.00	0.00	0.00	0.00	0.00	0.00	0.00	0.00	0.00	0.00	0.00	0.00	0.00	0	1
0.00	0.00	0.00	0.00	0.01	0.02	-0.02	0.00	0.00	0.02	-0.20	-0.06	0.06	0.20	0.16	0.26	0.85	-0.20	0	0
-0.13	-0.08	-0.14	0.52	-0.09	-0.02	-0.17	0.36	-0.54	-0.09	-0.13	0.47	0.05	0.24	-0.03	0.12	-0.17	-0.27	0	0

limited numeric precision, may result in a zero value in P_D misrepresented as a very small negative value in computer which does not make sense. For this reason, one should aim to compile the A matrix so that all entries are non-zero.

Now we have everything to estimate the evolutionary distance between two aligned amino acid sequences. We will first compile an A matrix from these two aligned sequences (Table 4.7). The best D is one that maximizes the log-likelihood (lnL):

$$\ln L = A_{ij} \ln(\pi_i P_{D.ij}) \tag{4.5}$$

where A_{ij} is in Table 4.7, π_i is the equilibrium frequencies typically approximated by the empirical amino acid frequencies, and matrix P_D is specified in Eq. (4.4). The maximum lnL is -1722.26665, achieved when $D = 0.03065$. To estimate D for another pair of sequences, we do not need to change U or U^{-1} in Eq. (4.4). We only need to replace D in the diagonal matrix Λ and find the best D that maximizes lnL in Eq. (4.5) for the new pair of sequences. For likelihood-based phylogenetic reconstruction, the transition probability matrix is needed to compute the likelihood for a given branch length or to find the branch length that maximizes lnL.

You are encouraged to take the A matrix in Table 4.2, work through the process to generate the Q matrix, and the eigenvalues and eigenvectors, and then compute the distance between APF46400 and ACT36649 with data shown in Table 4.7. If you use R to obtain eigenvalues and eigenvectors, remember to first transpose the Q matrix so that each column, instead of each row, sums up to 0. Also, because of the limited compilation in Table 4.2 with many 0 values, you may get 0 and small negative values in P_D in Eq. (4.4). You should ignore such values by using $P_{D.ij}$ values greater than 0 in computing lnL in Eq. (4.5).

4.1.3   PROBLEMS WITH THE EMPIRICAL AMINO ACID SUBSTITUTION MATRIX

There are three inherent difficulties with amino acid-based substitution models derived from empirical compilation of substitution patterns. The first is what I would call one-hat-doesn't-fit-all problem. Protein-coding genes often differ much in substitution patterns, and one can never be sure if any of the empirical matrices is appropriate for the protein sequences one is studying. While different amino acids tend to replace each other

TABLE 4.7 Empirical substitution matrix A from comparing two aligned HA protein sequences (GenBank accessions APF46400 and ACT36649). Because we cannot distinguish between substitutions such as Ala→Arg and Arg→Ala, the two corresponding off-diagonal values have been averaged.

	Ala	Arg	Asn	Asp	Cys	Gln	Glu	Gly	His	Ile	Leu	Lys	Met	Phe	Pro	Ser	Thr	Trp	Tyr	Val
Ala	32	0	0	0	0	0	0	0	0	0	0	0	0	0	0	0	1	0	0	0
Arg		18	0	0	0	0	0	0	0	0	0	0.5	0	0	0	0.5	0	0	0	0
Asn			40	0.5	0	0	0	0	0	0	0	0	0	0	0	2.5	0	0	0	0
Asp				25	0	0	0	0	0	0	0	0	0	0	0	0	0	0	0	0
Cys					15	0	0	0	0	0	0	0	0	0	0	0	0	0	0	0
Gln						15	0	0	0	0	0	0.5	0	0	0	0	0	0	0	0
Glu							33	0	0	0	0	1.5	0	0	0	0	0	0	0	0
Gly								40	0	0	0	0	0	0	0	0	0	0	0	0
His									15	0	0	0	0	0	0	0	0	0	0	0
Ile										35	0	0	0	0	0	0	0	0	0	0.5
Leu											46	0	0	0	0	0	0	0	0	0
Lys												39	0	0	0	0	0	0	0	0
Met													7	0	0	0	0	0	0	0
Phe														19	0	0	0	0	0	0
Pro															19	0	0	0	0	0
Ser																41	1	0	0	0
Thr																	36	0	0	0
Trp																		10	0	0
Tyr																			27	0
Val																				37

less frequently than similar amino acids, natural selection may favor drastic amino acid replacement in surface proteins of pathogens that are recognized by the host immune system. Such drastic changes allow the pathogen to evade host's immune defense. The hemagglutinin in Influenza A viruses is a surface protein and its substitution pattern is different from that of proteins compiled in the JTT matrix (Fig. 4.2). One could derive an amino acid substitution model based on the specific sequence (Adachi and Hasegawa, 1996; Kishino et al., 1990), but this is not only slow and tedious, but also plagued by insufficient amount of data.

Second, an amino acid replacement is effected by a nonsynonymous codon replacement. Two codons can differ by 1, 2, or 3 sites, and an amino acid replacement involving two codons differing by one site is expected to be more likely than that involving two codons differing by 3 sites. However, at the amino acid level, there is no information on whether an amino acid replacement results from a single nucleotide replacement or a triple nucleotide replacement. This is what I name as the missing-codon-link problem. Only a codon-based model can incorporate this information.

Third, while two similar amino acids are expected to, and do, replace each other more frequently than two different amino acids (Xia and Li, 1998), the similarity between amino acids is often difficult to define. For example, polarity may be highly conserved at some sites but not at others. Two very different amino acids rarely replace each other in functionally important domains but can replace each other frequently at unimportant segments. Moreover, the likelihood of two amino acids replacing each other also depends on neighboring amino acids (Xia and Xie, 2002). For example, whether a stretch of amino acids will form an α-helix may depend on whether the stretch contains a high proportion of amino acids with high helix-forming propensity, and not necessarily on whether a particular site is occupied by a particular amino acid. This third problem I name as the site-dependence problem.

4.2 CODON-BASED MODELS AND ASSOCIATED DISTANCES

One can approach codon-based models the same way as we did with nucleotide-based or amino acid-based models. The standard genetic code has 61 sense codons, and we will simply have a 61×61 P matrix and Q matrix instead of 4×4 matrices for nucleotides or 20×20 for amino acids. The codon-based substitution models (Goldman and Yang, 1994; Muse and Gaut, 1994) were proposed to overcome the first two of three problems in amino acid-based models.

4.2.1 PROBLEMS WITH CODON-BASED MODELS

While codon-based model may be useful in some cases, one should be aware of the potential problems, especially its simplifying assumptions.

4.2.1.1 MORE IS OFTEN LESS

Codon-based models have practical difficulties with a potentially large number of parameters in rates and frequencies inherent in codon-based models, and need to have two simplifying assumptions to reduce them. First, we cannot have the equivalent of GTR for nucleotide sequences (Lanave et al., 1984; Tavaré, 1986) because GTR for a 61×61 rate matrix (for standard genetic code with 61 sense codons) would demand too much data for reliable parameter estimation and too much computation power to do the estimation. Thus, simplifying assumptions have to be made, one involving the rate parameters and other the frequency parameters.

The first simplification in codon-based models is to lump different substitution rates into the same rate category, just like the F84 model that lumped six rates in a GTR model into two rate categories, with all transitions having the same rate and all transversions having the same rate. The typical specification of substitution rates for a codon-based model (Goldman and Yang, 1994; Muse and Gaut, 1994) is

$$
q_{ij} = \begin{cases}
0 & \text{if i and j differ at 2 or 3 codon sites} \\
\pi_j & \text{if i and j differ by a synonymous transversion} \\
\kappa\pi_j & \text{if i and j differ by a synonymous transition} \\
\omega\pi_j & \text{if i and j differ by a nonsynonymous transversion} \\
\omega\kappa\pi_j & \text{if i and j differ by a nonsynonymous transition}
\end{cases}
\tag{4.6}
$$

Such a specification implies that TTA(Leu)→CTA(Leu) and CTG(Leu)→CTA(Leu) have the same rate (i.e., $\kappa\pi_{CTA}$). Note that TTA→CTA involves a T→C transition and CTG→CTA involves a G→A transition. You may recall that A↔G and C↔T transitions are allowed to have different rates in TN93 (Tamura and Nei, 1993) which was proposed to accommodate the observation that the two types of transitions often have different rates.

However, no currently used codon-based model treat these two types of transitions differently. In this aspect, the codon-based model, as specified above, is already a step backwards.

The second simplifying assumption concerns the number of frequency parameters. A protein-coding gene typically has only a few hundred codons, and some codons may not be represented at all. So our problem is equivalent to applying a nucleotide-based substitution model to sequences containing only nucleotides A and G. To avoid such awkwardness, the F3 × 4 codon frequency model is frequently used (Yang, 2002; Yang and Nielsen, 2000) so that codon frequencies are inferred from nucleotide frequencies at each of the three codon sites. However, codon usage is affected by many factors, including differential ribonucleotide concentration (Xia, 1996), biased mutation (Chithambaram et al., 2014a, 2014b; Marin and Xia, 2008; Xia, 2005, 2015; Xia et al., 2006) and, in particular, tRNA-mediated selection (Bulmer, 1991; Ikemura, 1981a, 1992; Prabhakaran et al., 2015; Xia, 1998a, 2015). For example, the site-specific nucleotide frequencies are poor predictors of codon usage (Table 4.8, contrasting the observed N_{cod} and the expected N_{cod}' based on the nucleotide frequencies at each codon site) of highly expressed protein-coding genes in *Escherichia coli* K12. Although G is slightly more frequent than A at the third codon site (Table 4.8), AAA is used far more frequently than AAG for coding Lys (Table 4.8). The biased codon usage is easy to understand with the tRNA-mediated selection. *E. coli* K12 genome has six tRNA[Lys/UUU] genes (where UUU is the anticodon forming Watson-Crick base pair with codon AAA) but no tRNA[Lys/CUU] gene to pair with codon AAG. So AAA is favored by tRNA[Lys/UUU] against AAG. One should expect the F3 × 4 codon frequency model to perform poorly in such a situation.

TABLE 4.8 Site-specific nucleotide frequencies for A and G, and codon usage in lysine (Lys) codon family.

Nuc. freq. by codon sites (*CS*)				Codon freq.			
Base	CS_1	CS_2	CS_3	Codon	AA	N_{cod}	N_{cod}'
A	0.273	0.32	0.18	AAG	Lys	24	95
G	0.409	0.16	0.219	AAA	Lys	149	78

AA, amino acid; N_{cod} and N_{cod}', observed and expected (from nucleotide frequencies at three codon sites) number of codons. Results from eight highly expressed genes (*gapC, gapA, fbaB, ompC, fbaA, tufA, groS, groL*) from the *Escherichia coli* K12 genome (GenBank Accession: *NC_000913*).

4.2.1.2   CODON-BASED MODELS FOR TESTING POSITIVE SELECTION

Claiming positive selection from aligned codon sequences by running through certain programs was once very popular, and served as an efficient pipeline for generating publications. The approach seems to experience a resurrection lately. It is therefore important to point out the caveats concerning this approach.

Let me briefly outline the conceptual framework of selection and adaptation. Organisms evolve adaptation in response to natural selection. Suppose we have different bacteriophage species parasitizing two different bacterial hosts (Host A and Host B). Host A has a tRNA pool quite different that of Host B. It is known that highly expressed host genes would evolve codon usage maximizing the number of codons decoded by abundant tRNAs and minimizing the number of codons that have few tRNA decoding them (Gouy and Gautier, 1982; Ikemura, 1981a, 1981b, 1982, 1992). This tRNA-mediated codon-anticodon adaptation has been shown experimentally to increase translation efficiency (Haas et al., 1996; Kaishima et al., 2016; Ngumbela et al., 2008; Robinson et al., 1984; Sorensen et al., 1989). Given this, we would predict that bacteriophage genes should evolve codon usage similar to host highly expressed genes (Chithambaram et al., 2014a, 2014b; Prabhakaran et al., 2014, 2015). We may also predict that if one phylogenetic clade of phage species all parasitize Host A, but one member of the clade has switched to parasitize Host B, then this host-jumping phage would evolve codon usage more different from Host A and more similar to Host B relative to its sister species that are still parasitizing Host A. This last example with host-switching offers us a phylogenetic control to peek into the evolutionary process of codon adaptation. Testing and substantiating such hypotheses and predictions would constitute examples of codon usage adaptation.

If we dissect such a study, we can identify (1) differential selection pressure on codon usage mediated by different tRNA pools between Host A and Host B, (2) the directional changes in codon usage driven by the differential selection pressure between Host A and Host B, with tangible evolutionary benefit of codon adaptation leading to more efficient translation efficiency, and (3) the predicted directional changes in codon usage in response to different tRNA pools can be tested (and indeed have been tested and validated).

The approach of testing positive selection from aligned codon sequences is quite different. First, one has no idea what the claimed positive selection is. Second, one has no idea what directional (or non-directional) evolutionary changes are expected. Third, one claims positive selection not with any direct evidence, but by saying that a particular neutral model does not fit the data sufficiently, in particular by saying that there are more nonsynonymous substitutions observed at a particular site than expected from a particular neutral model (a higher than usual dN/dS ratio, where dN and dS are nonsynonymous and synonymous substitution rates, respectively). This kind of detecting positive selection is what Jody Hey (2000), in discussing on evidence for human mitochondrial recombination, labelled as conclusion through a backdoor. Hey argued that if one wishes to conclude that mitochondrial recombination has occurred, one needs to provide evidence that it occurred instead of claiming recombination by saying that an alternative mutation hypothesis is insufficient to explain the data. Following the same logic, one should not claim to have detected positive selection by saying that a particular neutral model is insufficient to explain the data. One should provide direct evidence as illustrated with the example of codon adaptation. The so-called "positive selection" could result from diverse "non-positive-selection" scenarios. This being said, the test implemented in CODEML is a far better test than McDonald–Kreitman test which does not even take codon frequencies into consideration.

Let me illustrate one case in which one could obtain higher than usual dN/dS ratio. Take, for example, AGR codons coding for Arginine. According to EMBOSS compilation, among 314 codons in highly expressed yeast genes, only one is AGG, and the other 313 are all AGA. This is understandable given the relative tRNA availability. There are 11 tRNA genes with anticodon UCU decoding AGA, but only 1 tRNA gene with anticodon CCU decoding AGG without wobble pairing. So it is beneficial to use more AGA codons than AGG codons. The dramatic difference in codon usage (313 AGA vs. 1 AGG) suggests a very strong purifying selection on synonymous substitutions (i.e., AGA→AGG is selected against). Similar pattern is observed for Lysine encoded by AAA and AAG codons, with AAG selected against. Thus, a codon site in a highly expressed yeast protein genes may have a high dN/dS ratios because AGA and AAA may replace each other frequently (Arg and Lys are both positively charged amino acids of roughly similar size) but dS is low due to negative (purifying) selection against AAG and AGG. CODEML does not take this into consideration and tends to report this as a positively selected sites.

4.2.2   CODON-BASED DISTANCES (LPB93)

Evolutionary distances associated with codon-based models measure the number of synonymous substitutions and nonsynonymous substitutions, often represented as K_S and K_A or d_S and d_N, respectively. Here I will illustrate the computation of K_S and K_A by the LPB93 method (Li, 1993; Pamilo and Bianchi, 1993). The method was criticized (Yang, 2006) because (1) the counting of 0-fold, 2-fold, and 4-fold sites needs to be implemented for each genetic code, and (2) it does not take into consideration the differences in codon frequencies. The first difficulty is not difficult to circumvent. There are currently 18 different genetic codes, but some differ only in the start codon usage. For example, the standard code and the genetic code 11 used by most bacterial species differ only in start codon usage. So it is not too much work to accommodate them individually and has indeed been accommodated in DAMBE (Xia, 2013b; Xia, 2017a). The second criticism is against the current implementation of the LBP93 method that uses the K80 model (Kimura, 1980) for correcting multiple substitutions at the same site, but this is not an inherent shortcoming of the method because one can use F84 (Felsenstein, 2004) or TN93 (Tamura and Nei, 1993) models for correction. This directly account for differential nucleotide usage at 0-fold, 2-fold, and 4-fold sites, and indirectly account for differential codon usage. One main reason for LBP93 implementation not using more realistic models such as F84 or TN93 is the possibility of having many cases where F84 and TN93 are inapplicable, especially when sequences are short or when one needs to compute K_S and K_A along a sliding window of limited width. However, in practice we almost always work with multiple sequences, which allows one to use the simultaneous estimation (SE) method (Tamura et al., 2004; Xia, 2009). SE will effectively eliminate inapplicable cases, although one could still concoct artificial cases where inapplicable cases exist even with SE. Here I will first illustrate the LPB93 method and then introduce the SE method that eliminates the inapplicable cases.

4.2.2.1 NUMERICAL ILLUSTRATION OF THE LPB93 METHOD

Suppose we have three aligned codon sequences from a vertebrate mitochondrial gene (Fig. 4.3) and wish to compute K_A and K_S between sequences *S1* and *S2*. This can be done with the LPB93 method in three steps. First, we count the number of 0-fold, 2-fold, and 4-fold sites. A 0-fold site in a codon is one where any nucleotide substitution is nonsynonymous. For example, the first two codon sites of a Gly GGA codon are 0-fold sites because the codon will not encode Gly any more if a nucleotide substitution occur at these two sites. In contrast, a 4-fold site is one that, when replaced by any other nucleotide, will not change what the codon encodes. For example, the third site of GGA is a 4-fold site because the codon will encode Gly when this site is occupied by any other nucleotides. A 2-fold site is one that can be occupied by two nucleotides without changing what the codon encodes. For example, the third site of Lys AAA codon is a 2-fold site because it can be occupied by two nucleotides (A and G) without changing what it encodes (Both AAA and AAG encode Lys). I have labelled which site is 0-fold, 2-fold, and 4-fold sites for *S1* in Figure 4.3. Note that whether a codon site is 0-fold, 2-fold, or 4-fold depends on genetic code. For this reason, K_A and K_S can only be computed between sequences sharing the same genetic code. If you use DAMBE, and have already read in a sequence file, you may see what vertebrate mitochondrial code looks like by clicking "Sequence|Change Seq. Type|Protein-coding sequences|2-Vertebrate mitochondrial|View code." You can view other genetic codes in the same way. DAMBE implements all 18 known genetic codes. You will find that vertebrate mitochondrial genetic code is different from invertebrate mitochondrial code. For this reason, you cannot compute synonymous and nonsynonymous distance for *COX1* gene between a vertebrate and an invertebrate species. This is what I name as the no-trade-without-common-currency problem in codon models.

```
     004 002 004 002 004 004 002 002 002 002 002 004 004 204 002 204 202 002 004 004
S1   CGU UGA CCA UUC UCU ACA AAC CAC AAA GAC AUU GGA ACA CUA UAC CUA UUA UUC GGC GCA
     Arg Trp Pro Phe Ser Thr Asn His Lys Asp Ile Gly Thr Leu Tyr Leu Leu Phe Gly Ala
S2   CGU UGC CUA UUC UCA ACA AAC CAU ACA GAC AUA GGG ACC CUU UAU CUG CUA UUU GGU ACU
     Arg Cys Leu Phe Ser Thr Asn His Thr Asp Met Gly Thr Leu Tyr Leu Leu Phe Gly Thr
S3   CGC UGG CUA UUC UCA ACC CAC CAU ACA GAA AUU GGU ACC CUU UAU CUA CUA UUU GGU GCU
     Arg Trp Leu Phe Ser Thr His His Thr Glu Ile Gly Thr Leu Tyr Leu Leu Phe Gly Ala
     **  **  *  *  *** **   **      ** **   *  **  **  **  **  **  **  **  ** **  **     *
```

FIGURE 4.3 Three aligned vertebrate mitochondrial sequences for illustrating the LPB93 method.

The number of 0-fold, 2-fold, and 4-fold sites for *S1*, designated as N_0, N_2, and N_4, are 37, 13, and 10, respectively. The corresponding numbers for *S2* are 37, 11, and 12, respectively. The mean numbers of 0-fold, 2-fold, and 4-fold sites for *S1* and *S2* are 37, 12, and 11, respectively (L_i in Table 4.9a). The average numbers may not be integers.

TABLE 4.9 Detailed output for computing synonymous and nonsynonymous distances with LPB93 method.

(a)	*S1..S2*			(b)	*S1..S3*			(c)	*S2..S3*		
i-fold	0	2	4		0	2	4		0	2	4
L	37	12	11		37	12	11		37	11	12
S	2	5	3		1	5	2		1	1	2
V	1	1	4		2	1	6		1	2	2
P	0.05405	0.41667	0.27273		0.02703	0.41667	0.18182		0.02703	0.09091	0.16667
Q	0.02703	0.08333	0.36364		0.05405	0.08333	0.54545		0.02703	0.18182	0.16667
A	0.05870	1.19687	0.87413		0.02860	1.19687	N/A		0.02839	0.11300	0.24521
B	0.02778	0.09116	0.64964		0.05721	0.09116	N/A		0.02778	0.22599	0.20273

Second, we count the number of transitions and transversions (designated as s_i and v_i where the subscript i is 0, 2, and 4 for 0-fold, 2-fold, and 4-fold sites) between *S1* and *S2*. These observed s_i and v_i values (Table 4.9a) do not correct for multiple hits, so we need to estimate the number of transitions and transversions from them. For the K80 model, the expected number of transitions and transversions, designated A_i and B_i, respectively, are simply αt and $2\beta t$ that we have derived before:

$$A_i = \alpha t_i = -\frac{\ln(1 - 2P_i - Q_i)}{2} + \frac{\ln(1 - 2Q_i)}{4}$$

$$B_i = 2\beta t = -\frac{\ln(1 - 2Q_i)}{2}$$

(4.7)

where P_i and Q_i are proportion of transitions and transversions at the i-fold site, e.g., $P_0 = s_0/L_0 = 2/37 = 0.054054$ (Table 4.9). The A_i and B_i values are also listed in Table 4.9. You may have noticed a much stronger transition bias at 2-fold sites than at the 0-fold and 4-fold sites. This is because transitions at the 2-fold sites in vertebrate mitochondrial code are all synonymous but transversions at the 2-fold sites are all nonsynonymous. At 0-fold sites, both transitions and transversions are nonsynonymous; at 4-fold sites, both transitions and transversions are synonymous. Thus,

transition bias at the 0-fold and 4-fold sites are attributed mainly to mutation bias (Xia et al., 1996). In contrast, transition bias at 2-fold sites results
from both mutation bias and purifying selection against nonsynonymous
substitutions (Xia et al., 1996).

The last step is to compute K_A and K_S based on the following two
equations:

$$K_S = \frac{L_2 A_2 + L_4 A_4}{L_2 + L_4} + B_4$$

$$K_A = \frac{L_0 B_0 + L_2 B_2}{L_0 + L_2} + A_0 \tag{4.8}$$

Note that, for vertebrate mitochondrial code, transitions at 2-fold sites
are all synonymous and transversions at 2-fold sites are all nonsynonymous. LPB93 method assumes that synonymous transitions at 2-fold sites
and 4-fold sites, being synonymous, occur at the same rate. Consequently,
their rate is estimated by the weighted average as shown in the first term
for K_S in Eq. (4.8). Similarly, transversions at the 2-fold site and 0-fold
sites, both being nonsynonymous, are assumed to have the same rate and
estimated as the weighted average as shown in the first term for K_A in
Eq. (4.8). In short, K_S is the sum of transversions at the 4-fold sites plus
transitions at the 2-fold and 4-fold sites. K_A is the sum of transitions at the
0-fold sites plus transversions at the 0-fold and 2-fold sites.

The equations above assumes (1) that all transitions at the 2-fold sites
are synonymous, which is true for vertebrate mitochondrial code and nearly
true for all other genetic codes, (2) synonymous transition rates at the
2-fold and 4-fold sites are the same, and are best estimated by a weighted
average, (3) transversions at the 2-fold sites are all nonsynonymous, which
is also true for vertebrate mitochondrial genetic code and nearly true for
all other genetic codes, and (4) nonsynonymous transversions at the 2-fold
sites and at 0-fold sites have the same rate which is best estimated by
a weighted average. These assumptions appear reasonable, although a
previous study (Xia, 1998b) showed that nonsynonymous transversions
at 2-fold sites involve amino acids more similar than nonsynonymous
transversions at 0-fold sites.

The estimated K_S and K_A are 1.69216 and 0.1020, respectively. The
approximate formula for variance of K_S and K_A can be obtained by
using the delta method (Xia, 2018a, Appendix). However, a more robust

estimation is by resampling (bootstrapping or jackknifing). Both methods are implemented in DAMBE.

4.2.2.2 THE UGLINESS OF INAPPLICABLE CASES IN CORRECTING FOR MULTIPLE HITS

We will find the method above inapplicable when we attempt to compute K_A and K_S between $S1$ and $S3$. The basic counts such as N_i, s_i, v_i are listed in Table 4.9b, but we cannot compute A_4 and B_4. This is because Eq. (4.7) needs $\ln(1 - 2Q_4)$, but $Q_4 = 0.54545$ between $S1$ and $S3$ (Table 4.9b) leads to $(1 - 2Q_4) = (1 - 2*0.54545) < 0$ (Table 4.9). Logarithm is undefined for a number smaller than or equal to 0. This evil of inapplicable cases is frequently associated with independent estimation (IE), i.e., when the correction for multiple hits is based on information only from two sequences.

The original program for computing LPB93, as written by Andrey Zharkikh, would fall back to JC69 model when K80 becomes inapplicable. Other programs do the same simply because there is no other alternative. This has often generated seemingly inexplicable K_A and K_S values when two highly divergence sequences have smaller K_A and K_S values than two less divergent sequences. The cause for this peculiarity is that K80 is inapplicable for the high-divergence sequence pair and K_A and K_S values are then calculated with JC69 correction, whereas the two less divergent sequences have their K_A and K_S values calculated with the K80 correction. Because the JC69 correction typically results in severe underestimation relative to the K80 correction, the more divergent sequence pair ends up having smaller K_A and K_S values than the less divergent sequences. Strangely, this problem, which could be fixed by using simultaneous estimation (SE) illustrated below, is not fixed in all programs except in DAMBE (version 7 and newer) for calculating LPB93 distances.

4.2.2.3 TWO APPROACHES TO AVOID INAPPLICABLE CASES

The first approach to avoid the inapplicable cases is to replace IE by simultaneous estimation (SE) in correcting for multiple hits in estimating A_i and B_i. I will use the K80 model (Kimura, 1980) to illustrate the principle of SE distance estimation based on the likelihood framework. The K80 model, as shown in a previous chapter on nucleotide substitution models, has two parameters, which can be expressed either as αt and βt, or as D and κ. With three sequences $S1$, $S2$, and $S3$, we have three sequence pairs. The expected proportions of transitions and transversions for sequences i and j, designated by EP_{ij} and EQ_{ij} and expressed in D_{ij} and κ, respectively, are

$$EP_{ij} = \frac{1}{4} + \frac{1}{4}e^{-\frac{4D_{ij}}{\kappa+2}} - \frac{1}{2}e^{-\frac{2D_{ij}(\kappa+1)}{\kappa+2}}$$

(4.9)

$$EQ_{ij} = \frac{1}{2} - \frac{1}{2}e^{-\frac{4D_{ij}}{\kappa+2}}$$

We will illustrate with the 4-fold sites, and extracted relevant data for 4-fold sites from Table 4.9 and present them in Table 4.10. Let $N_i = N - N_s - N_v$, the log-likelihood function for the SE method is:

$$\begin{aligned} \ln L = &N_{s.12}\ln[EP_{12}] + N_{v.12}\ln[EQ_{12}] + N_{i.12}\ln[1 - EP_{12} - EQ_{12}] \\ &+ N_{s.13}\ln[EP_{13}] + N_{v.13}\ln[EQ_{13}] + N_{i.13}\ln[1 - EP_{13} - EQ_{13}] \\ &+ N_{s.23}\ln[EP_{23}] + N_{v.23}\ln[EQ_{23}] + N_{i.23}\ln[1 - EP_{23} - EQ_{23}] \end{aligned}$$

(4.10)

TABLE 4.10 Counting data for 4-fold sites extracted from Table 4.9, with N being the number of 4-fold sites, and N_s and N_v being the number of transitions and transversions observed at 4-fold sites. D is the estimated distance and is partitioned into transitional and transversional contributions A and B, respectively, $\kappa = 2.50260762$.

Seq. pair	N_s	N_v	N	D	A	B
$S1$ vs $S2$	3	4	11	1.4909455	0.82869	0.66226
$S1$ vs $S3$	2	6	11	32. 8469259	18.25675	14.59018
$S2$ vs $S3$	2	2	12	0.4492651	0.24971	0.19956

We could take partial derivative of lnL with respect to D_{12}, D_{13}, D_{23}, and κ, set them to zero and solve the four simultaneous equations for the four unknowns or use one of the ready-to-use algorithms in Press (1992) to obtain the four parameters that maximize lnL. The resulting estimates are shown in Table 4.10, with the maximized lnL equal to -33.49298986.

Note that $D = \alpha t + 2\beta t$ for the K80 model, and $\kappa = \alpha/\beta$, so that the proportion of D due to transition is $\alpha t/(\alpha t + 2\beta t) = \kappa\beta t/(\kappa\beta t + 2\beta t) = \kappa/(\kappa+2)$, and the rest is due to transversion. This partitions D to A (transitions) and

B (transversions) as shown in Table 4.10. We do the same for 0-fold and 2-fold sites to obtain their *A* and *B*, and K_A and K_S are then computed from Eq. (4.8) as before. Thus, SE estimation allows us to eliminate the inapplicable case encountered when computing K_a and K_s between *S1* and *S3* (Table 4.9).

The K80 model does not account for codon frequencies. Using the F84 or TN93 model would directly account for the nucleotide frequencies at the 0-fold, 2-fold, and 4-fold sites and indirectly (and partially) account for codon usage bias. To use F84 model, we simply replace EP_{ij} for K80 in Eq. (4.10) by the equivalent terms for F84 which have already been derived in the chapter on nucleotide substitution models. To obtain A and B in Eq. (4.7):

$$A = D_{F84} \frac{R_{F84}}{R_{F84} + 1}; B = D_{F84} - A$$

$$R_{F84} = \frac{\pi_T \pi_C (1 + \kappa / \pi_Y) + \pi_A \pi_G (1 + \kappa / \pi_R)}{\pi_Y \pi_R} \qquad (4.11)$$

where D_{F84} is the evolutionary distance between two sequences based on the F84 model, R_{F84} is the expected number of transitions over the expected transversions after correcting for multiple hits, T, C, A, and G are the four nucleotide frequencies, R = A+G, and Y = C+T.

The SE approach does not completely eliminate the inapplicable cases. For example, we may have only two sequences such as *S1* and *S3* and wish to obtain K_A and K_S from them, or several extremely divergent sequences that happen to all have pairwise $Q_{ij} \geq 0.5$ or $(1 - 2P_{ij} - Q_{ij}) \leq 0$ at 4-fold sites. One way to avoid such inapplicable cases is to adopt the same formulation as specified in Eq. (4.6) by assuming the same κ at the 0-fold sites (where all substitutions are nonsynonymous and presumably have similar fixation probability) and 4-fold sites (where all substitutions are synonymous and presumably also have the same fixation probability), so we estimate the same κ for this two categories of sites. That is, $\kappa_{0\text{-}fold} \approx \kappa_{4\text{-}fold} \approx \kappa$. Because 0-fold sites will almost never experience full substitution saturation, and because there are always more 0-fold sties than 4-fold sites, we generally should not encounter inapplicable cases.

Now we have covered four different versions of the LPB93 method to estimate K_A and K_S: (1) K80 correction with IE (K80+IE), (2) K80 correction with SE (K80+SE), (3) F84 correction with SE (F84+SE), and (4)

F84 correction with SE but with the same κ for 0-fold and 4-fold sites (F84+SE, $\kappa_{0\text{-}fold} = \kappa_{4\text{-}fold}$). Figure 4.4 contrasts these four versions with mitochondrial *COX1* sequences from eight vertebrate species in a file VertCOI.fas that comes with DAMBE installation (Xia, 2018b). K80+IE is the original LPB93, with two prominent features different from the rest. First, K_A/K_S ratio is high (Fig. 4.4a) relative to the other three versions (Fig. 4.4c,d,e). Just replacing IE with SE results in substantially smaller K_A/K_S ratio (e.g., contrasting Fig. 4.4a and Fig. 4.4b). Replacing K80 by F84 leads to even smaller K_A/K_S ratio. There is little change in K_A between K80+SE and F84+SE, K_S is much greater with F84 than with K80 (Fig. 4.4b vs. Fig. 4.4c). Thus, accounting for frequency differences by F84 alleviates the effect of underestimating K_S by the K80 correction, which I validated with simulated sequences.

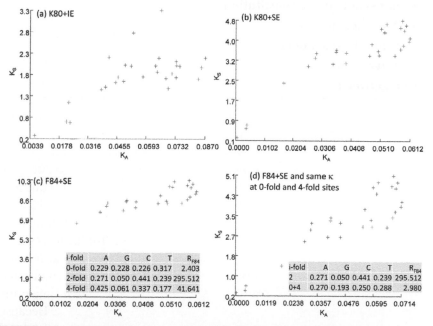

FIGURE 4.4 Contrasting the four versions of the LPB93 method: (a) K80 correction with IE (K80+IE), (b) K80 correction with SE (K80+SE), (c) F84 correction with SE (F84+SE), and (d) F84 correction with SE but with the same κ for 0-fold and 4-fold sites (F84+SE, $\kappa_{0\text{-}fold} = \kappa_{4\text{-}fold}$). Nucleotide frequencies at *i*-fold sites are shown for (c) and (d).

Forcing the same κ at 0-fold and 4-fold sites (Fig. 4.4d) results in a reduction in estimated K_S (contrasting Figs 4.4c and 4.4d), partly because it obscures the differences in nucleotide frequencies between 0-fold and 4-fold sites. While nucleotide frequencies for this set of mitochondrial COI sequences are roughly equal at 0-fold sites, they are AC-biased at the 4-fold sites. However, for aligned sequences with a well-established topology that can be assumed to be the true tree, substitutions obtained from F84+SE recovers the true tree less frequently than (F84+SE, $\kappa_{0\text{-}fold} = \kappa_{4\text{-}fold}$) which is DAMBE's default implementation of LPB93.

KEYWORDS

- **synonymous substitution**
- **nonsynonymous substitution**
- **AA-based model**
- **codon-based model**
- **eigenvalue**
- **eigenvector**

CHAPTER 5

Substitution Rate Heterogeneity Over Sites

ABSTRACT

Rate heterogeneity over sites refers to the observation of differential evolutionary rates among different sites in aligned sequences. For protein-coding sequences, third codon sites are mostly 2-fold and 4-fold degenerate, whereas the second codon sites are invariably nonsynonymous, leading to much faster evolutionary rate at third codon position than at second codon position. For RNAs forming stem-loop secondary structure, stem regions are typically much more conserved than loop regions. Rate heterogeneity over sites can strongly affect evolutionary distance and branch length estimation and needs to be modeled, typically by gamma-distributed rates. I explore factors affecting rate heterogeneity, present a simple method for estimating the alpha parameter of the gamma distribution, and apply the estimation method to study rate heterogeneity among the three codon sites. Finally, I emphasize the point that the shape parameter of the gamma distribution used to describe rate heterogeneity over site, as estimated from sequences, may depend on topology as well as on sequences.

The substitution models we have learned in the previous chapters assume all sites in a set of aligned sequences to evolve independently at the same rate. However, many factors are known to contribute to rate heterogeneity over sites. Here we (1) outline a few biological factors contributing the rate heterogeneity, (2) list several evolutionary distances based on the assumption that the evolutionary rates over sites are drawn from a gamma distribution, (3) present a simple and fast method for estimating the shape parameter of the gamma distribution, and (4) emphasize the point that the shape parameter of the gamma distribution, as estimated from aligned sequences, may not necessarily be a property of the sequences because its value may vary dramatically among competing topologies.

5.1   CAUSES FOR RATE HETEROGENEITY OVER SITES

For protein-coding genes, the substitution rate at the three codon positions, designated by r_1, r_2, and r_3, respectively, are typically in the order of $r_3 > r_1 > r_2$. This rate heterogeneity over codon positions has been attributed to two factors (Xia, 1998b). First, substitutions are always nonsynonymous at the second codon position, mostly nonsynonymous at the first codon positions, and frequently synonymous at the third codon position. Second, nonsynonymous substitutions at the second codon position involve very different amino acid, whereas those at the third codon position involve similar amino acids. This rate heterogeneity over codon sites depends on the intensity of purifying selection. For functionally unimportant genes, with pseudogenes as an extreme case, the difference among r_1, r_2, and r_3 is small. For functionally important genes such as ribosome protein genes or histone genes, the difference becomes dramatic.

There are rate heterogeneity even among synonymous substitutions, mediated by differential selection imposed by differential tRNA availability (Xia, 2018a, Chapter 9). For example, in highly expressed yeast (*Saccharomyces cerevisiae*) genes compiled in EMBOSS (Rice et al., 2000), we observe 314 AGA codons and only a single AGG codon. Both codons encode amino acid Arg. The difference in their usage can be attributed mainly to differential tRNA availability. The yeast genome encodes 11 tRNA[Arg/UCU] to decode AGA but only a single tRNA[Arg/CCU] to decode AGG without wobble pairing. This tRNA-mediated selection would favor G→A replacement at third site of AGR codons. However, another codon family, e.g., AAR for Lys, may not have such differential tRNA availability and consequently does not favor G→A replacement at third site of AAR codons. Differential codon usage and adaptation have been observed not only in sense codons (Akashi, 1994; Ikemura, 1981a, 1981b, 1982, 1992; Moriyama and Powell, 1997; Ran and Higgs, 2012; Xia, 1998a, 2008) but also in stop codons mediated by differential concentration of release factors that decode stop codons (Wei et al., 2016; Wei and Xia, 2017).

Protein genes have functionally important and unimportant domains that evolve at different rates. Some proteins (e.g., human insulin) are processed in such a way that some part of the polypeptides are discarded and do not appear in the mature protein, with those discarded segments having higher evolutionary rates than those retained in the mature protein. Such rate heterogeneity among functional domains can often be detected by measuring the K_A/K_S ratio (nonsynonymous substitutions over synonymous substitutions) over a sliding window (Xia and Kumar, 2006).

RNA genes such as rRNA and tRNA genes need to maintain a stable stem-loop secondary structure for their normal function. The stem regions are typically conserved and the loop regions evolve rapidly (Wang et al., 2006). The 18S rRNA has highly conserved and variable domains with both indel and nucleotide substitution events occurring predominantly in the eight variable domains (Van de Peer et al., 1993).

5.2   GAMMA DISTRIBUTION AND GAMMA DISTANCES

Empirical studies of nucleotide substitution patterns (Gu and Zhang, 1997; Tamura and Nei, 1993; Wakeley, 1994; Yang, 1994) suggest that rate heterogeneity over sites is well approximated by gamma distribution defined as

$$f(x) = \frac{x^{\alpha-1}\beta^{\alpha}e^{-\beta x}}{\Gamma(\alpha)}; \quad \alpha, \beta > 0; 0 \le x \le \infty \tag{5.1}$$

where α determines the shape of the gamma distribution and β is a scaling parameter. Gamma distances have been derived from commonly used substitution models such as JC69, K80, F84, and TN93. Application of these distances requires a known α. We will present a simple method for estimating α (Gu and Zhang, 1997) in the next section.

The gamma distance for the JC69 model (Golding, 1983; Nei and Gojobori, 1986; Rzhetsky and Nei, 1994b), subscripted with Γ, is given below:

$$D_{JC69.\Gamma} = \frac{3\alpha}{4}\left[\left(1 - \frac{4p}{3}\right)^{-1/\alpha} - 1\right] \tag{5.2}$$

where p is the proportion of sites differing between the two alignment sequences from which D is desired. Contrasting Eq. (5.2) with the regular D_{JC69} below, we see a regularity pointed out before (Yang, 2006) that $\ln(y)$ in the regular D_{JC69}, where y is $(1 - 4p/3)$, is replaced by $-\alpha(y^{-1/\alpha} - 1)$ in $D_{JC69.\Gamma}$.

$$D_{JC69} = -\frac{3}{4}\ln\left(1 - \frac{4p}{3}\right) \tag{5.3}$$

The gamma distance for K80 (Jin and Nei, 1990; Nei, 1991) is given below together with the regular D_{K80}, derived in a previous chapter on substitution models, for comparison:

$$D_{K80.\Gamma} = \frac{\alpha}{2}[(1 - 2P - Q)^{-1/\alpha} - 1] + \frac{\alpha}{4}[(1 - 2Q)^{-1/\alpha} - 1] \tag{5.4}$$

$$\kappa_\Gamma = \frac{2[1 - 2P - Q)^{-1/\alpha} - 1]}{(1 - 2Q)^{-1/\alpha} - 1} - 1 \tag{5.5}$$

$$D_{K80} = -\frac{\ln(1 - 2P - Q)}{2} - \frac{\ln(1 - 2Q)}{4} \tag{5.6}$$

$$\kappa = \frac{2\ln(1 - 2P - Q)}{\ln(1 - 2Q)} - 1 \tag{5.7}$$

where P and Q are proportions of sites differing by a transition and a transversion, respectively, between two aligned sequences from which a distance is desired. We again see that $D_{K80.\Gamma}$ can be obtained by replacing $\ln(y)$ in the regular D_{K80} by $-\alpha(y^{-1/\alpha} - 1)$. Here we have $y_1 = 1 - 2P - Q$, and $y_2 = 1 - 2Q$. We replace $\ln(y_1)$ by $-\alpha(y_1^{-1/\alpha} - 1)$ and $\ln(y_2)$ by $-\alpha(y_2^{-1/\alpha} - 1)$ to get $D_{K80.\Gamma}$ and κ_Γ.

We can do the same to replace $\ln(y)$ by $-\alpha(y^{-1/\alpha} - 1)$ to obtain the gamma distance for F84 (Yang, 1994). The regular $DF84$ needs αt and βt which were derived in a previous chapter on substitution models. We now use y_1 and y_2 to represent the arguments of the logarithms:

$$\alpha t = -\ln\left|1 - \frac{S}{2(\pi_C\pi_T/\pi_Y + \pi_A\pi_G/\pi_R)} - \frac{(\pi_C\pi_T\pi_R/\pi_Y + \pi_A\pi_G\pi_Y/\pi_R)V}{2(\pi_C\pi_T\pi_R + \pi_A\pi_G\pi_Y)}\right| = -\ln(y_1) \tag{5.8}$$

$$\beta t = -\ln\left|1 - \frac{V}{2\pi_R\pi_Y}\right| = -\ln(y_2) \tag{5.9}$$

For $D_{F84.\Gamma}$, we will express αt and βt in the format of $-\alpha(y^{-1/\alpha} - 1)$. To avoid confusion between the α in αt and the shape parameter of the gamma distribution, I will use *at* and *bt* in equations below for αt and βt in Eqs. (5.8)–(5.9), respectively.

$$at = \alpha\left(y_1^{-1/\alpha} - 1\right)$$

$$bt = \alpha\left(y_2^{-1/\alpha} - 1\right)$$

(5.10)

The equation for $D_{F84.\Gamma}$ is of the same form as the regular D_{F84}:

$$D_{F84.\Gamma} = 2at\left(\frac{\pi_C\pi_T}{\pi_Y} + \frac{\pi_A\pi_G}{\pi_R}\right) - 2bt\left(\frac{\pi_C\pi_T\pi_R}{\pi_Y} + \frac{\pi_A\pi_G\pi_Y}{\pi_R} - \pi_Y\pi_R\right)$$ (5.11)

We do the same to obtain the gamma distance for TN93 (Tamura and Nei, 1993). The regular D_{TN93} needs $\alpha_R t$, $\alpha_Y t$, and βt that have been derived in a previous chapter. We now use y_1, y_2, and y_3 to represent the arguments for the logarithms:

$$\alpha_R t = -\ln\left(1 - \frac{\pi_R S_R}{2\pi_A\pi_G} - \frac{V}{2\pi_R}\right) = -\ln(y_1)$$ (5.12)

$$\alpha_Y t = -\ln\left(1 - \frac{\pi_Y S_Y}{2\pi_C\pi_T} - \frac{V}{2\pi_Y}\right) = -\ln(y_2)$$ (5.13)

$$\beta t = -\ln\left(1 - \frac{V}{2\pi_R\pi_Y}\right) = -\ln(y_3)$$ (5.14)

To obtain $D_{TN93.\Gamma}$, we rewrite

$$a_R t = \alpha\left(y_1^{-1/\alpha} - 1\right)$$ (5.15)

$$a_Y t = \alpha\left(y_2^{-1/\alpha} - 1\right)$$ (5.16)

$$bt = \alpha\left(y_3^{-1/\alpha} - 1\right)$$ (5.17)

$D_{TN93.\Gamma}$ is of the same form as for regular D_{TN93}:

$$D_{TN93} = \frac{2\pi_A \pi_G}{\pi_R}\left(a_R t - \pi_Y bt\right) + \frac{2\pi_C \pi_T}{\pi_Y}\left(a_Y t - \pi_R bt\right) + 2\pi_R \pi_Y bt \quad (5.18)$$

These distances have been implemented in DAMBE (Xia, 2013b; Xia, 2017a) together with distance-based phylogenetic methods.

5.3 ESTIMATING THE SHAPE PARAMETER OF A GAMMA DISTRIBUTION

We need to estimate α from empirical substitution data in order to compute the gamma distances in the previous section. The method by Gu and Zhang (Gu and Zhang, 1997) is very fast and reasonably accurate, and is available in DAMBE (Xia, 2013b; Xia, 2017a). The estimation takes a set of aligned sequences and is done in three steps: (1) construct a phylogenetic tree from the aligned sequences and reconstruct ancestral sequences at internal nodes of the tree, (2) perform pairwise comparisons along the tree between two nodes on each side of a branch to obtain observed number of substitutions per site and then apply correction for multiple hits to get the estimated number of substitutions per site, and (3) estimate the shape parameter (α) using the following probability density function (Johnson and Kotz, 1969):

$$f(k) = \frac{\Gamma(\alpha+k)}{\Gamma(k+1)\Gamma(\alpha)}\left(\frac{\bar{k}}{\bar{k}+\alpha}\right)^k \left(\frac{\alpha}{\bar{k}+\alpha}\right)^\alpha \quad (5.19)$$

where k, instead of being integers, is replaced by the estimated number of substitutions per site, and, $\bar{k}$ is mean k. Eq. (5.19) differs from that in Gu and Zhang (Gu and Zhang, 1997) in that they wrote $\Gamma(k + 1)$ as $k!$ which is confusing because k is typically not an integer after correction for multiple substitutions. Another minor difference is that they used D for $\bar{k}$. The advantage of using the probability density function in Eq. (5.19) over that in Eq. (5.1) is that, when $k = 0$ (for monomorphic sites with no substitution), $f(k)$ cannot be computed as defined in Eq. (5.1) for $\alpha < 1$. Below I will illustrate in detail these steps which are all automated in DAMBE (Xia, 2013b; Xia, 2017a).

5.3.1   CONSTRUCTING A TREE AND INFER ANCESTRAL SEQUENCES AT INTERNAL NODE

Suppose we use the aligned sequences in the file VertCOI.fas (Fig. 5.1a) that comes with DAMBE installation (Xia, 2013b; Xia, 2017a). The file contains mitochondrial COI sequences from eight vertebrate species, with 1512 aligned sites and no indels. We will learn molecular phylogenetic methods for building trees with distance-based, maximum parsimony and maximum likelihood methods later, but any of these methods will generate the same topology in Figure 5.1b.

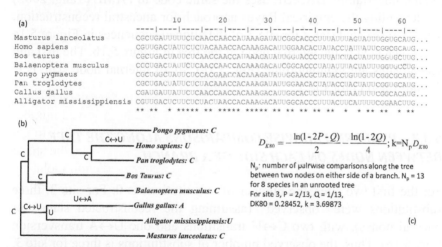

FIGURE 5.1   Phylogenetic reconstruction and estimation of site-specific number of substitutions. (a) Aligned mitochondrial COI sequences from eight vertebrate species (shown partially) in file VertCOI.fas that comes with DAMBE installation (Xia, 2013b; Xia, 2017a). (b) Phylogenetic tree with reconstructed ancestral states for site 3 in the aligned sequences. (c) Correcting for multiple hits by using K80 distance. k (=3.69873) is the estimated number of substitutions at site 3.

Reconstructing ancestral states started with the application of the maximum parsimony algorithm (Fitch, 1971; Hartigan, 1973). The approach was popularized by MacClade (Maddison and Maddison, 2000) and PAUP (Swofford, 1993; Swofford, 2000) which included many options for handling nonuniqueness of reconstructed states. More recent approaches include empirical Bayes for nucleotide and amino acid sequences (Yang et al., 1995) and for amino acid sequences with options to incorporate structural information (Koshi and Goldstein, 1996). A web server taking the empirical Bayes approach is available (Ashkenazy et al., 2012) for reconstructing ancestral nucleotide, amino acid, and codon sequences. The empirical Bayes approach assumes that the tree and branch lengths are correctly estimated. Because the tree and branch lengths in reality are uncertain, a more general hierarchical Bayesian approach (Huelsenbeck and Bollback, 2001; Pagel et al., 2004) has been investigated by using Markov chain Monte Carlo techniques for sampling phylogenetic trees and associated parameters. However, the reconstructed states from this general approach are similar to those from empirical Bayes except with greater uncertainty. DAMBE uses the same code in PAML (Yang, 2002) implementing the empirical Bayes approach for ancestral reconstruction. The reconstructed states for site 3 of the aligned sequences in Figure 5.1a are shown next to the internal node of the tree in Figure 5.1b. The first and second sites are monomorphic (Fig. 5.1a), so all internal node state is C for site 1 and G for site 2.

5.3.2   PERFORM PAIRWISE COMPARISONS ALONG THE TREE BETWEEN NODES ON EACH SIDE OF A BRANCH

For the first two sites, the number of substitutions is 0. For site 3, three substitutions were "observed" (assuming the reconstructed states for internal nodes), with two C↔U transitions and one U↔A transversion (Fig. 5.1b). Thus, the observed number of substitutions is three for site 3. Correcting for multiple hits by using the K80 model (Fig. 5.1c) results in the estimated number of substitutions being k (=3.69873). Note that the K80 distance calculated this way uses only one site of information. A more robust correction is to use all sites to estimate the transition/transversion ratio and estimate k by using this fixed transition/transversion ratio for all sites. I illustrate these two approaches with the K80 model from which the expected proportion of transitions and transversions are

$$E(P) = \frac{1}{4} + \frac{1}{4}e^{-(4D/(\kappa+2))} - \frac{1}{2}e^{-((2D(\kappa+1))/\kappa+2)}$$

$$E(Q) = \frac{1}{2} - \frac{1}{2}e^{-(4D/(\kappa+2))}$$

$$(5.20)$$

For site 3, the observed P and Q are 2/13 and 1/13, respectively (Fig. 5.1c). Replacing $E(P)$ and $E(Q)$ by the observed P and Q allow us to solve for D and κ. This approach using only one site of information may often lead to inapplicable cases when D_{K80} cannot be estimated, especially when there are only eight or fewer sequences. In particularly, the inapplicable cases will increase with more complicated but more realistic substitution models, e.g., F84.

We can combine information from all sites to perform simultaneous estimation. We rewrite Eq. (5.20) slightly differently to indicate that each site i has its site-specific D_i but all share the same κ:

$$E(P_i) = \frac{1}{4} + \frac{1}{4}e^{-(4D_i/(\kappa+2))} - \frac{1}{2}e^{-((2D_i(\kappa+1))/(\kappa+2))}$$

$$E(Q_i) = \frac{1}{2} - \frac{1}{2}e^{-(4D_i/(\kappa+2))}$$

(5.21)

Now we can estimate all D_i and κ by maximizing the following log-likelihood:

$$\ln L = \sum_{i=1}^{N}\left\{N_{s,i}\ln\left[E(P_i)\right] + N_{v,i}\ln\left[E(Q_i)\right] + N_{I,i}\ln\left[1 - E(P_i) - E(Q_i)\right]\right\}$$

(5.22)

where N is the number of branches, $N_{s,i}$, $N_{v,i}$, and $N_{I,i}$ are recorded number of transitional difference, transversional difference, and no difference from pairwise comparisons along the tree between nodes on each side of each branch ($N = N_{s,i} + N_{v,i} + N_{I,i}$). For example, $N_{s,3} = 2$, $N_{v,3} = 1$, and $N_{I,3} = 10$ (Fig. 5.1b). The resulting D_i is then multiplied by N_p (Fig. 5.1c) to obtain k_i. This simultaneous estimation is implemented in version 7 of DAMBE (Xia, 2013b; Xia, 2017a) with the F84 substitution model.

5.3.3 ESTIMATE THE SHAPE PARAMETER (α)

Of the 1512 aligned sites, 869 sites are monomorphic ($k = 0$). On the other extreme, one site recorded five transitions and two transversions, with $k = 11.5642$ (Table 5.1). The log-likelihood function for estimating α, following the notation in Table 5-1, is

$$\ln L = \sum N_i \ln\left[f(k_i)\right]$$

(5.23)

where $f(k)$ is defined in Eq. (5.19). For any given α value, we can obtain the column of $f(k)$ value according to Eq. (5.19). Summing up the $N \times \ln[f(k)]$

column in Table 5.1 gives ln$L$. The largest ln$L$ is -1942.924472, arrived when $\alpha = 0.4977$ which is therefore the maximum likelihood estimate of α. With k and N columns in Table 5.1, one can easily solve for α by using Solver in Microsoft EXCEL or the optimize function in R.

TABLE 5.1   Estimated k and the number sites with the same k value (N). $f(k)$ is defined in Eq. (5.19) with values for $\alpha = 0.4977$.

k	N	$f(k)$	$N \times \ln[f(k)]$	k	N	$f(k)$	$N \times \ln[f(k)]$
0	869	0.5494	-520.5370	4.7909	3	0.0870	-7.3256
1.0429	121	0.1889	-201.6587	5.1005	10	0.0256	-36.6657
1.0962	60	0.1863	-100.8256	5.4592	34	0.0409	-108.7124
2.1799	107	0.1075	-238.5962	5.8814	15	0.0732	-39.2279
2.2996	59	0.1136	-128.3390	6.3893	2	0.0256	-7.3332
2.4340	50	0.1217	-105.3292	7.2630	2	0.0143	-8.4925
3.4244	50	0.0825	-124.7452	7.8998	1	0.0414	-3.1835
3.6278	41	0.0992	-94.7368	8.6969	4	0.0211	-15.4428
3.8594	64	0.1240	-133.5730	10.2276	1	0.0042	-5.4681
4.1260	18	0.0408	-57.5806	11.5642	1	0.0058	-5.1513

When $\alpha \leq 1$, the distribution of k is L-shaped (Fig. 5.2) with a strong right skew. Such a plot sometimes helps us appreciate the rate heterogeneity over sites. Some sites hardly change but some other sites could have experienced nearly 12 substitutions (Table 5.1).

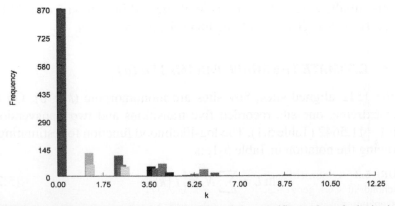

FIGURE 5.2   Frequency distribution of k (estimated site-specific number of substitutions). Output from DAMBE (Xia, 2013b; Xia, 2017a).

5.4   CONTRASTING RATE HETEROGENEITY OVER SITES AMONG THREE CODON POSITIONS

The three codon positions are expected to exhibit different heterogeneity (Xia, 1998b). Substitutions at the third codon positions are mostly synonymous and expected to occur at similar rates approximating neutral substitutions (Xia, 2009; Xia and Yang, 2011). Consequently, there should be relatively little rate heterogeneity at the third codon position. Substitutions at the first and second codon positions are almost all nonsynonymous. While substitutions at some functionally unimportant site might be close to neutral ones, some sites are expected to be strongly conserved. Thus, their rate differences among sites would span from nearly neutral rate at unimportant sites to almost no substitution at functionally constrained sites. This implies greater rate heterogeneity at the first and second codon positions than at the third codon position. This expectation is substantiated by empirical data illustrated here with the aligned mitochondrial COI sequences from eight vertebrate species in the VertCOI.fas file that comes with DAMBE (Fig. 5.3). The rate heterogeneity is small at the third codon position (Fig. 5.3c) relative to those at the first and second codon positions (Fig. 5.3a,b). The third codon position also evolves in a more clock-like manner than the first and second codon positions (Xia, 2009; Xia and

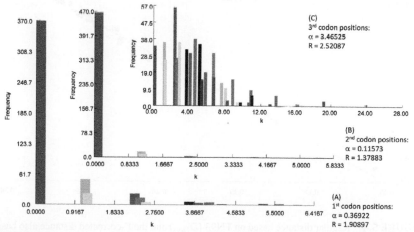

FIGURE 5.3   Contrast of rate heterogeneity among three codon positions of the vertebrate mitochondrial COI gene, together with estimated shape parameter α and transition/transversion ratio (R) for the F84 model used in DNAML. Output from DAMBE (Xia, 2013b; Xia, 2017a).

Yang, 2011). The α value is the smallest for the 2nd codon position (Fig. 5.3b), which may be attributable to the observation that nonsynonymous substitutions at the 2nd codon position involve substantially more different amino acids than at the 1st codon position (Xia, 1998b).

5.5 COMPARISON OF DISTANCES WITH OR WITHOUT Γ-CORRECTION

Evolutionary distances with or without Γ-correction are typically highly correlated and generate very similar phylogenetic trees. Figure 5.4 shows a plot of the regular TN93 distance (D_{TN93}) versus the Γ-corrected TN93 distance ($D_{TN93.\Gamma}$), calculated from the aligned mitochondrial COI sequences from the eight vertebrate species in the file VertCOI.fas that comes with DAMBE (Xia, 2013b; Xia, 2017a). D_{TN93} and $D_{TN93.\Gamma}$ are highly correlated and both generate the same topology in Figure 5.1b. However, with highly diverged sequences, $D_{TN93.\Gamma}$ fluctuates quite wildly and is definitely not a robust distance.

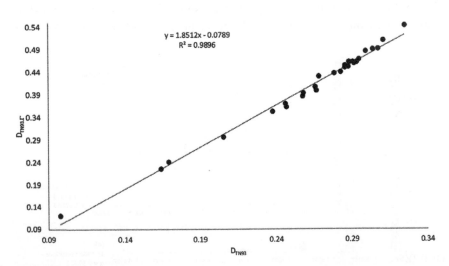

FIGURE 5.4 Regular distance based on TN93 (D_{TN93}) and the Γ-corrected distance also based on TN93 ($D_{TN93.\Gamma}$).

5.6   SHAPE PARAMETER α AND TOPOLOGY

So far we have discussed rate heterogeneity over sites as a sequence property. However, when rate heterogeneity over sites is modeled by a gamma distribution with the shape parameter α estimated from aligned sequences as a description of rate heterogeneity over sites, it is no longer just a sequence property, but also depends on tree topology. An intuitive understanding of this dependence of rate heterogeneity over sites on topology is perhaps best illustrated by a set of four sequences (Fig. 5.5a) from a parsimony perspective. With a star tree (Fig. 5.5b), each of the three sequence sites will require a minimum of two independent substitutions, so there is no rate heterogeneity over sites. However, for a resolved tree in Figure 5.5c, one site (with identical nucleotides between sister groups such as the first site in Fig. 5.5a) would require a minimum of only one substitution, but two other sites (with different nucleotides between sister groups such as the 2nd and 3rd sites in Fig. 5.5a) would require a minimum of two independent substitutions. Thus, sites 2 and 3 evolve faster than site 1, giving rise to rate heterogeneity. This is the same with the likelihood method or Bayesian inference that use a substitution model to correct for multiple hits. Thus, with a star tree, we will find no rate heterogeneity over sites, with a very large estimated α typically equal to 10,000 which is the upper limit of most computer programs implementing substitution models with gamma-distributed rates. In contrast, if we allow a resolved tree, then the estimated α may be equal or even smaller than 1 indicating very strong rate heterogeneity.

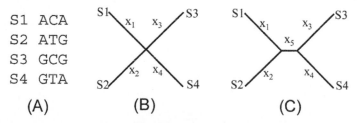

S1	ACA
S2	ATG
S3	GCG
S4	GTA

(A)   (B)   (C)

FIGURE 5.5   Estimated shape parameter α depends on tree topology.

In phylogenetic literature, one frequently finds interpretations of a small α as evidence of strong rate heterogeneity over sites and of strong purifying selection constraining certain sites but not others. The dependence of the

α parameter on both sequences and the tree topology cautions us against such an interpretation unless we are sure that the phylogeny is correct (of which we are almost never sure).

KEYWORDS

- **rate heterogeneity over sites**
- **gamma distribution**
- **fast estimation method**
- **gamma distances**
- **shape parameter**
- **rate heterogeneity among codon sites**

CHAPTER 6

Maximum Parsimony Method in Phylogenetics

ABSTRACT

A phylogenetic tree offers a simple way of visualizing evolutionary history. Out of many possible trees that one can draw to connect different species, we must have a criterion to choose the best tree, just as we need a criterion to choose the best alignment (the highest alignment score given the scoring scheme) or the best substitution model (the smallest information-theoretic indices). Maximum parsimony (MP) is one of the criteria for choosing the best phylogenetic tree, i.e., the tree that requires the smallest number of changes to account for the sequence variation is the best tree. This chapter details two frequently used algorithms used in the MP framework to obtain the minimum number of changes: The Fitch algorithm, which assumes all nucleotides or amino acids replacing each other with equal frequency, and the Sankoff algorithm, which uses the cost matrix to accommodate differential substitution rate among different nucleotides or different amino acids. The Fitch algorithm uses phylogenetic signals only in the so-called informative sites, but the Sankoff algorithm can use information beyond informative sites. Both belong to the dynamic programming algorithm we were first exposed to in the chapter on sequence alignment. The long-branch attraction problem, which is associated not only with the MP method but also with other methods that do not correct, or insufficiently correct, for multiple substitutions, is numerically illustrated in detail. Two different ways of reporting statistical support for a phylogenetic tree are presented: The resampling method (bootstrapping and jackknifing) and the statistical test of alternative topologies. Various ways of improving the power of the statistical tests are included and discussed.

6.1   INTRODUCTION

Phylogenetics has two main objectives. The first is to build phylogenetic relationships among operational taxonomic units (OTUs, which could be a group of species or a gene family with duplicated genes). The second is to date speciation or gene duplication events. There are four categories of methods that can contribute to the first objective, maximum parsimony, distance-based, maximum likelihood method, and Bayesian inference, but only the last three can contribute to the second objective.

The maximum parsimony method (MP), as well as the maximum likelihood (ML) method that will be covered in a later chapter, is character-based. Its great success, facilitated by the excellent program PAUP (Swofford, 1993; Swofford, 2000), resulted in a rapid expansion of the field and development of alternative and better phylogenetic methods that eventually ended with its decreasing popularity in recent years. It is still useful for a variety of purposes and often serves as an entry point for molecular phylogenetics. Excellent sources of references on the theory and application of MP include Hillis et al. (1996) and Brooks and McLennan (1991).

MP uses a parsimonious criterion to choose the best tree, i.e., the tree that can account for the sequence variation with the smallest number of substitutions or the smallest substitution cost is the best tree. MP does not specify an explicit substitution model or make any explicit effort in correcting for multiple hits. For this reason, it has the inherent assumption of a slow rate of evolution (so slow that multiple hits are negligible). Because molecular phylogenetics is moving toward resolving deep phylogenies which typically involve sequences with multiple substitutions at the same site, MP has gradually faded away, like an old soldier.

MP remains popular among phylogeneticists working on plants, but much less so among those working on animals. There is a good reason for this difference. Historically, most phylogenies were reconstructed with mitochondrial sequences. Animal mitochondrial genomes evolve very rapidly (Xia, 2012c) and violate a key assumption of MP (i.e., slow evolution rate). In contrast, most plant mitochondrial genomes evolve extraordinarily slowly, even slower than plant nuclear genomes (Drouin et al., 2008; Wolfe et al., 1987). Thus, MP is bad for animal mitochondrial sequences but is not bad for plant mitochondrial sequences. MP is particularly powerful in cladistics analysis of morphological, physiological, embryological, or paleontological characters (Brooks and McLennan, 1991) whose changes are slow because of functional constraints and whose rates of change cannot be rendered into a substitution model. These nonsequence data represent the last stronghold of MP. Other phylogenetic methods have sounded their trumpets around the MP castle, but the latter has so far refused to come tumbling down.

For aligned molecular sequences, two key algorithms have been used in phylogenetic reconstruction with MP: the Fitch algorithm (Fitch, 1971) and the Sankoff algorithm (Sankoff, 1975). The Fitch algorithm further assumes that all nucleotides or amino acids replace each other with equal frequencies. This is equivalent to the JC69 model but without correcting for multiple substitutions at the same site. The Sankoff algorithm makes use of a step matrix to accommodate different substitution rates among different nucleotides or among different amino acids. The step matrix is sometimes also called a cost matrix with different values for different types of substitutions.

The Sankoff algorithm, through the step matrix, is advantageous over the Fitch algorithm in two ways. First, it uses more information. For example, in a four-taxon case with a site having A, C, G, and T for the four taxa, respectively, the site is not informative for the Fitch algorithm, but is informative if transitions (A↔G or C↔T) occur at a different rate from transversions (R↔Y). Take for example four sequences ($S1$ to $S4$) with nucleotides A, G, C, and T, respectively, at site i. If we assign a cost of 1 to a transition but a cost of 2 to a transversion, then the Sankoff algorithm will favor the grouping of ($S1,S2$) with A and G, and ($S3,S4$) with C and T, whereas such a site pattern is not informative with the Fitch algorithm. Second, the step matrix alleviates the long-branch attraction problem (Felsenstein, 1978a) because frequent substitutions can be assigned a smaller cost than rare substitutions. Impossible changes will have substitute cost equal to ∞.

I will first present numerical illustrations of the Fitch and Sankoff algorithms, followed by a brief introduction on the branch-and-bound algorithm which is guaranteed to find the best topology without exhaustive searching through the tree space. Exhaustive searching and branch-and-bound algorithm are possible with MP because MP is fast, especially in comparison with computation-intensive maximum likelihood or Bayesian method. However, even with the fast MP, the exhaustive and the branch-and-bound searches can be applied to only a small number (~20) of OTUs.

The illustration of the Fitch and the Sankoff algorithms is followed by an illustration of the long-branch attraction problem which has plagued MP when the method is misapplied to molecular sequences that have experienced a high degree of substitution saturation. An advocate of the MP method can argue that it is unfair to criticize MP with the long-branch attraction problem because MP does not correct for multiple hits and, therefore, is not supposed to be used where long-branches (which implies substitution saturation) exist. However, phylogeneticists do frequently run MP on highly diverged sequences and it is only fair to highlight the long-branch attraction problem. The last section of the chapter details MP-related statistical tests (both parametric and non-parametric) for alternative topologies. Some materials in this chapter have been presented in Xia (2018a).

Both Fitch and Sankoff algorithms can reconstruct ancestral sequences. While such a reconstruction is often not unique, hence reducing its value, methods have been developed to take alternative ancestral reconstructions as initial hypotheses and evaluate them further with other methods.

6.2   THE FITCH ALGORITHM

The Fitch algorithm (Fitch, 1971) takes a topology and a set of aligned sequences, and find the minimum number of steps (nucleotide or amino acid changes). The algorithm is implemented in all programs with an MP phylogenetic function. Such a program will generate a large number of trees and let the Fitch algorithm to evaluate each. A topology with the smallest number of changes, or multiple topologies with the same minimal number of changes, will be reported as MP tree(s).

The Fitch algorithm is illustrated for the six aligned sequences in Figure 6.1. We will first focus on the first site (in bold in Fig. 6.1). There are six leaf nodes labeled $S1$ to S6, and five internal nodes labeled 7–11 (Fig. 6.1). Each node is represented by a set of characters. For example, each of the six leaf nodes is represented by a set with a single character, with $S1$ having {A}, $S2$ having {A}, and so on. For each site, the ancestral node is represented by a set that is either the intersection of the two daughter sets if the intersection is not empty, or the union of the daughter sets if the intersection is empty. For example, the ancestral node 8 has daughter nodes with {A} and {G}. The intersection of these two nodes is empty, so internal node 8 will have the union of the two daughter sets, i.e., {A,G}, represented by a single character {R} for purine. We now move to internal node 9 whose two daughter sets are {A} and {A,G}. The intersection of these two sets is not empty, so internal node 9 will be represented by the intersection of the two daughter sets, which is {A}. Now we move to internal node 10 whose two daughter sets are {A} and {C,T}, respectively. The intersection of these two daughter sets is again empty, so the ancestral state is then the union of {A} and {C,T}. This results in {A,C,T}, represented by H (Table 2.2) according to the International Union of Pure and Applied Chemistry (IUPAC), at internal node 10 (Fig. 6.1).

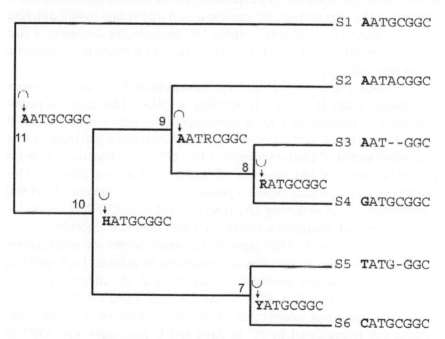

FIGURE 6.1 Reconstructing ancestral sequence states along the tree with the first site illustrated. "R" stands for purine, "Y" for pyrimidine and "H" for either A, C, or T.

We progress from the leaf node to the root and count the number of union operations each representing a nucleotide substitution. The first site in Figure 6.1 has three union operations, which means that a minimum of three nucleotide substitutions is required to explain sequence evolution at the first site given the topology. We can do the same with other sites. In this particular case, sites 2, 3, 6, 7, and 8 are monomorphic (i.e., no variation), and therefore require 0 substitutions. If we ignore sites 4 and 5 which contain indels, then the total number of steps is simply $3+0+0+0+0+0 = 3$. We now take the same approach to obtain the number of steps (nucleotide substitutions for other 6-OTU trees. The tree with the smallest number of steps is the MP tree.

We do feel a bit uneasy about ignoring sites 4 and 5. Unfortunately, MP does not have a satisfactory way of handling gaps. We surely can treat it as a fifth state, but it is unreasonable to consider the occurrence of an indel as equally likely as a nucleotide substitution. Furthermore, $S3$ has two consecutive gaps. Should we treat the two gaps equally or give differential cost to gap open and gap extension? In the Sankoff algorithm that is covered in the next section, we can use a step matrix and assign different costs to different types of substitutions. For example, we can assign a cost of 1 to a transition, 2 to a transversion, and 3 to a difference between a nucleotide and a gap.

To illustrate with site 4 (Fig. 6.1), internal node 8 is a union between two daughter sets {G} and {-}, resulting in {G,-}. This union is penalized by 3 in contrast to 1 for a union operation between two different nucleotides. That is, a union involving a nucleotide and a gap incurs a cost equivalent to that of 3 unions involving two different nucleotides. Internal node 9 is a union of {A} (site 4 of $S2$) and {G,-} (site 4 of Node 8). This results in {A,G,-}, which implies a probability of 0.5 of having {A,G} and a probability of 0.5 of having {A,-}, so the cost would be $0.5 \times 1 + 0.5 \times 3 = 2$. However, such treatment is rarely used with the Fitch algorithm.

The simplicity of the Fitch algorithm of using unions and intersections allows programmers to use bitwise operations to achieve high speed in computation. First, we represent nucleotides and the ambiguous codes ACMGR...N by 1, 2, 3, 4, 5, ..., 15 as shown in Table 6.1. We can now obtain the union and intersection by using two bitwise operations, the bitwise OR (represented by "|" in Java and C languages and "OR" in Visual Basic) and bitwise AND (represented by "&" in Java and C and "AND" in Visual Basic). Thus, the union of A (represented in binary as 00000001, Table 6.1) and G (represented in binary as 00000100, Table 6.1) is 00000001 | 00000100 = 00000101, which equals a decimal value of 5 for R (for either A or G according to the IUPAC coding). Similarly, the union of C and T is 00000010 | 00001000 = 00001010, which equals a decimal value of 10 for Y (for either C or T according to IUPAC coding).

The union of R and Y is N (any of the four nucleotides), obtained by 00000101 | 00001010 = 00001111 which equals the decimal value of 15.

TABLE 6.1 Nucleotides (Nuc), their ASCII code, assigned decimal (binary) values, and their meanings.

Nuc	ASCII	Value	Meaning
A	65	1 (00000001)	A
C	67	2 (00000010)	C
M	77	3 (00000011)	A or C
G	71	4 (00000100)	G
R	82	5 (00000101)	A or G
S	83	6 (00000110)	C or G
V	86	7 (00000111)	A or C or G
T	84	8 (00001000)	T
W	87	9 (00001001)	A or T
Y	89	10 (00001010)	C or T
H	72	11 (00001011)	A or C or T
K	75	12 (00001100)	G or T
D	68	13 (00001101)	A or G or T
B	66	14 (00001110)	C or G or T
N	78	15 (00001111)	G or A or T or C

Similarly, the intersection can be obtained by using the bitwise AND, which combines corresponding bits of two binary numbers in such a way that the result is 1 if both operand bits are 1 and is 0 otherwise. Thus, the intersection of A (00000001) and R (00000101) is 00000001 (= A & R) which means A (Table 6.1), and the intersection of Y (00001010, representing C or T) and H (00001011, representing A, C, or T) is 00001010, i.e., Y (=Y & H). Bitwise operations are extremely fast for any programming languages.

6.3 THE SANKOFF ALGORITHM

The Sankoff algorithm will take as input (1) a step matrix (C, whose elements are c_{ij} with i and j taking the value of A, C, G, T for nucleotide sequences or the 20 amino acids for the amino acid sequences), (2) a topology, and (3) a multiple sequence alignment (Fig. 6.2, which shows only a single site of an alignment with six OTUs) and will evaluate the substitution cost (or number of steps) of the topology. A computer program implementing the MP method will systematically generate a large number of topologies, feed it individually to Sankoff algorithm for evaluation and then report the topology with the smallest substitution cost as the MP tree. In reality, most published MP trees are not real MP trees because they are typically the result of a heuristic search which does not guarantee that the final tree is, in fact, the MP tree (Xia, 2007b).

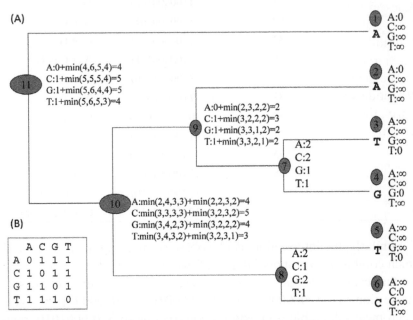

FIGURE 6.2 Computing the minimum number of changes for one site of a multiple sequence alignment using the Sankoff algorithm (A) with step matrix C in (B). All nodes are numbered sequentially, with a 4-element step vector (S) for each node.

The step matrix has dimension 4×4 for nucleotide sequences and 20×20 for amino acid sequences (or 5×5 and 21×21 if we include indel as an additional state). Its diagonal elements are zero and off-diagonal elements typically increase with the rarity of substitutions between nucleotides or amino acids. If all off-diagonal elements of a step matrix is 1, it means that all four nucleotides or all 20 amino acids replace each other with the same frequency. In this case, the Sankoff algorithm is reduced to the Fitch algorithm. However, transitions typically occur more frequently than transversions during the evolution of nucleotide sequences and are consequently given a lower value in the step matrix than transversions. Similarly, replacement between similar amino acids such as Ala and Gly will be given a smaller cost than replacement between two very different amino acids such as Gly and Arg. A step matrix represents an attempt of the MP method to approximate a substitution model used in model-based phylogenetic methods, such as the distance-based, maximum likelihood, or Bayesian methods. The main problem is that there is no objective way of assigning values in the step matrix, although an empirical substitution matrix from closely related species can be used as a guide. For example, if transitions occur three times as frequent as transversions, then we may assign a cost of 1 for a transition substitution and 3 for a transversional substitution.

The step matrix (C) in Figure 6.2B has $c_{ij} = 1$ (which means that a nucleotide substitution is counted as one step) and $c_{ii} = 0$. For such a C matrix, the results from the Sankoff algorithm are exactly the same as the Fitch algorithm. For this reason, Sankoff algorithm, which is slower than the Fitch algorithm, should be used only when we give c_{ij} different values, e.g., when a transition, such as A↔G, is given $c_{A,G} = 1$ and a transversion, such as A↔T, is given $c_{A,T} = 2$ (which means that a transversion is counted as two steps and a transition as one step). For amino acid sequences, a Trp↔Gly substitution is very rare and should have a large $c_{Trp,Gly}$, whereas an Asp↔Glu substitution is very common and $c_{Asp,Glu}$ should be small. We will first illustrate the Sankoff algorithm with the C matrix in Figure 6.2B and then with a C matrix of unequal c_{ij} ($i \neq j$).

The Sankoff algorithm, just as the Fitch algorithm, is site-based, i.e., the evaluation is done to obtain the minimum number of steps (of changes) for each site. For the Fitch algorithm, the minimum number of steps at site j (designated by L_j) is the minimum number of substitutions needed to account for the nucleotide (or amino acid) variation at site j. After evaluating all sites, the total number of steps for the tree, often designated as tree length (TL), is

$$TL = \sum_{j=1}^{N} L_j \tag{6.1}$$

where N is the number of sites in the multiple alignment. These designations are also used for the Sankoff algorithm, although here a step is typically not equivalent to a nucleotide or amino acid substitution unless the step matrix is the same as that in Figure 6.2B. The MP tree is the one with the smallest *TL*.

In contrast to the Fitch algorithm where each node can be represented by a single character, the Sankoff algorithm represents each node (either a leaf node or an internal node) by a cost vector (*S*). *S* would have 4 elements for nucleotide sequences or 20 for amino acid sequences. For simplicity, I will illustrate the algorithm with nucleotide sequences with the four elements in *S* in the order of A, C, G, and T (Fig. 6.2). For terminal nodes (leaves) with character *i*, the element corresponding to character *i* is assigned a cost of 0 and other elements are assigned ∞ (Fig. 6.2). This means, in a probabilistic sense, that the probability of the character remaining the same is 1 in a time interval of 0 (i.e., there should be no cost/penalty). Similarly, the probability of a nucleotide becoming a different one is 0 (impossible) when there is no time to change and should be given the maximum cost. In short, higher costs are associated with less likely substitutions.

For an internal node (say a, where a = 7, 8, …, or 11 in Fig. 6.2) with two daughter nodes, each element in the cost vector is the summation of two parts, one from each of the daughter nodes, according to the following equation:

$$S_a(i) = \min_j[c_{ij} + S_l(j)] + \min_k[c_{ik} + S_r(k)] \qquad (6.2)$$

where c_{ij} is the cost between characters *i* and *j* specified in Figure 6.2B, and the subscripted *l* and *r* represent the two daughter nodes of node a, following my own programming convention of representing two daughter nodes as left (*l*) and right (*r*) nodes. According to Eq. (6.2), to get $S_7(A)$ with node 7 (which has daughter nodes 3 and 4 with characters "T" and "G," respectively, Fig. 6.2), we first compute four values based on S_3:

$$
\begin{aligned}
c_{AA} + S_3(A) &= 0 + \infty = \infty \\
c_{AC} + S_3(C) &= 1 + \infty = \infty \\
c_{AG} + S_3(G) &= 1 + \infty = \infty \\
c_{AT} + S_3(T) &= 1 + 0 = 1
\end{aligned}
\qquad (6.3)
$$

The minimum of the four values in Eq. (6.3) is 1, which simply means that it will incur a cost of 1 to go from an A at node 7 to a T at node

3. Similarly, we compute the four values based on the leaf node 4. The minimum value out of these four values is also 1, obtained as $c_{AG}+S_4(G)$. Summing up the two minimum values gives us $S_7(A) = 2$, which means that, if we have A at node 7, it will take a cost of 2 to account for the two daughter nodes with T and G, respectively, necessitated by an A↔T and an A↔G substitutions (Fig. 6.2). We do the same to obtain $S_7(C) = 2$, $S_7(G)$ = $S_7(T) = 1$. The S vector for node 8 is obtained in exactly the same way. For $S_9(A)$ with daughter nodes 2 and 7 in Figure 6.2, the minimum of the four values based on node 2 is 0. The four values based on node 7 are

$$
\begin{aligned}
c_{AA} + S_7(A) &= 0 + 2 = 2 \\
c_{AC} + S_7(C) &= 1 + 2 = 3 \\
c_{AG} + S_7(G) &= 1 + 1 = 2 \\
c_{AT} + S_7(T) &= 1 + 1 = 2
\end{aligned}
\tag{6.4}
$$

You must have noted that each equation above are made of two terms, the first being the cost to go from nucleotide i in the parental node 9 to nucleotide j in the daughter node 7, and the second is the cost already accumulated at the daughter node 7. So $S_9(A) = 0 + 2 = 2$. In the same way, we obtain $S_9(C) = 3$, $S_9(G) = S_9(T) = 2$ (Fig. 6.2). We progress all the way to node 11 to obtain the score vector (4, 5, 5, 4). L_j in Eq. (6.1) for this site is the minimum of these four values (= 4). For a C matrix in Figure 6.2B, L_j is the minimum substitutions required to account for the nucleotide variation at the site in Figure 6.2. In other words, mapping the first nucleotide site to the topology requires a minimum of four nucleotide substitutions. We will do the same for all other sites and then add all L_j values to obtain TL for the topology. The same is then done for all other alternative topologies. The most parsimonious tree is the one with the smallest TL.

The strength of the Sankoff algorithm is that it allows a variety of cost matrices to be used. In some mammalian mitochondrial sequences where transitions occur about 40 times higher than transversions (Xia et al., 1996), one can specify a much high cost for transversions than transitions. In single-stranded DNA viruses where C↔T mutations occur more frequently than A↔G mutations (Chithambaram et al., 2014a, 2014b; Frederico et al., 1990; Kreutzer and Essigmann, 1998), one can assign a higher cost to A↔G substitutions than C↔T substitutions. Such a C matrix can alleviate the problem of substitution saturation and the long-branch attraction problem that is particularly pronounced in the maximum parsimony method. I will numerically illustrate the long-branch attraction problem later.

The computational details involving a C matrix with a higher cost for transversions than for transitions is illustrated in Figure 6.3. The final vector for node 11 is (6,8,7,7). The L_j value in Eq. (6.1) for this site is the minimum of the vector (= 6) when the character at node 11 is A. This cost, obtained with different c_{ij} values, does not have the same straightforward interpretation as that obtained with all $c_{ij} =1$ (in which case the cost is the number of nucleotide substitutions). A cost of 6, in this case, could result from 6 transitional substitutions or two transitional plus two transversional substitutions or just three transversional substitutions. One of the possible reconstruction of ancestral nodes, shown in Figure 6.5, requires two transitions and two transversions. Note that such a reconstruction of ancestral nodes is not unique. For example, node 7 could be A or G and node 8 could be C or T without increasing the total cost of 6.

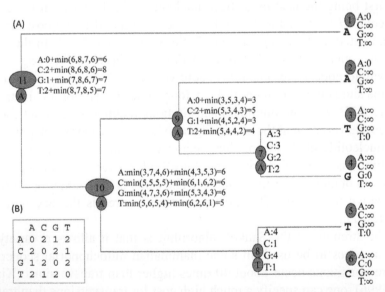

FIGURE 6.3 Computing substitution cost for the same nucleotide site as in Figure 6.2 using the Sankoff algorithm (A) with the cost of 2 for transversions and 1 for transitions (B). All nodes are numbered sequentially, with an S vector associated with each node. The circled nucleotides at internal nodes represent one of several possible ancestral reconstructions.

The benefit of accommodating differential substitution rates may be illustrated with a practical example. Here, I compare the Fitch and Sankoff algorithms with sequence data in Figure 6.4 which was part of simulated data along Topology T_1 (Fig. 6.4) based on the K80 model (Kimura, 1980) with $\alpha/\beta = 4$ (where α and β stand for transitional and transversional rates, respectively). Because the Fitch algorithm assumes equal rates among all substitutions, we expect it to be less likely to recover the true tree (which is Topology T_1 that is used to simulate the sequence data). In contrast, the Sankoff algorithm allows us to give a higher cost to transversional substitutions than to transitional substitutions and, therefore, should be more appropriate for analyzing the data set than the Fitch algorithm. Indeed, the Fitch algorithm recovered Topology T_2 as the most parsimonious tree ($TL_{2F} = 10$, smaller than TL_{1F} and TL_{3F}, where the subscripted 'F' stands for Fitch algorithm, Fig. 6.4), whereas the Sankoff algorithm with the step matrix in Figure 6.3B recovered T_1 ($TL_{1S} = 14$, smaller than TL_{2S} and TL_{3S}, where the subscripted 'S' stands for Sankoff algorithm, Fig. 6.4). Analogously, if we use either the distance-based methods or maximum likelihood with the JC69 model (Jukes and Cantor, 1969) that does not accommodate the transition bias, then topology T_2 will be recovered as the best tree. However, if a substitution model that accommodates the transition bias, such as K80, F84 (Felsenstein and Churchill, 1996; Kishino and Hasegawa, 1989) or TN93 (Tamura and Nei, 1993) is used, then both the distance-based or maximum likelihood methods will recover tree T_1 (the true tree) as the best tree. Numerous studies have shown that judicious use of a step matrix in MP can often alleviate the long-branch attraction problem and result in improved accuracy in phylogenetic analysis.

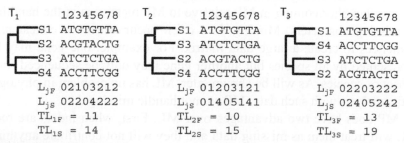

FIGURE 6.4 Maximum parsimony evaluation of tree lengths (TL) for the three possible topologies (T_1, T_2, and T_3) with four aligned sequences ($S1$ to $S4$). L_{jF} and L_{jS} are substitution cost at site j evaluated with the Fitch algorithm and Sankoff algorithm (with the step matrix in Figure 6.3B), respectively. TL_{iF} and TL_{iS} are tree length for tree i from the Fitch algorithm and from the Sankoff algorithm, respectively.

The MP criterion cannot identify the root, although the trees in Fig. 6.2 and Fig. 6.3 are presented in a rooted form. We can take any internal node as the root node and *TL* will be the same, i.e., topologies rerooted with any alternative internal node are equally parsimonious trees. For this reason, a phylogenetic tree is often rooted by an outgroup in contrast to an ingroup which is a group of OTUs whose phylogenetic relationship needs to be resolved. An outgroup is an OTU that is not a descendant from the most recent common ancestor of the ingroup. An ideal outgroup is one that not only does not belong to the ingroup, but also is the closest phylogenetically to the ingroup. That is, it is a sister taxon of the ingroup. If an ingroup consists of primate species, we should not use a bacterial species as an outgroup because it would be too distant to identify the root of the ingroup. Thus, a bacterial species, while being a valid outgroup to the ingroup of mammalian species, is not a good one.

6.4   CONTRASTING MP AND ML

The illustration above suggests the paramount importance of a good substitution model in phylogenetic analysis. Because values in a step matrix are quite subjective and do not have the statistical rigor of a substitution model, it is impossible to know if a step matrix provides a good approximation to the substitution process or to evaluate statistically different step matrices to see which one is the best. In contrast, one can use likelihood ratio test for nested models or information-theoretic indices, such as AIC (Akaike, 1973), BIC (Schwarz, 1978), or Bayes factor (Kass and Raftery, 1995) to choose the best-fitting substitution model.

Another shortcoming in MP relative to ML method is in the handling of missing characters. Missing data often occur when we concatenate sequences to create a large data matrix. For example, one gene may be represented by all species but another gene may only be sequenced for a subset of species. As will be shown later, ML has no problem in phylogenetic analysis with such data. MP cannot handle missing data.

MP does have two advantages over ML. First, when indels are real, ML will treat them as missing data and they will not contribute anything to phylogenetic resolution. However, if two homologous sequences share a unique stretch of indels, they should be considered more closely related, everything else being equal. MP can incorporate the indels as the fifth states in nucleotide sequences or 21st states in amino acid sequences by expand the step matrix. Thus, in the step matrix, we may assign a cost of 1 to transitions, a cost of 2 to transversions, and a cost of 5 to indels. Such assignment can be made more objective if we count the number of transitions, transversions, and indels in closely related species and give higher cost to less frequent events. So far MP is the only phylogenetic method that can handle indels as indels instead of as missing data.

Second, because MP is much faster, and can search the tree space much more thoroughly than ML, a published MP tree tends to be a real MP tree, but a published ML tree is often not a true ML tree simply because practical ML implementations typically search through only a limited tree space and may never encounter the true ML true. I once evaluated a few published MP and ML trees and the MP trees actually have higher log-likelihood than the reported ML tree. This suggests that the ML search that generated the published "ML" tree had never encountered the MP tree that has higher likelihood. Thus, some of the discrepancies between published MP and ML trees are just artifacts of insufficient ML search.

6.5 THE UPHILL SEARCH AND BRANCH-AND-BOUND SEARCH ALGORITHMS

The number of possible topologies (Felsenstein, 1978b) increases very quickly with the number of OTUs (n), with the number of rooted and unrooted topologies, designated as N_R and N_U, respectively, being

$$N_R = \frac{(2n-3)!}{2^{n-2}(n-2)!}$$

$$N_U = \frac{(2n-5)!}{2^{n-3}(n-3)!}$$

(6.5)

Searching through all possible topologies is called exhaustive search. It is often computationally impossible to search all possible trees with a large n. Two faster alternatives are commonly used. The first is the uphill search which does not guarantee that the resulting tree is the most parsimonious. The second is the branch-and-bound approach which does guarantee the finding of the most parsimonious tree. Obviously, the uphill search is much faster than the exhaustive search which evaluates all possible topologies.

The shortcoming of the uphill search is that it may miss the most parsimonious tree (which may be among those discarded without being evaluated).

The branch-and-bound algorithm for the MP method (Hendy and Penny, 1982) starts by generating an initial tree with fast algorithms such as the uphill search. Designate the tree length of this initial tree as TL_i, with the subscripted 'i' for initial tree. TL_i is now the upper bound of TL for the true MP tree because TL for the true MP tree will be either smaller or equal to TL_i. One may also use the neighbor-joining method (Saitou and Nei, 1987) to generate a topology and then evaluate the topology to obtain TL_i. The resulting distance-based tree also allows us to know which OTUs exhibit the highest divergence. This information is crucial for an efficient branch-and-bound search.

The next step is to start with four most divergent sequences and evaluate their TL. If only one topology is shorter than TL_i, then we can safely discard the two other topologies with $TL > TL_i$ because TL will only get longer with more OTUs added to the tree. This is why we always add more divergent OTUs to the growing tree first because this increases the chance of having subtrees with a $TL > TL_i$ so that such subtrees get eliminated early. If we take four closely related species to start, then none of the three topologies will have $TL > TL_i$ and we would have to keep them all, leading to a very inefficient branch-and-bound algorithm. If no 4-OTU topology is eliminated (i.e., their TL are all shorter than TL_i), then we have to evaluate all 5-OTU topologies derived from them. Again, we evaluate all these 5-OTU topologies and eliminate anyone that has $TL > TL_i$. This process is continued until we have added all OTUs and declare with confidence that our final tree is the true MP tree.

The efficiency of the branch-and-bound algorithm depends much on the initial topology. If the initial topology is good (i.e., with TL_i being very close to TL of the true MP tree), then many non-MP alternatives get eliminated early. If TL_i is unduly long, then the algorithm will be nearly as slow as the exhaustive search.

6.6   THE LONG-BRANCH ATTRACTION PROBLEM

The MP method is known to be inconsistent (Felsenstein, 1978a; Takezaki and Nei, 1994) as a result of long-branch attraction. Consistency is an important criterion for a good estimator, the others being unbiased and efficient (with small variance of the parameter). A consistent estimator is one that, biased or not, will converge to the true parameter (e.g., the true tree) with increasing probability when sample size increases (e.g., longer and longer sequences). An inconsistent estimator is one that will become increasingly more likely to converge to a wrong parameter value with increasing sample size. Thus, an estimator that is inconsistent is deemed unacceptable. I will provide a simple demonstration here by using trees in Figure 6.5. With four species, we have three possible unrooted topologies, designated T_k (k = 1, 2, 3), with T_1 being the correct topology.

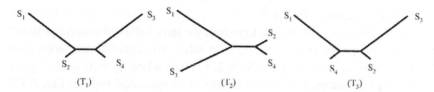

FIGURE 6.5   The long-branch attraction problem in the maximum parsimony methods.

Let X_{ij} be nucleotide at site j for species S_i. For simplicity, we specify three conditions: 1) nucleotide frequencies are equal to 0.25, 2) the lineages leading to S_1 and S_3 have experienced substitution saturation so that the probability of any site being A, C, G, or T is 0.25, i.e., $P(X_{1j} = X_{ij}) = 0.25, P(X_{3j} = X_{ij}) = 0.25,$, and 3) proportion of sites identical between S_2 and S_4 is 0.8, i.e., $P(X_{2j} = X_{4j}) = 0.8$.. These specifications are in fact compatible with a star tree or any of the trees in Fig. 6-5. The illustration below is to shown that T_2, with the two long branches clustered together, will receive more support than the two alternative topologies (T1 and T3) with the long branches separated by an internal node.

We now consider the proportion of informative sites supporting the three alternative topologies (T_1, T_2 and T_3) in Fig. 6-5. Let us start with T_1 which groups S_1 and S_2 together. Suppose we pick a site which happens to be nucleotide A for S_1. The nucleotide for S_2 is either A, C, G, or T, with equal probabilities because of conditions 1 and 2 specified above. When S_1 = A, then T_1 will have a chance of being supported only when S_2 = A, i.e, when nucleotides for S_1 and S_2 are of the {S_1=A, S_2=A} combination which I will abbreviate at {A,A}. We consider what fraction from this {A,A} combination will support T_1.

Given the {A,A} combination for S_1 and S_2, we now consider the nucleotide combination at S_3 and S_4. Let i be the nucleotide at S_3, i being A, C, G, or T with equal probability following conditions 1 and 2 specified above. Given S_2 = A, the probability of S_4 = A is 0.8 (condition 3), and that of (S_4 = $\bar{A}$) is 0.2 ($\bar{A}$ means "not A"). Obviously, an {A, A, i, A} combination for S_1 to S_4 does not support T_1. Only certain combinations within $\{A, A, i, \bar{A}\}$ would support T_1. There are 12 $i\bar{A}$ combinations, with three (CC, GG and TT), or 3/12 (=1/4), supporting T_1 and the rest do not. Therefore the fraction of sites support T_1 is

$$P(T_1) = \left(\frac{1}{4}\right) \times 0.2 \times \left(\frac{1}{4}\right) = 0.0125 \qquad (6.6)$$

which is also equal to $P(T_3)$.

For T_2 that groups S_1 and S_3 together, we may follow the same protocol to obtain the proportion of supporting sites. We against start with $S_1 = A$. The chance of having A for S_3 is 1/4. Only when $S_2 = S_4$ will T_2 have a chance to be supported. Given condition 3 specified before, i.e., $P(S_2 = S_4) = 0.8$, there are four combinations of $S_2 = S_4$, of which the $\{A,A\}$ combination ($S_2 = A$, $S_4 = A$) will not support T_2, but $\{C,C\}$, $\{G,G\}$, and $\{T,T\}$ combinations will, so the proportion of sites supporting T_2 is

$$P(T_2) = \left(\frac{1}{4}\right) \times 0.8 \times \left(\frac{3}{4}\right) = 0.15 \qquad (6.7)$$

If sequence length is 1000, then we expect 12.5 sites supporting T_1 and 150 sites supporting T_2. Therefore, in spite of T_1 being the true topology, we should have, on average, only about 12.5 informative sites favoring T_1 and T_3, but 150 sites supporting the wrong tree T_2. This is one of the several causes for the familiar problem of long-branch attraction (Hendy and Penny, 1989) or short-branch attraction (Nei, 1996) depending on one's perspective. Because it is the two short branches that contribute a large number of informative sites supporting the wrong tree, "short-branch attraction" seems a more appropriate term for the problem than "long-branch attraction." However, because the problem is mainly caused by the failure of correcting for multiple hits in long-branches, naming it long-branch attraction also makes sense. I wish to emphasize again that long-branch attraction problem is not unique in MP. It occurs in distance-based, maximum likelihood and Bayesian inference methods as well when multiple hits are not corrected properly. For example, if sequences evolve with a strong transition bias but we choose the JC60 model which will not correct multiple substitutions as a consequence of strong transition bias, then all model-based methods will also exhibit the long-branch attraction problem.

Inconsistency in statistical estimation is never a good thing. Some advocates of the MP method have gone so far as to claim that long-branch attraction problem could be a good thing because lineages with long branches tend to be sister lineages, so a bias favoring their grouping together will, in fact, give MP greater efficiency to arrive at the true tree. Such increased efficiency due to bias or inconsistency is purchased with illegal statistical currency (Xia, 2014). However, as I have illustrated before, using a step matrix with different costs for different substitutions can often dramatically alleviate the long-branch attraction problem.

6.7   STATISTICAL TESTS OF ALTERNATIVE TOPOLOGIES

It is often useful to test if alternative topologies are significantly different from each other. In order to have a powerful test, it is crucial to consider (1) what sites are relevant to the test, (2) what OTUs are relevant to the test, and (3) when to include sites as a random effect.

6.7.1   WHAT SITES ARE RELEVANT TO THE TEST?

Suppose I have four species and wish to evaluate relative statistical support for the three alternative topologies. I will use cow (*Bos taurus*), orangutan (*Pongo pygmaeus*), chimpanzee (*Pan troglodytes*), and human (*Homo sapiens*) mitochondrial *COX1* gene to illustrate the test. These are taken from the VertCOI.fas file that comes with software DAMBE (Xia, 2013b) and contains 1512 aligned sites of mitochondrial COI genes with no indels. We can use either the Fitch algorithm or Sankoff algorithm to evaluate L_j (minimum number of steps for site j) for each of the three possible topologies (T_1, T_2, and T_3) to obtain the site-specific steps in a table (Fig. 6.6). This table can then be used to evaluate relative statistical support of alternative topologies with the null hypothesis being that the three column averages for T_1, T_2, and T_3, respectively in the table in Figure 6.6 are equal. Given the data configuration in Figure 6.6, the simplest test is a one-way ANOVA with three groups (i.e., three columns of data shown in Fig. 6.6). Here we consider which site should be included in the test.

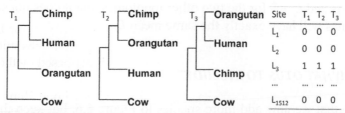

FIGURE 6.6   Three topologies for illustrating statistical tests of alternative topologies. Tree length is 540, 563, and 563 for T_1, T_2, and T_3, respectively. Four aligned sequences have 1512 sites with no indels.

It makes no sense to include all 1512 sites in the significance tests. For sequences with little divergence, most sites will be monomorphic (i.e., featuring a single nucleotide) and have $L_j = 0$ for all three topologies. A large number of shared 0's will obscure true differences among the three topologies. For example, if we subject the table in Figure 6.6 to a one-way ANOVA, we will see no significant difference among the three topologies (F = 0.2947, DF1 = 2, DF2 = 4533, p = 0.7448). You can use alternative statistical tests other than ANOVA but the point here is to illustrate that, regardless of what statistical test you use, including irrelevant sites, will reduce the power of the test.

If we exclude all monomorphic sites, then the p value becomes 0.1505. However, this is still not appropriate. For example, a large number of sites could be autapomorphic with only one species differing from the other three species. Such sites will have $L_j = 1$ for all three topologies. A large number of shared 1's will also obscure true differences among the three topologies. Excluding all these autapomorphic sites leaves us with only 145 sites but these sites yield a highly significant difference among the three topologies (F = 6.8246, DF1 =2, DF2 = 432, p = 0.001207758).

We can refine the test even further. The tabled L_j values in Figure 6.6 are evaluated by the Fitch algorithm for which only informative sites matters. An informative site contains at least two nucleotides with each nucleotide represented by at least two OTUs. Thus, for these L_j values generated from the Fitch algorithm, we should use only informative sites in the significance tests. There are 83 informative sites. Applying one-way ANOVA to these sites gives us F = 10.2307, DF1 = 2, DF2 = 246, p = 0.000054). Both T_2 and T_3 are highly significantly worse than T_1 (p = 0.0001 for both comparisons between T_1 and T_2 and between T_1 and T_3).

There is no point in considering sites as a random effect with only four species because, when we use only informative sites, all sites will have the same steps. An informative site will have $L_j = 1$ for the topology that it supports and $L_j = 2$ for the two other topologies that it does not support. So, all sites will have exactly the same mean L_j.

6.7.2   WHAT OTUS TO INCLUDE?

Suppose that we now add more species to Figure 6.6, but keep the same biological question of testing the three alternative topologies featuring different relationships among the three hominids (Fig. 6.7). The three topologies (Fig. 6.7) are the same except for the different relationships among the three hominids. We again use the Fitch algorithm to evaluate the 473 informative sites and I have made available the L_j values for the three topologies at http://dambe.bio.uottawa.ca/teach/VertCOI.txt, but it is easy to generate these values yourself.

We now subject these L_j values to a one-way ANOVA. To our surprise, there is no significant difference among the three topologies ($F = 0.2804$, DF1 = 2, DF2 = 1416, $p = 0.7555$), in contrast to our previous results of highly significant differences among the three topologies in Figure 6.6, also based on the informative sites. The reason for this discrepancy is that, when we add more species, we added 390 (=473−83) informative sites that, while contributing to the resolution of other parts of the tree, contribute nothing to resolving the three topologies in Figure 6.7. That is, these 390 informative sites all add exactly the same number of steps to the three topologies. In short, there are informative sites that support T_1 against T_2 and T_3 (Fig. 6.7), but their effect is now diluted by the addition of a large number of sites that support the three topologies equally.

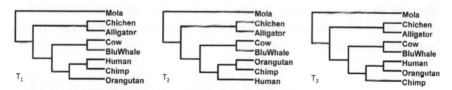

FIGURE 6.7 Three topologies for illustrating the effect of adding irrelevant species in testing alternative topologies. Tree length is 1427, 1446, and 1445 for T_1, T_2, and T_3, respectively.

The rule of thumb in phylogenetics is that, if you wish to resolve phylogenetic controversies among great apes, you can include the lesser apes as outgroup species but not remote relatives such as fish or worms or even bacteria. The addition of these taxa remotely related to the ingroup will add many informative sites that are irrelevant to the resolution of the ingroup. The outgroup provides you with a perspective to see which ingroup species is close to the root. If the outgroup is very far from the ingroup, then all ingroup species will become blurry.

6.7.3   INCLUDE SITES AS A RANDOM EFFECT IN A MIXED MODEL

We mentioned that there is no point to include sites as a random effect when we use informative sites with only four OTUs because all sites will have the same mean L_j values. With more than four OTUs, including sites as a random effect will increase the power of statistical tests if there is heterogeneity among sites, i.e., L_j depends on both topology (TREE) and sites (SITE). There are specialized programs for mixed models, but in our case, just a two-way ANOVA with no replication (which is an extension of the paired-sample t-test, just as a one-way ANOVA is an extension of the unpaired two-sample t-test) would suffice. Note that we cannot test TREE*SITE interactions. In R, one would specify lm(L_j ~TREE+SITE). The result shows highly significant differences in tree length among the three topologies ($p = 0.002129$) and among sites ($p < 0.000001$). If one uses the lmer function in R, fits a model with both TREE and SITE and a reduced model without TREE but with SITE, then a likelihood ratio test will yield a $p = 0.002129$, i.e., the tree lengths of the three topologies are significantly different from each other. This is a demonstration that a mixed model with SITE as a random effect could dramatically increase the power in phylogenetic tests. I expect such models to be implemented in all phylogenetic analysis that is site-based (e.g., maximum parsimony and maximum likelihood).

6.8   BOOTSTRAPPING AND DELETE-HALF JACKKNIFING

Resampling methods, such as bootstrapping and delete-half jackknifing (Efron, 1982), were introduced into phylogenetics by Felsenstein (Felsenstein, 1985a). Figure 6.8 shows a bootstrapped tree with support values at the internal nodes. Bootstrapping and jackknifing methods serve two purposes. First, they give us an intuitive measure of data consistency. If all sites in a set of aligned sequences contain the same phylogenetic signal, then we will have high support values. If sites contain conflicting signals, then the support values will be small. Second, they provide an easily interpretable measure of our confidence in a tree or its subtrees. Figure 6.8 shows that there are conflict phylogenetic signals over sites concerning *Bos Taurus* and *Balaenoptera musculus,* with a support value of only 66%.

The bootstrap resampling involves the site-wise resampling of the aligned sequences with replacement, so that a set of aligned sequences of N sites long will be resampled N times to generate a new set of aligned sequences of the same length (a pseudosample), with some sites in the original sequences, sampled one or more times while some other sites do not get sampled at all. In short, to obtain each pseudosample, one generates N random integers between 1 and N, e.g., 3, 1, 101, ..., and put sites 3, 1, 101, ..., in the new pseudosample. In molecular phylogenetics, one typically will generate at least 500 pseudosamples, so we will reconstruct 500 trees, each from a pseudosample, and obtain a consensus tree expressing our confidence in the subtrees (Fig. 6.8). A bootstrap value of 93 for the three great apes (*Pongo pygmaeus, Homo sapiens,* and *Pan troglodytes*) means that 93% of the trees group the three species together as a monophyletic taxon. Note that the bootstrapping values will be similar but not identical if one repeats the procedure to regenerate another bootstrapped tree.

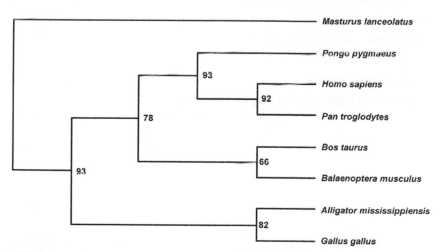

FIGURE 6.8 A maximum parsimony tree of eight vertebrate species with bootstrap support values. Generated from DAMBE (Xia, 2013b; Xia, 2017a).

The delete-half jackknifing technique will randomly purge off half of the sites from the original sequences to generate a pseudosample, so that the new set of aligned sequences in the pseudosample will be half as long as the original. The rest is the same as with bootstrapping.

Although the bootstrap and the jackknife generally produce similar results, there are some subtle differences. Suppose that we have a set of aligned sequences of N sites long. For the bootstrap resampling, the probability of each site being sampled is $1/N$, and the mean number of times a site gets sampled in each bootstrapping resampling is simply one. Thus, a site gets sampled 0, 1, 2, ..., N times, with the associated probability mass following a Poisson distribution with a mean equal to one. The proportion of sites that will not be sampled will then be $p(0) = e^{-1} = 0.368$ which means that 36.8% of the sites will not be sampled with bootstrapping, while 63.2% of the sites will be sampled at least once. In jackknifing, we have 50% of the sites not sampled and the other 50% of the sites sampled just once.

KEYWORDS

- **rate heterogeneity over sites**
- **gamma distribution**
- **fast estimation method**
- **gamma distances**
- **shape parameter**
- **rate heterogeneity among codon sites**

CHAPTER 7

Distance-Based Phylogenetic Methods

ABSTRACT

Distance-based phylogenetic methods are fast and remain popular in molecular phylogenetics, especially in the big-data age when researchers often build phylogenetic trees with hundreds or even thousands of leaves. A distance-based method has two components: The evolutionary distance matrix typically derived from a substitution model and the tree-building algorithm that constructs a tree from the distance matrix. Evolutionary distances differ not only by substitution models but also by whether they are estimated independently (based on information only between two aligned sequences) or simultaneously (based on information from all pairwise comparisons). Simultaneously estimated distances perform much better in molecular phylogenetics than independently estimated distances. Frequently used tree-building algorithms include neighbor-joining which clusters two taxa by weighing two measures: How close they are to each other and how far they jointly are from all other taxa. Another class of methods with a global optimization criterion is based on the least-squares framework. They first evaluates alternative topologies by the least-squares method and then choose the best tree by either the least-square criterion or the minimum evolution criterion. Distance-based dating methods are also illustrated numerically, with both fossil-calibrated dating and tip-dating, together with the estimation of variation in the inferred dates by resampling.

7.1 INTRODUCTION

Distance-based methods aim to achieve the two objectives of molecular phylogenetics, phylogenetic tree reconstruction, and dating. For the first objective, we need a distance matrix and a tree-building algorithm making use of the distance matrix. For dating, we need calibration points to convert branch lengths to geological time. There are two commonly used calibration methods, one by using the fossil record to calibrate internal nodes and the other by differential sampling times for rapidly evolving viral lineages, e.g., RNA viruses such as HIV-1. This latter calibration method is commonly known as tip-dating (Drummond et al., 2003a; Drummond et al., 2003b). The conceptual framework of tip-dating was proposed in the 1980s (Buonagurio and Fitch, 1986; Li et al., 1988; Saitou and Nei, 1986).

Distance-based phylogenetic methods, especially those based on the least-squares (LS) criterion, are widely used in evolutionary studies and featured in major textbooks on molecular phylogenetics (Felsenstein, 2004; Li, 1997; Nei and Kumar, 2000; Yang, 2006). The least-square method for phylogenetic reconstruction is generally consistent when the distance is estimated properly (Felsenstein, 2004; Gascuel and Steel, 2006; Nei and Kumar, 2000). However, even when the distance is over- or underestimated, the resulting phylogenetic bias is generally quite small (Xia, 2006).

7.1.1 DISTANCES: SIMULTANEOUS ESTIMATION AND INDEPENDENT ESTIMATION

The conceptual framework of deriving evolutionary distances from substitution models has been covered extensively in a previous chapter on substitution models, illustrated with commonly used substitution models such as JC69 (Jukes and Cantor, 1969), K80 (Kimura, 1980), F84 (used in DNAML since 1984 Hasegawa and Kishino, 1989; Kishino and Hasegawa, 1989), HKY85 (Hasegawa et al., 1985), TN93 (Tamura and Nei, 1993), and GTR (Lanave et al., 1984; Tavaré, 1986) models. Distances derived from these models are respectively referred to as JC69 distance, K80 distance, and so on.

There are independently estimated (IE) and simultaneously estimated (SE) distances, with the latter performs much better than the former in phylogenetic analysis. IE distances are estimated from two aligned sequences without using information from other sequence pairs. In contrast, SE distances are estimated by using information from all sequence pairs. IE distances suffer from three problems. The first involves inapplicable cases where the distance often cannot be computed for highly diverged sequences (Rzhetsky and Nei, 1994b; Tajima, 1993;

Zharkikh, 1994). For example, the K80 distance cannot be computed when $(1 - 2Q \leq 0)$ or $(1 - 2P - Q \leq 0)$. The second is internal inconsistency. Again, take the K80 model for example. The substitution process between sequences A and B would have a substitution rate ratio κ_{AB} but that between sequences A and C would have a rate ratio κ_{AC} that can be quite different from κ_{AB} (Felsenstein, 2004, p 200; Yang, 2006, pp 37–38). These two problems are exacerbated by limited sequence length with large stochastic effects. The third problem is insufficient use of information because the computation of pairwise distances ignores information in other sequences that should also contain information about the substitution process involving the two compared sequences (Felsenstein, 2004, p 175; Yang, 2006, p 37). Because of these problems, distance-based phylogenetic methods are generally considered as quick and dirty methods, used either in situations where high phylogenetic accuracy is not particularly important or as a first step to generate preliminary candidate trees for subsequent more rigorous phylogenetic evaluation by maximum likelihood (ML) methods (Ota and Li, 2000, 2001). However, these problems can be eliminated, or at least dramatically alleviated, by SE distances.

SE distances are based on information from all pairs of sequences and are generally much more robust than IE distances. There are two approaches for estimating SE distances, the LS approach and the ML approach that will be numerically illustrated later. In addition to distances based on stationary substitution processes, I have also included the paralinear (Lake, 1994) and LogDet (Lockhart et al., 1994) distances which are similar to each other and presumably suitable for nonstationary substitution processes. These distances have been implemented in my program DAMBE (Xia, 2001; Xia, 2013b; Xia and Xie, 2001).

Evolutionary distances typically cannot be estimated between two sequences that do not share any homologous sites. For example, if we concatenate a number of mitochondrial genes into a supermatrix, we may have OTU1 represented by *COX1* only, and OTU3 by *CytB* only. Because *COX1* and *CytB* genes are not homologous, we cannot compute evolutionary distance between OTU1 and OTU3. However, assuming the same substitution process, we can impute the distance between OTU1 and OTU3 based on their distances to other OTUs that have both *COX1* and *CytB* (Xia 2018c). Distance imputation is numerically illustrated later.

7.1.2   RATIONALE OF DISTANCE-BASED PHYLOGENETIC METHODS

Two frequently used distance-based phylogenetic methods are used in practice. Given a distance matrix and a topology, the first uses LS method to evaluate branch lengths, sums up all branches as the tree length (TL), and then choose the tree that has the shortest TL. Computer programs implementing this method will generate N topologies and obtain TL_1, TL_2, ..., TL_N. Tree i whose TL_i is the smallest is the best tree. This criterion of choosing the tree is known as the minimum-evolution criterion. The method was made popular by the FastME program (Desper and Gascuel, 2002, 2004). This function is also available in DAMBE, together with SE distances.

The other frequently used method is neighbor-joining (NJ) by Saitou and Nei (1987). It represents a significant extension of the UPGMA method that has been numerically illustrated elsewhere (Xia, 2018a, pp. 129–144). UPGMA algorithm will simply cluster OTUs i and j if d_{ij} is the smallest. NJ method will also consider whether OTUs i and j are both far away from the other OTUs. This makes intuitive sense. If OTUs i and j have a small d_{ij} and they are both pretty far from other OTUs, then it makes sense that they should be grouped together.

7.1.3   PHYLOGENETICS BY PAIRWISE ALIGNMENT ONLY

The distance-based method has one advantage not shared by other phylogenetic methods. That is, it can be done with pairwise alignment only. Phylogenetic reconstruction becomes difficult with deep phylogenies, mainly due to the difficulty in obtaining reliable multiple sequence alignment (MSA) (Blackburne and Whelan, 2013; Edgar and Batzoglou, 2006; Herman et al., 2014; Kumar and Filipski, 2007; Lunter et al., 2008; Wong et al., 2008). In contrast to pairwise sequence alignment (PSA) by dynamic programming which is guaranteed to generate, for a given scoring scheme, the optimal alignment or at least one of the equally optimal alignments, MSAs of highly divergent sequences are often poor, especially those obtained from a progressive alignment with a poor guide tree. Although an iterative approach (Feng and Doolittle, 1990; Hogeweg and Hesper, 1984; Katoh et al., 2009; Thompson et al., 1994) is typically used for MSA in which a guide tree is used to generate an alignment which is then used to construct a new guide tree to guide the next round of progressive alignment, such as approach still often produces poor alignment for deeply diverged sequences. A poor alignment typically leads to bias and inaccuracy in phylogenetic estimation (Blackburne and Whelan, 2013; Kumar and Filipski, 2007; Wong et al., 2008).

One way to avoid problems associated with poor MSA is simply not to do MSA, i.e., by phylogenetic analysis based on PSA only as pioneered by Thorne and Kishino (1992). However, Thorne and Kishino (1992) did not actually implement the method and evaluate it against the ML method. It is only recently that the method, termed PhyPA for phylogenetics from pairwise alignment, has been implemented in DAMBE (Xia, 2016). PhyPA outperforms ML methods for highly diverged sequences.

This chapter has three sections. I first introduce the SE distances and the paralinear/LogDet distances. This is followed by numerical illustration of phylogenetic algorithms building trees from distances. The distance-based dating methods (Xia and Yang, 2011; Xia, 2013b) are then illustrated. The last part details methods for imputing missing distances (Xia, 2018c).

7.2 EVOLUTIONARY DISTANCES

7.2.1 SIMULTANEOUSLY ESTIMATED DISTANCES

There are two approaches to derive SE distances. The first is the quasi-likelihood approach (Tamura et al., 2004), referred to as the maximum composite likelihood distance in MEGA (Tamura et al., 2007) and MLComposite in DAMBE (Xia, 2009, 2013b; Xia, 2017a), respectively. MEGA implemented the distance only for the TN93 model (Tamura and Nei, 1993), whereas DAMBE implemented it for both the TN93 and the F84 models, referred as MLCompositeTN93 and MLCompositeF84, respectively. The inclusion of MLCompositeF84 is to facilitate comparison between distance-based method against DNAML in the PHYLIP package (Felsenstein, 2014). The second approach for deriving SE distances is the LS or weighted least-squares (WLS) approach that has been implemented in DAMBE for F84, TN93, and GTR models.

7.2.1.1   SIMULTANEOUS ESTIMATION OF DISTANCES WITH THE QUASI-LIKELIHOOD APPROACH

I will use the K80 model (Kimura, 1980) to illustrate the principle of SE distance estimation based on the likelihood framework. The K80 model, as we have learned from the chapter on nucleotide substitution models, has two parameters, which can be expressed either as αt and βt or as D and κ. The expected proportions of transitions and transversions, designated by $E(P)$ and $E(Q)$ and expressed in D and κ, respectively, are

$$E(P) = \frac{1}{4} + \frac{1}{4}e^{-\frac{4D}{\kappa+2}} - \frac{1}{2}e^{-\frac{2D(\kappa+1)}{\kappa+2}}$$

$$E(Q) = \frac{1}{2} - \frac{1}{2}e^{-\frac{4D}{\kappa+2}}$$

(7.1)

Suppose we have three aligned sequences, $S1$, $S2$, and $S3$, with sequence length $N (= 100)$. The observed number of sites with transitional and transversional differences are shown in Table 7.1, used for contrasting the IE and SE estimation of distances. For IE estimation, one simply substitute $E(P)$ and $E(Q)$ in Eq. (7.1) by the observed P and Q (which equal N_s/N and N_v/N, respectively) and then solve for D and κ. You will encounter the frustration that you cannot estimate D between $S1$ and $S3$ (Table 7.1).

TABLE 7.1   Observed number of sites with transitional and transversional differences (N_s and N_v, respectively) from pairwise comparisons among three sequences ($S1$, $S2$, and $S3$) of length 100. Independently estimated k80 distances (D_{IE}) and simultaneously estimated K80 distances (D_{SE}) from the maximum likelihood (ML) and least-squares (LS) frameworks are included. Note that K80 distance cannot be computed for $S1$ and $S3$ using independent estimation method (labeled as 'Inapplicable').

Seq. pair	N_s	N_v	D_{IE}	$D_{SE,ML}$	$D_{SE,LS}$
$S1$ vs $S2$	9	4	0.1451	0.1464	0.1473
$S1$ vs $S3$	40	30	Inapplicable	2.0914	2.0725
$S2$ vs $S3$	20	10	0.4024	0.4116	0.4131

For the SE method, we assume the same κ but different D_{ij} (i.e., D_{12}, D_{13}, and D_{23}) and maximize the following lnL:

$$\begin{aligned}
\ln L = &\, N_{s.12}\ln[E(P_{12})] + N_{v.12}\ln[E(Q_{12})] + N_{i.12}\ln[1 - E(P_{12}) - E(Q_{12})] \\
&+ N_{s.13}\ln[E(P_{13})] + N_{v.13}\ln[E(Q_{13})] + N_{i.13}\ln[1 - E(P_{13}) - E(Q_{13})] \quad (7.2) \\
&+ N_{s.23}\ln[E(P_{23})] + N_{v.23}\ln[E(Q_{23})] + N_{i.23}\ln[1 - E(P_{23}) - E(Q_{23})]
\end{aligned}$$

where $N_i = (N - N_s - N_v)$, e.g., $N_{i.12} = (100\text{-}9\text{-}4)$. We take the partial derivative of lnL with respect to D_{12}, D_{13}, D_{23}, and κ, set them to zero and solve the four simultaneous equations for the four unknowns. This leads to $\kappa = 6.2382$ and the three D_{ij} values shown in Table 7.1. There is no problem for the SE method to estimate D_{13} which was not possible with the IE method.

7.2.1.2   SIMULTANEOUS ESTIMATION OF DISTANCES WITH THE LS APPROACH

The LS method uses one of a class of models differing in the form of weight. The general form is to minimize the following residual sum of squares (RSS):

$$RSS = \sum \left[\frac{\left(o_{ij} - e_{ij} \right)^2}{w_{ij}^m} \right] \tag{7.3}$$

where o_{ij} and e_{ij} are the observed and expected values, w_{ij} is the weight typically equal to o_{ij} or e_{ij}, and m is an integer typically taking the value of 0, 1, or 2. If $m = 0$, Eq. (7.3) becomes an ordinary least-squares (OLS) method. If $m > 0$, then RSS represents WLS method. If $m = 1$ and $w_{ij} = e_{ij}$, RSS is the familiar chi-square (χ^2). Thus, parameter estimation by minimizing the chi-square function is a special case of the WLS method. The Fitch–Margoliash method (Fitch and Margoliash, 1967) for reconstructing phylogenies from a distance matrix has $m = 2$ and $w_{ij} = o_{ij}$ (where o_{ij} is the estimated evolutionary distance between species i and j, and e_{ij} is the patristic distance along the path linking species i and j on the tree.)

I illustrate the WLS method for estimating D and κ by specifying $m = 1$ and $w_{ij} = e_{ij}$, i.e., RSS in Eq. (7.3) is χ^2. For IE estimation of D_{12}, we would minimize the following χ^2:

$$\chi_{12}^2 = \frac{[P_{12} - E(P_{12})]^2}{E(P_{12})} + \frac{[Q_{12} - E(Q_{12})]^2}{E(Q_{12})} + \frac{\{1 - P_{12} - Q_{12} - [1 - E(P_{12}) - E(Q_{12})]\}^2}{1 - E(P_{12}) - E(Q_{12})} \tag{7.4}$$

where $P_{12} = N_{s.12}/N$ and $Q_{12} = N_{v.12}/N$ (values in Table 7.1). Minimizing χ^2_{12} would result in $D_{12} = 0.1451$ and $\kappa = 4.9596$.

For the SE method with N species and $N*(N-1)/2$ pairwise distances, we will again assume the same κ but different D_{ij} values and minimize the following

$$\chi^2 = \sum_{i=1}^{N-1} \sum_{j=i+1}^{N} \chi_{ij}^2$$

$$\chi_{ij}^2 = \frac{[P_{ij} - E(P_{ij})]^2}{E(P_{ij})} + \frac{[Q_{ij} - E(Q_{ij})]^2}{E(Q_{ij})} + \frac{\{1 - P_{ij} - Q_{ij} - [1 - E(P_{ij}) - E(Q_{ij})]\}^2}{1 - E(P_{ij}) - E(Q_{ij})} \quad (7.5)$$

which leads to $\kappa = 6.276273961$ and D_{12}, D_{13}, and D_{23} values shown in Table 7.1. These four parameters are close to those estimated in the likelihood framework (also shown in Table 7.1).

7.2.2   PARALINEAR AND LOGDET DISTANCES

All substitution models that I have covered are time-reversible stationary models in which the change of a nucleotide or an amino acid to another is balanced by the reverse change so that the nucleotide or amino acid frequencies remain the same along the lineages. However, substitution rates may also change over time. For example, some bacterial lineages have several CpG-specific methyltransferases, with consequent high rate of methylated C changing to T leading to low frequency of C as well as CpG deficiency (Xia, 2003). However, genes encoding such CpG-specific methyltransferases may lose during evolution, with descendent lineages regaining C and CpG dinucleotides (Xia, 2003). This is a case of nonstationary substitution process. Phylogeneticists are all aware of such processes but generally avoided the topic because it is too complicated to implement nonstationary substitution process in phylogenetics. It is easy to say that substitution rates are not constant and should be represented as functions of time but it is difficult to express substitution rates as functions of time.

Paralinear (Lake, 1994) and LogDet (Lockhart et al., 1994) distances were suggested to be relevant to the nonstationary process. For two nucleotide or amino acid sequences, the paralinear distance (Lake, 1994) between sequences 1 and 2 is defined as

$$D_{12} = -\frac{1}{N} \ln \frac{|J_{12}|}{\sqrt{\prod_{i=1}^{N} F_{1i} \prod_{i=1}^{N} F_{2i}}} \qquad (7.6)$$

where N is 4 for nucleotide sequences and 20 for amino acid sequences, J_{12} is the observed substitution matrix between sequences 1 and 2, F_1 and F_2 are nucleotide frequencies (counts, not proportions) for sequences 1 and 2, respectively, derived from J_{12}. For data in Table 7.2, the matrix determinant $|J_{12}|$ = 544202788, denominator = 1843167240, and D_{12} = 0.30498. Note that we did not average the two corresponding off-diagonal elements (e.g., A→G and G→A) in Table 7.2. In time-reversible models, forward and backward substitutions such as A→G and G→A are assumed to be the same. Any difference between the two numbers (40 and 35 in our case in Table 7.2) is assumed to be due to stochastic sampling of the same variable. The substitution model underlying LogDet and paralinear distances assumes the difference to be real. That is, there are more A→G substitutions (40) than G→A substitutions (35), so the two numbers should not be averaged.

TABLE 7.2 Observed nucleotide substitution patterns from comparing two aligned sequences 1 and 2, for illustrating the calculation of paralinear and LogDet distances. The J_{12} matrix is in bold. F_1 and F_2 are the column and row sums of J_{12}.

	A	G	C	T	F_2	p_2
A	**100**	**40**	**8**	**12**	160	0.186047
G	**35**	**200**	**11**	**8**	254	0.295349
C	**9**	**9**	**250**	**15**	283	0.32907
T	**11**	**12**	**20**	**120**	163	0.189535
F_1	155	261	289	155	860	1
p_1	0.180233	0.303488	0.336047	0.180233		

The LogDet distance (Lockhart et al., 1994) is the same as the paralinear distance except for two minor details. It defines J_{12} as proportions summing up to 1, i.e., with each value in the 4×4 J_{12} matrix in Table 7.2 divided by the sum (= 860) and replaces F_1 and F_2 by p_1 and p_2 which are proportions summing up to 1. If p_1 and p_2 are calculated from F_1 and F_2 as in Table 7.2, then LogDet distance would be the same as paralinear distance. However, there are some reasons for one to use p_1 and p_2 different from those in Table 7.2. One of the reasons may be illustrated with 18S and 23S rRNA sequences which have conserved and variable domains. First, both substitution and indel events have occurred almost exclusively in just a few variable domains of the 18S rRNA sequences (Van de Peer et al., 1993) but the variable domains have nucleotide frequencies different from those of the conserved domains in the 18S rRNA gene and in the 28S rRNA gene (Xia et al., 2003a). In phylogenetic analyses involving distance and maximum-likelihood methods, frequency parameters most appropriate for the underlying substitution model should be used. The most appropriate estimate of the frequency parameters should be from the sites where substitutions occur, i.e., from the variable domains. However, variable domains in the 18S rRNA sequences are poorly represented in the aligned sites because of the presence of many indels in these domains (indel-containing sites are often ignored in distance calculation). Thus, p_1 and p_2, as calculated in Table 7.2, are dominated by conservative domains and consequently are not appropriate for phylogenetic recon-struction. For this reason, one might use p_1 and p_2 calculated from all sequences instead of those site pairs entered in J_{12} (Xia et al., 2003a). Obviously, if one computes LogDet distances by uses p_1 and p_2 that are different from those in Table 7.2, then such distances will be different from paralinear distances.

The paralinear and LogDet distances are typically smaller than GTR distances or even TN93 distances. This is intuitively understandable. Suppose a new evolutionary lineage has acquired CpG methylation which dramatically elevated C→T substitution rate to such an extent that T→C substitution rate is negligible in comparison. When we observe many such C→T transitions and take a time-reversible perspective, we may think that some of these observed C→T substitutions may result from C→T→C→T. Time-reversible models, such as GTR and TN93, will indeed aim to correct these presumed multiple hits which did not happen because we have already specified the non-time-reversible process to have high C→T but negligible T→C substitution rate. In short, GTR distance will be greater than paralinear and LogDet distances because it has added such multiple hits that did not occur.

7.2.3   OTHER DISTANCES NOT FROM ALIGNED SEQUENCES

Evolutionary distances can be computed from a variety of data other than molecular sequence data. Conventional data includes 1D and 2D gel protein electrophoresis, DNA hybridization, restriction fragment length polymorphism, and gene frequency data (especially microsatellite data which accumulate rapidly in human biology and molecular ecology). In recent years, the availability of genomic data for a variety of species has resulted in the development of new types of distances derived from whole genomes for molecular phylogenetic reconstruction. This latter category includes genome BLAST distances (Auch et al., 2006; Deng et al., 2006; Henz et al., 2005), breakpoint distances based on genome rearrangement (Gramm and Niedermeier, 2002; Herniou et al., 2001), distances based on the relative information between unaligned/unalignable sequences (Otu and Sayood, 2003), distances based on the sharing of oligopeptides (Gao and Qi, 2007), and composite distances incorporating several whole-genome similarity measures (Lin et al., 2009). Some of the whole-genome-based distances are necessary for constructing phylogenies of bacterial species because of three complications. The first is the rampant occurrence of horizontal gene transfer leading to difficulties in identifying orthologous genes. The second is that the leading strand and lagging strand in bacterial genomes typically have very different mutation patterns (Marin and Xia, 2008), yet bacterial genes frequently switch between strands and consequently would experience different substitution patterns. The third is the frequent loss or gain of genomic DNA methylation affecting both genomic CpG dinucleotides and genomic GC content (Xia, 2003). Both the second and third complications lead to heterogeneity in the evolutionary process even among orthologous gene lineages. All these genome-based distances mentioned above have been used in molecular phylogenetic reconstruction but whether they are proportional to divergence time has never been studied. This hinders their use in molecular phylogenetics in general and dating speciation events or gene duplication events in particular (Xia, 2009).

7.2.4   CONTRASTING PERFORMANCE OF DIFFERENT DISTANCES

Distance estimation becomes difficult with deep phylogeny. I will use the third codon site of the VertCOI.fas file that comes with DAMBE for such illustration. The file contains mitochondrial COI sequences from eight vertebrate species. The third codon sites are highly diverged and are equivalent to data from a deep phylogeny. The same data were then subject to tree reconstruction by the same FastME method (Desper and Gascuel, 2002, 2004) available in DAMBE. The first tree (Fig. 7.1a) was reconstructed with likelihood-based SE TN93 distance (MLCompositeTN93 in DAMBE), the second (Fig. 7.1b) with IE TN93 distance and the last (Fig. 7.1c) with LogDet distance. MLCompositeTN93 and LogDet distances recovered the true tree but the bootstrap support values are substantially higher with MLCompositeTN93 distance than with LogDet distance. The IE TN93 distance (Fig. 7.1b) recovered a wrong tree. Such differences in performance are generally true for all 13 mitochondrial genes in vertebrate mtRNA.

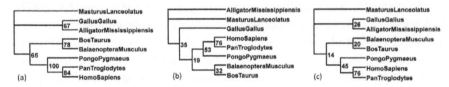

FIGURE 7.1 Contrasting phylogenetic performance among three distances, with the third codon sites only from a set of mitochondrial COI sequences from eight vertebrate species. Values next to internal nodes are bootstrap support values. (a) Likelihood-based simultaneously estimated TN93 distances. (b) Independently estimated TN93 distances. (c) LogDet distance.

7.3   DISTANCE-BASED PHYLOGENETIC ALGORITHMS

Distance-based phylogenetic reconstruction has two components, the first being the distance and the second being the algorithm of building trees from a distance matrix. Representatives of tree-building algorithms include UPGMA (Sneath, 1962), the neighbor-joining (NJ) method (Saitou and Nei, 1987), and FastME (Desper and Gascuel, 2002) with the last two accounting for almost all published distance-based phylogenies. The UPGMA method is an average-linkage clustering method and has already been numerically illustrated elsewhere (Xia, 2018a, pp. 129–144). Most frequently used distance-based tree-building algorithms are NJ and LS-based method with global optimization. I will numerically illustrate these methods in detail in this chapter. These algorithms have also been implemented in my program DAMBE (Xia, 2013b; Xia, 2017a, 2018b) which also imputes distances between two OTUs whose sequences do not share homologous sites by using the computable distances between these OTUs and other OTUs in the data set (Xia, 2018c).

7.3.1   LEAST-SQUARE METHODS AND MINIMUM EVOLUTION CRITERION

Distance-based tree reconstruction with the minimum evolution (ME) criterion involves two steps. The first is branch-length evaluation given a topology, which is typically done with LS method. The second is to choose the best tree among all trees based on *TL*. The tree with the shortest *TL* is the best tree. This criterion is mostly consistent with the LS criterion which chooses the tree with the smallest sum of squared residuals. However, one may occasionally encounter conflicts between the two criteria, especially when negative branch lengths are allowed. All these will become quite clear after numerical illustration below.

Let us start with a tree with only three OTUs (operational taxonomic units). There is only one unrooted tree with three OTUs (*S1*, *S2*, and *S3* in Fig. 7.2A), so we only need to evaluate branch lengths by using the following equation:

$$\hat{d}_{12} = x_1 + x_2$$
$$\hat{d}_{13} = x_1 + x_3 \qquad (7.7)$$
$$\hat{d}_{23} = x_2 + x_3 .$$

where $\hat{d}_{ij}$ is the expected distance between OTUs i and j, and x_1, x_2, and x_3 are branch lengths (Fig. 7.2A). After replacing the three expected distances by the observed distances (d_{ij}) computed from a set of aligned sequences, we have three equations with three unknowns, so x_1, x_2, and x_3 can be easily obtained by solving the simultaneous equations, i.e.,

$$x_1 = \frac{d_{12} + d_{13} - d_{23}}{2}; x_2 = \frac{d_{12} + d_{23} - d_{13}}{2}; x_3 = \frac{d_{13} + d_{23} - d_{12}}{2} \qquad (7.8)$$

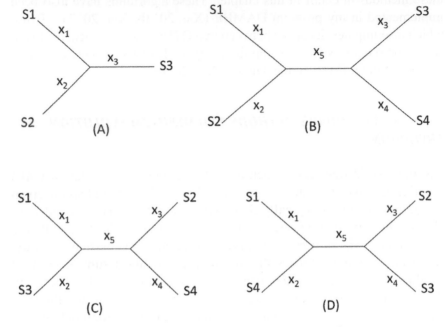

FIGURE 7.2   Topologies for illustrating the distance-based methods.

For the four-OTU tree in Figure 7.3B, we can write down the equations in the same way as in Eq. (7.7), i.e.,

$$\hat{d}_{12} = x_1 + x_2$$
$$\hat{d}_{13} = x_1 + x_5 + x_3$$
$$\hat{d}_{14} = x_1 + x_5 + x_4$$
$$\hat{d}_{23} = x_2 + x_5 + x_3 \qquad (7.9)$$
$$\hat{d}_{24} = x_2 + x_5 + x_4$$
$$\hat{d}_{34} = x_3 + x_4$$

where $\hat{d}_{ij}$ is the expected distance between OTUs i and j (i.e., distance computed from aligned sequences) as the summation of branch lengths linking OTUs i and j). $\hat{d}_{ij}$ is known as patristic distance.

If we now replace $\hat{d}_{ij}$ by the observed d_{ij}, we will have six equations for five unknowns (x_1 to x_5), so we will not be able to solve for x_1 to x_5 exactly.

The OLS method finds the x_i values that minimize the residual sum of squared deviations (RSS),

$$RSS = \sum \left(d_{ij} - \hat{d}_{ij} \right)^2 = \left[d_{12} - \left(x_1 + x_2 \right) \right]^2 + \dots + \left[d_{34} - \left(x_3 + x_4 \right) \right]^2 \quad (7.10)$$

Recall that OLS is a special case of WLS method which is expressed as

$$RSS = \frac{\sum \left(d_{ij} - \hat{d}_{ij} \right)^2}{w_{ij}^m} \quad (7.11)$$

where w_{ij} is the weight, typically equal to either d_{ij} or $\hat{d}_{ij}$, m is an integer typically equal to either 0, 1, or 2. When $m = 0$, we have OLS. When $m = 1$ and $w_{ij} = \hat{d}_{ij}$, we have RSS = χ^2. For numerical illustration, we will stay with OLS.

By taking the partial derivatives of RSS in Eq. (7.10) with respect to x_i, setting the derivatives to zero and solving the resulting simultaneous equations, we get

$$
\begin{aligned}
x_1 &= d_{13}/4 + d_{12}/2 - d_{23}/4 + d_{14}/4 - d_{24}/4 \\
x_2 &= d_{12}/2 - d_{13}/4 + d_{23}/4 - d_{14}/4 + d_{24}/4 \\
x_3 &= d_{13}/4 + d_{23}/4 + d_{34}/2 - d_{14}/4 - d_{24}/4 \\
x_4 &= d_{14}/4 - d_{13}/4 - d_{23}/4 + d_{34}/2 + d_{24}/4 \\
x_5 &= - d_{12}/2 + d_{23}/4 - d_{34}/2 + d_{14}/4 + d_{24}/4 + d_{13}/4 .
\end{aligned}
\quad (7.12)
$$

If we have $d_{12} = 0.3$, $d_{13} = 0.4$, $d_{23} = 0.5$, $d_{14} = 0.4$, $d_{24} = 0.6$, $d_{34} = 0.6$, then $x_1 = 0.075$, $x_2 = 0.225$, $x_3 = 0.275$, $x_4 = 0.325$, $x_5 = 0.025$. The summation of all branch lengths is termed TL:

$$TL = \sum_{i=1}^{2n-3} x_i \quad (7.13)$$

where n is the number of OTUs. For our topology in Figure 7.2, TL = 0.925. With four OTUs, there are three unrooted trees, so we need to repeat the above procedure to obtain x_1 to x_5 for the other two trees in Figure 7.2C and Figure 7.2D. We will designate TL for topologies in Figure 7.2B, 7.2C, and 7.2D as TL_B, TL_C, and TL_D, respectively.

Once we have evaluated the branch lengths and computed TL_B, TL_C, and TL_D, the ME criterion (Rzhetsky and Nei, 1992, 1994a) will choose the tree with the shortest TL as the best tree. This is conceptually analogous to the maximum parsimony criterion, i.e., the best tree is the one that requires the simplest explanation.

7.3.2 NEIGHBOR-JOINING METHOD

NJ method and UPGMA are related. UPGMA clusters two OTUs with the shortest distance in the distance matrix. In contrast, NJ takes into consideration two pieces of information: (1) The distance between the two OTUs and (2) how far these two OTUs are from other species. Two OTUs should be clustered if they have a short distance between them and jointly are far from the rest of the OTUs. This makes good sense.

Suppose we have a tree with four species (*S1* to *S4*) and labeled branch lengths shown in Figure 7.3A. We can estimate the distance between each species pair from aligned molecular sequences. Suppose we have estimated the distances shown in Figure 7.3B. How would the NJ method infer the tree from the distance matrix?

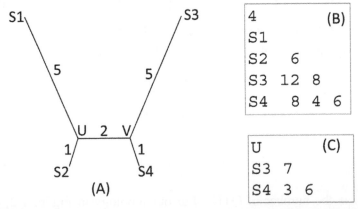

FIGURE 7.3 A presumed true tree (A) with branch lengths labeled, together with an observable distance matrix (B), for illustrating a neighbor-joining method that takes the matrix (B) to infer the tree (A). The matrix (B) is directly derived from the tree (A), which is equivalent to having perfectly accurate distance estimates. The two internal nodes are labeled *U* and *V*. The NJ method progressively reduces the distance matrix to smaller ones, e.g., from the 4 × 4 matrix in (B) to 3 × 3 matrix in (C).

The first step of NJ is to compute the "total distance" for species i (r_i) as

$$r_i = \sum_{j=1, j \neq i}^{N} d_{ij} \tag{7.14}$$

For our four species,

$$\begin{aligned}
r_1 &= d_{12} + d_{13} + d_{14} = 26 \\
r_2 &= d_{12} + d_{23} + d_{24} = 18 \\
r_3 &= d_{13} + d_{23} + d_{34} = 26 \\
r_4 &= d_{14} + d_{24} + d_{34} = 18
\end{aligned} \tag{7.15}$$

Now for each pair of species i and j, we calculate an index (M_{ij}) that will help us decide which two species should be clustered:

$$M_{ij} = d_{ij} - \frac{r_i + r_j}{N - 2} \tag{7.16}$$

where N ($= 4$) is the number of OTUs in the distance matrix.
For our four species with six species pairs,

$$\begin{aligned}
M_{12} &= d_{12} - \frac{r_1 + r_2}{N - 2} = 6 - \frac{26 + 18}{2} = -16 \\
M_{13} &= M_{14} = M_{23} = M_{24} = -14, M_{34} = -16
\end{aligned} \tag{7.17}$$

Note that $M_{12} = M_{34} = -16$, and the other four M_{ij} values are -14. The difference is 2, which means that, if we cluster $S1$ and $S2$, or $S3$ and $S4$, then the branch length between the two ancestors (i.e., the two internal nodes) is 2. If the branch length between the two internal nodes is zero (i.e., a star tree), then all six M_{ij} values will be equal, or vice versa.

Now we choose the smallest M_{ij} and cluster species i and j together. Note that we would have UPGMA if $M_{ij} = d_{ij}$ and would have wrongly clustered species 2 and 4 because d_{24} ($= 4$) is the smallest distance, leading to failure to recover the true tree in Figure 7.3A. With NJ, we found M_{12} and M_{34} to be the smallest, so we may cluster either $S1$ and $S2$ together or $S3$ and $S4$ together. This is a nonconflicting situation and we may choose either M_{12} or M_{34}. A conflict occurs if M_{12} and M_{13} are both the smallest.

Suppose we have chosen M_{12} to cluster $S1$ and $S2$, which has a common ancestor U (Fig. 7.3). We need to compute the branch lengths linking species 1 and U and species 2 and U:

$$b_{1U} = \frac{d_{12}}{2} + \frac{r_1 - r_2}{2(N-2)} = 5$$

$$b_{2U} = d_{12} - b_{1U} = 1 = \frac{d_{12}}{2} + \frac{r_2 - r_1}{2(N-2)}$$

(7.18)

Recall that UPGMA would have $b_{1U} = d_{12}/2$. In NJ, a species with a large r will have a longer branch to the ancestor than the sister species with a small r. This again makes intuitive sense. Note that the numerator is $(r_1 - r_2)$ for computing b_{1U} but $(r_2 - r_1)$ for computing b_{2U}.

Now that we have node U representing $S1$ and $S2$, we need to compute the distances between U and $S3$ and between U and $S4$:

$$d_{U3} = \frac{d_{13} + d_{23} - d_{12}}{2} = 7$$

$$d_{U4} = \frac{d_{14} + d_{24} - d_{12}}{2} = 3$$

(7.19)

which are the same equations we used in Eq. (7.8) for three OTUs. These two distances, together with the original d_{34}, are shown in Figure 7.3C where $S1$ and $S2$ have been replaced by U.

Now we have only three OTUs (U, $S3$, and $S4$) with their pairwise distances shown in Figure 7.3C. We can now directly apply Eq. (7.8) to obtain the three remaining branch lengths. This yields $b_{UV} = 2$, $b_{3V} = 5$ and $b_{4V} = 1$. However, had we started with 10 OTUs, we would now have 9 OTUs remaining. To illustrate the general approach, we will pretend to have more than 3 remaining OTUs. We repeat the process by computing r_U, r_3, and r_4 as well as M_{U3}, M_{U4}, and M_{34}:

$$r_U = d_{U3} + d_{U4} = 10, \, r_3 = 13, \, r_4 = 9$$

$$M_{U3} = d_{U3} - \frac{r_U + r_3}{N-2} = -16 = M_{U4} = M_{34}$$

(7.20)

where N again is the number of OTUs, but now reduced from 4 to 3 as we see in Figure 7.3C.

Note that r_3 and r_4 in Eq. (7.20) are different from those in Eq. (7.15). Also note that, with three OTUs ($N = 3$), we will always have equal M_{ij} values which are equal to

$$M_{12} = M_{13} = M_{23} = -(d_{12} + d_{13} + d_{23}) \qquad (7.21)$$

This is because we have only one unrooted tree with three OTUs and we will always get to this same tree no matter which two OTUs are clustered.

Now we need to compute the branch lengths from S_3 and S_4 to their common ancestor (internal node V in Fig. 7.3A):

$$b_{UV} = \frac{d_{U3}}{2} + \frac{r_U - r_3}{2(N-2)} = \frac{7}{2} + \frac{10-13}{2(3-2)} = 2 = \frac{d_{U4}}{2} + \frac{r_U - r_4}{2(N-2)}$$

$$b_{3V} = d_{U3} - b_{UV} = 5 = \frac{d_{U3}}{2} + \frac{r_3 - r_U}{2(N-2)} = \frac{d_{34}}{2} + \frac{r_3 - r_4}{2(N-2)} \qquad (7.22)$$

$$b_{4V} = d_{34} - b_{3V} = 1 = \frac{d_{U4}}{2} + \frac{r_4 - r_U}{2(N-2)} = \frac{d_{34}}{2} + \frac{r_4 - r_3}{2(N-2)}$$

where $N = 3$. Now we have fully reconstructed the tree in Figure 7.3A from the distance matrix in Figure 7.3B. We can apply the LS method to the distance matrix in Figure 7.3B and obtain exactly the same result. However, as we have mentioned before, UPGMA will fail to reconstruct the tree because it will start by cluster $S2$ and $S4$ together because $d_{24} (= 4)$ is the smallest of all pairwise distances.

You might be wondering why in computing M_{ij} in Eqs. (7.17) and (7.20), the denominator in the second term is $(N-2)$. Why not $(N-1)$ or $(N-3)$? Let us focus on the three-OTU case and pretend that we do not know if the denominator should be $(N-1)$, $(N-2)$ or $(N-3)$. We will just use $(N-x)$ and then infer the value of x.

We now have expressions of M_{ij} as

$$M_{12} = d_{12} - \frac{r_1 + r_2}{N-x};$$

$$M_{13} = d_{13} - \frac{r_1 + r_3}{N-x}; \qquad (7.23)$$

$$M_{23} = d_{23} - \frac{r_2 + r_3}{N-x}$$

We know that there is only one tree with three OTUs, which implies that clustering *S1* and *S2*, or *S1*, and *S3*, or *S2* and *S3* together will all arrive at the same tree. This implies that $M_{12} = M_{13} = M_{23}$, which is satisfied only when $x = 2$.

We can also use the 3-OTU case to explain why in computing branch lengths in Eq. (7.18), we have $(N-2)$ in the denominator of the second term. Take the 3-OTU tree in Figure 7.2A for example. We have already obtained x_1, x_2, and x_3 in Eq. (7.8). Suppose we now need to compute x_1 using NJ, and not sure if the denominator should have $(N-1)$, $(N-2)$, or $(N-3)$. So, we just use $(N-x)$:

$$x_1 = \frac{d_{12}}{2} + \frac{r_1 - r_2}{2(3-x)} \qquad (7.24)$$

We can set this x_1 in Eq. (7.24) equal to the x_1 in Eq. (7.8) and solve for x. This leads to $x = 2$.

7.3.3   CONSEQUENCE OF OVER- AND UNDERESTIMATED DISTANCES

Whether a distance-based method will recover the true tree depends critically on the accuracy of the distance estimates. Distances typically cannot be estimated accurately for a variety of reasons, such as substitution saturation that erode historical information, stochastic effect, differential selection operating at different sites, etc. It is, therefore, important to understand the consequences of overestimated and underestimated distances. We will briefly examine the bias in the distance-based methods, by using both the ME criterion and the LS criterion.

Let TL_A and TL_B be the tree length for Trees A and B in Figure 7.4. Suppose that OTUs 1 and 3 have diverged from each other so much as to have experienced substitution saturation (Xia et al., 2003b) to cause difficulty in estimating the true D_{13}. Let pD_{13} be the estimated D_{13}, where p measures the degree of underestimation ($p < 1$) or overestimation ($p > 1$).

$$TL_A - TL_B = \frac{d_{12} + d_{34} - (pd_{13} + d_{24})}{4}. \qquad (7.25)$$

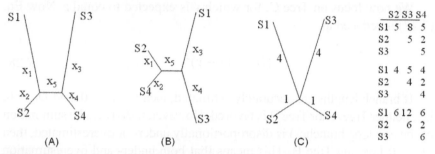

FIGURE 7.4   Topologies for illustrating bias in distance-based methods.

With the ME criterion for choosing the best tree, Tree A is better than Tree B if $TL_A < TL_B$ and worse than Tree B if $TL_A > TL_B$. Simple distances such as the p-distance or JC69 distance tend to have $p < 1$ and consequently increase the chance of having $TL_A > TL_B$. This is equivalent to the long-branch attraction problem, first recognized in the maximum parsimony method (Felsenstein, 1978a). Evolutionary distances corrected with gamma-distributed rates over sites (Golding, 1983; Jin and Nei, 1990; Nei and Gojobori, 1986; Tamura and Nei, 1993) tend to have $p > 1$ when the shape parameter is underestimated, and consequently would tend to favor Tree A over Tree B, leading to long-branch repulsion (Waddell, 1995).

The LS criterion chooses the tree with the smallest SS defined below.

$$SS = \sum_{i=1}^{n-1} \sum_{j=i+1}^{n} \frac{\left(d_{ij} - \hat{d}_{ij}\right)^2}{d_{ij}^P} \tag{7.26}$$

where n is the number of OTUs, d_{ij} and $\hat{d}_{ij}$ are respectively the observed and expected distances between species i and j, and P often takes the value of 0, 1 or 2.

Let SS_A and SS_B be SS in Eq. (7.26) for Trees A and B, respectively. With $P = 0$ in Eq. (7.26) and letting $D_{SS} = SS_A - SS_B$, we have

$$4D_{SS} = (d_{13} + d_{24})^2 - (d_{12} + d_{34})^2 + 2(d_{14} + d_{23})[(d_{12} + d_{34}) - (d_{13} + d_{24})]$$
$$= x^2 - y^2 + 2z(y - x) \tag{7.27}$$

where $x = d_{13} + d_{24}$, $y = d_{12} + d_{34}$ and $z = d_{14} + d_{23}$.

We now focus on Tree C, for which y is expected to equal z. Now Eq. (7.27) is reduced to

$$4D_{SS} = (x - y)^2 \qquad (7.28)$$

If branch lengths are accurately estimated, then $x = y = 10$, and $D_{SS} = 0$, i.e., neither Tree A nor Tree B is favored. However, if d_{13} (i.e., the summation of the two long branches) is disproportionally under- or overestimated, then $D_{SS} > 0$ favoring Tree B. This means that both under- and overestimation of the distance between divergence taxa will lead to long-branch attraction with the LS criterion. This can be better illustrated with a numerical example with Tree C in Figure 7.4 which also displays three distance matrices. The first one is accurate, the second one has genetic distances more underestimated for more divergent taxa and the third has genetic distances more overestimated for more divergent taxa (e.g., when gamma-distributed rates are assumed with an underestimated shape parameter). Note that Tree A and Tree B converge to Tree C when $x_5 = 0$. Table 7.3 shows the results by applying the ME and LS criterion in analyzing the three distance matrices.

When the distances are accurate, the application of both the ME criterion and the LS criterion recovers Tree C (the true tree) with $x_5 = 0$, $TL = 10$, and $SS = 0$. However, ME criterion favors Tree B when long branches are underestimated ($TL_B < TL_A$, Table 7.3) and Tree A when long branches are overestimated ($TL_A < TL_B$). In contrast, the LS criterion favors Tree B with both under- and overestimated distances (Table 7.3) when negative branch lengths are allowed. One may explore such biases further by analyzing simulated sequences.

TABLE 7.3   Effect of under- and overestimation of genetic distances for more divergent taxa.

	Correct		Underestimation		Overestimation	
	TreeA	TreeB	TreeA	TreeB	TreeA	TreeB
TL	10	10	7.75	7.5	12.5	13
SS	0	0	0.25	0	1	0
x_5	0	0	−0.25	0.5	0.5	−1

Sometimes one may be able to identify the bias in distance estimation by careful examination of the aligned sequences. Take, for example, 18S rRNA which has highly conserved and variable domains. Both indel and nucleotide substitution events have occurred predominantly in the eight variable domains (Van de Peer et al., 1993). If some sequences have experienced a number of deletions at their variable domains and if the genetic distance between the two sequences is calculated by using all homologous sites between the two sequences, then the genetic distance involving the shortest sequences, i.e., the one with the shortest variable region, will be relatively underestimated (Van de Peer et al., 1993).

7.4 DATING SPECIATION AND GENE DUPLICATION EVENTS

Although the molecular clock concept was proposed on the basis of evolutionary distances (Zuckerkandl and Pauling, 1965) and the conceptual framework for distance-based dating has been in place for many years (Chakraborty, 1977; Drummond and Rodrigo, 2000; Takezaki et al., 1995), it is only recently (Xia, 2013b; Xia, 2017a; Xia and Yang, 2011) that statistical methods and software for dating speciation and gene duplication events by using evolutionary distances have become available. This is partly due to the existence of more sophisticated methods based on Bayesian inference. However, there are two reasons to illustrate distance-based dating. First, it is simpler to explain the conceptual framework of dating by using distance-based methods than by using Bayesian inference. Second, there are still cases where distance-based methods represent a good contender in dating, just as there are still cases where distance-based methods are a good choice in phylogenetic reconstruction. This section outlines the rationale of the distance-based dating, numerically illustrated with both fossil-calibrated internal nodes for conventional dating and with tip-dating for rapidly evolving genomes such as retroviruses (Drummond et al., 2003a; Drummond et al., 2003b).

I will first detail the approach involving a single gene with one or more calibration points and with global and two versions of local clocks. This is followed by approaches for dating with multiple genes and estimating the variation of the divergence time by resampling methods, such as bootstrapping and jackknifing (Felsenstein, 2004, pp 335–363). The accuracy of the distance-based dating method is illustrated by applying it to dating with two datasets, one with seven great ape species (Rannala and Yang, 2007) and the other with 35 mammalian species including major mammalian lineages (Yang and Yoder, 2003).

7.4.1 THE LEAST-SQUARES METHOD FOR CONVENTIONAL INTERNAL-NODE-CALIBRATED DATING

The statistical framework of the least-square dating method has been presented independently in matrix form twice before (Chakraborty, 1977; Drummond and Rodrigo, 2000). Here we illustrate the mathematical rationale as well as the extensions including multiple calibration points and tip-dating, two versions of local clocks and the computation of confidence limits by resampling methods. The method is implemented in DAMBE (Xia, 2013b; Xia, 2017a; Xia and Yang, 2011).

7.4.1.1 DATING WITH ONE CALIBRATION POINT

Given the evolutionary distances d_{ij} and the topology in Figure 7.5, with the time to the root known as T_1, we need to estimate t_2, t_3, and r (the substitution rate). Assuming a global clock, we minimize the following RSS based on the OLS method:

$$RSS = (d_{12} - 2rt_3)^2 + (d_{13} - 2rt_2)^2 + (d_{23} - 2rt_2)^2 + ... + (d_{34} - 2rT_1)^2 \quad (7.29)$$

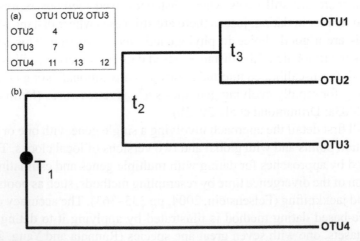

(a)	OTU1	OTU2	OTU3
OTU2	4		
OTU3	7	9	
OTU4	11	13	12

FIGURE 7.5 Rooted Tree with four OTUs (numbered 1–4) for illustrating the distance-based least-squares method for dating speciation events. T_1 is known and used to calibrate the molecular clock and t_2 and t_3, as well as the substitution rate r, are to be estimated.

Note that Eq. (7.29) is expressed as squared residuals between the observed distance (d_{ij}) and the expected distance ($2rt_i$). One can also express it as squared residuals in time such as

$$RSS = (\frac{d_{12}}{r} - 2t_3)^2 + (\frac{d_{13}}{r} - 2t_2)^2 + (\frac{d_{23}}{r} - 2t_2)^2 + ... + (\frac{d_{34}}{r} - 2T_1)^2 \quad (7.30)$$

To derive formulae for t_2, t_3, and r, we take the partial derivatives of RSS with respect to r, t_2, and t_3, equate the three partial derivatives to zero, and solve the three resulting simultaneous equations. This will give us

$$r = \frac{d_{14} + d_{24} + d_{34}}{6T_1}$$

$$t_2 = \frac{3(d_{13} + d_{23})T_1}{2(d_{14} + d_{24} + d_{34})} = \frac{d_{13} + d_{23}}{4r} \quad (7.31)$$

$$t_3 = \frac{3d_{12}T_1}{d_{14} + d_{24} + d_{34}} = \frac{d_{12}}{2r}$$

In general, when there is only one calibration point (T) for an internal node, then r is expressed as

$$r = \frac{\sum_{i=1}^{n}\sum_{j=1}^{m} d_{ij}}{2nmT} \quad (7.32)$$

where n is the number of children in one descendent clade of the node with calibration time T, m is the number of children in the other descendent clade of the node, and d_{ij} is the evolutionary distance from i^{th} leaf in one descendent clade to j^{th} leaf in the other descendent clade. In the four OTU case with T_1 known (Fig. 7.5), $n = 1$ (OTU 4) and $m = 3$ (OTUs 1, 2 and 3), and d_{ij} values are d_{14}, d_{24}, and d_{34}.

7.4.1.2   DATING WITH MULTIPLE CALIBRATION POINTS

With multiple calibration points, the method will be essentially the same except that we have fewer parameters to estimate. For example, if both T_1 and T_3 are known, then we only need to estimate r and t_2, which are

$$r = \frac{T_3 d_{12} + T_1 d_{14} + T_1 d_{24} + T_1 d_{34}}{2\left(T_3^2 + 3T_1^2\right)}$$

$$t_2 = \frac{(d_{13} + d_{23})\left(T_3^2 + 3T_1^2\right)}{2\left(T_3 d_{12} + T_1 d_{14} + T_1 d_{24} + T_1 d_{34}\right)} = \frac{d_{13} + d_{23}}{4r} \tag{7.33}$$

When N_c calibration points are available, then the LS estimate of r is

$$r = \frac{\displaystyle\sum_{k=1}^{N_c} T_k \sum_{i=1}^{n_k} \sum_{j=1}^{m_k} d_{ijk}}{2 \displaystyle\sum_{k=1}^{N_c} n_k m_k T_k^2} \tag{7.34}$$

For example, with the tree in Figure 7.5, but with both T_1 and T_3 known, then r is

$$r = \frac{T_1(d_{14} + d_{24} + d_{34}) + T_3 d_{12}}{2(3T_1^2 + T_3^2)} \tag{7.35}$$

The method above with multiple calibration points provides the flexibility for the user to further optimize the time estimates. This is done with three steps. The first is to construct a tree with an imposed clock and the LS criterion, without reference to the calibration time. This results in a set of internal nodes with estimated path lengths (D) to descendent leaves. The second step is to minimize the following RSS after constructing a tree with an imposed clock:

$$RSS = \sum_{i=1}^{N_c} (D_i - rT_i)^2 \tag{7.36}$$

where N_c is the number of nodes having calibration time T_1, T_2, ..., T_{Nc} and D_i is the distance from the node with calibration time T_i to the tip, i.e., the path length from the node with calibration time T_i to a descendent leaf (Note that the node has equal path length to any of its descendent leaves when a global clock is assumed). Solving for r leads to

$$r = \frac{\sum\limits_{i=1}^{N_c} D_i T_i}{\sum\limits_{i=1}^{N_c} T_i^2} \qquad (7.37)$$

The third, and final, step is to rescale all D_i values by r, i.e., converting D_i to divergence time. This rescaling includes the nodes with calibration time T_i. The approach of rescaling fossil dates by the LS criterion is termed soft-calibrated dating.

Note that r is an unbiased estimate of the true evolutionary rate (γ) only when T_i is an unbiased estimate of the true divergence time τ_i and D_i is an unbiased estimate of $\gamma\tau_i$. While D_i could arguably be an unbiased estimate of $\gamma\tau_i$ for molecular sequence data when the substitution model is correct and stochastic effect negligible, T_i is typically an underestimate of τ_i, i.e., $T_i = \tau_i - \varepsilon_{fossil.i}$, where ε_{fossil} is the bias in the fossil date. This implies that the estimated r is typically an overestimate of γ, with the bias (designated by h_{fossil}) being

$$h_{fossil} = \frac{\gamma - r}{\gamma} = -\frac{\sum\limits_{i=1}^{N_c} \varepsilon_{fossil.i} T_i}{\sum\limits_{i=1}^{N_c} T_i^2} \qquad (7.38)$$

When D_i is also uncertain, e.g., due to limited data or due to substitution saturation in molecular sequences (which typically leads to D_i underestimating $\gamma\tau_i$), we have $D_i = \gamma\tau_i - \varepsilon_{data,i}$, and the bias in the estimated r, designated by $h_{fossil+data}$, becomes

$$h_{fossil+data} = \frac{\gamma - r}{\gamma} = \frac{\sum\limits_{i=1}^{N_c} \varepsilon_{data.i} T_i - \gamma \sum\limits_{i=1}^{N_c} \varepsilon_{fossil.i} T_i}{\gamma \sum\limits_{i=1}^{N_c} T_i^2} \qquad (7.39)$$

Eq. (7.39) shows clearly that the estimated r (as well as the estimated divergence time) contains two sources of uncertainty, one due to ε_{fossil} and one due to ε_{data}. These two sources of uncertainty have not been distinguished in published papers on dating. It is important to keep in mind that, while unlimited amount of good sequence data for estimating D_i can reduce ε_{data} to 0, no amount of sequence data can reduce ε_{fossil}.

7.4.1.3   DATING WITH MULTIPLE GENES WITH ONE OR MORE CALIBRATION POINTS

The method can be easily extended to perform a combined analysis with multiple distance matrices, e.g., when there are two or more genes, when each distance is obtained from each of the three codon positions in a protein-coding gene or when one has one distance matrix from sequence data and another from DNA hybridization data. With two genes A and B and two corresponding distance matrices whose individual elements are represented by $d_{A.ij}$ and $d_{B.ij}$, respectively, we can perform a combined analysis to estimate jointly t_2, t_3, r_A, and r_B (where r_A and r_B are the substitution rate for genes A and B, respectively) in two steps. First, we obtain $k = r_B / r_A$ by using a simple linear regression with the regression model $d_B = k{\cdot}d_A$ (i.e., forcing the intercept to 0). Second, we rewrite Eq. (7.29) as follows:

$$RSS_1 = (d_{A.12} - 2r_A t_3)^2 + (d_{A.13} - 2r_A t_2)^2 + ... + (d_{A.34} - 2r_A T_1)^2$$
$$RSS_2 = (d_{B.12} - 2kr_A t_3)^2 + (d_{B.13} - 2kr_A t_2)^2 + ... + (d_{B.34} - 2kr_A T_1)^2 \qquad (7.40)$$
$$RSS = RSS_1 + RSS_2$$

Now r_A, t_2, and t_3 can be estimated just as before, and r_B can be estimated as $k{\cdot}r_A$. With the topology in Figure 7.5, the LS solutions for the unknowns are

$$r_A = \frac{C}{6T_1(1+k^2)}$$
$$t_2 = \frac{3(d_{A.13} + d_{A.23} + kd_{B.13} + kd_{B.23})T_1}{2C}$$
$$t_3 = \frac{3(d_{A.12} + kd_{B.12})T_1}{C} \qquad (7.41)$$
$$C = d_{A.14} + d_{A.24} + d_{A.34} + kd_{B.14} + kd_{B.24} + kd_{B.34}$$

If the two genes evolve at the same rate so that $d_{A.ij} = d_{A.ij}$ and $k = 1$, then r_A, t_2, and t_3 are reduced to the same expressions as those in Eq. (7.31).

One potential problem with this approach is that, if $k \gg 1$ (i.e., when gene B evolves much faster than gene A), the estimation will depend on $d_{B.ij}$ much more than $d_{A.ij}$. Similarly, if $k \ll 1$, the estimation will depend on $d_{A.ij}$ much more than $d_{B.ij}$. For example, the third codon position evolves much faster than codon positions 1 and 2. Applying Eq. (7.41) will result in estimates dominated by the distance matrix from the third codon position.

An alternative approach is to first scale RSS$_2$ in Eq. (7.40) by dividing values within each parenthesis in RSS$_2$ by k, so Eq. (7.40) becomes

$$RSS_1 = (d_{A.12} - 2rt_3)^2 + (d_{A.13} - 2rt_2)^2 + ... + (d_{A.34} - 2rT_1)^2$$

$$RSS_2 = (d_{B.12}/k - 2rt_3)^2 + (d_{B.13}/k - 2rt_2)^2 + ... + (d_{B.34}/k - 2rT_1)^2 \qquad (7.42)$$

$$RSS = RSS_1 + RSS_2$$

Neither this scaled approach nor the unscaled approach specified in Eq. (7.40) is well-reasoned. A better approach is to see which gene or which site partition conforms to the molecular clock better than others and then weigh them accordingly. Two approach can be used, preferably jointly, in evaluating the suitability of genes for dating. The first is by testing the clock hypothesis based on distances (Xia, 2009) and the second, when multiple high-quality calibration points are available, is to test which gene or site partition are consistent with the calibration points. The third codon position, less constrained by natural selection, should provide better estimates of evolutionary time as long as substitution saturation (Xia and Lemey, 2009; Xia et al., 2003b) is not an issue. In addition, the third codon position exhibits little heterogeneity in substitution rate over sites relative to the first and second codon positions, which is a highly desirable property in molecular phylogenetic reconstruction (Xia, 1998b). In other words, the third codon position may deserve a greater weight than codon positions 1 and 2 for dating evolutionary events and should not be scaled to have the same weight as codon positions 1 and 2. On the other hand, if the third codon position have all experienced multiple substitution, then it will have little information left for dating. An ideal case is when distances estimated from the three codon positions are all highly positively and linearly correlated.

In general, for the same period of evolutionary time, the fast-evolving gene (i.e., the one generating large pairwise distances) is expected to conform to neutral evolution better than a slow-evolving gene subject to functional constraints. For this reason, the unscaled method seems more justifiable. Following this reasoning, we can perform a simple combined analysis involving N_g genes by generating a new distance matrix with d_{ij} computed as a weighted average:

$$d_{ij} = \frac{\sum_{k=1}^{N_g} d_{ijk} \bar{d}_k}{\sum_{k=1}^{N_g} \bar{d}_k} \tag{7.43}$$

where $\bar{d}_k$ is the mean of all the pairwise distances from gene k.

7.4.1.4   DATING WITH LOCAL CLOCKS

Molecular sequence data violating a global clock have long been known (Britten, 1986; Li and Tanimura, 1987; Li et al., 1987; Li and Wu, 1987; Wu and Li, 1985) and it is rare for a large tree to have a global clock operating along all lineages (Pereira and Baker, 2006; Smith et al., 2006; Tinn and Oakley, 2008). Relatively fast-evolving lineages will have overestimated divergence times if a global clock is imposed. Although protocols are available to eliminate offending lineages that do not conform to the global clock (Rambaut and Bromham, 1998; Takezaki et al., 1995) and to generate linearized trees, such treatments lead to inefficient use of data and are practical only when the majority of the lineages conform to the global clock. For this reason, local clocks are often necessary for practical dating.

There are three general approaches for local clock dating with distance-based methods. The first is when specific lineages are a priori known to evolve differently from others and can, therefore, be explicitly modeled. Several approaches have been proposed to solve this local clock dating problem (Kishino and Hasegawa, 1990; Yoder and Yang, 2000).

The second approach to local clock dating is the rate-smoothing pioneered by Sanderson (1997), based on the inference that the evolution rate is autocorrelated along lineages (Gillespie, 1991). This constraint of rate autocorrelation will penalize dramatic changes in evolutionary rate along lineages. Thus, for rapidly evolving lineages, this approach will result in a divergence time smaller than that from the global clock approach but larger than that from the first approach without the constraint of rate autocorrelation. We will illustrate both approaches for comparative purposes.

The third approach is sister taxa scaling. It involves two steps. First, given a bifurcating tree with branch lengths, we start from the root to scale the two sister taxa to have the same mean branch lengths from the root. We continue to traverse the nodes to scale the two sister taxa to have the same mean branch lengths from their parental node. Second, convert branch to time by using fossil calibration of internal nodes. This approach is implemented in DAMBE (Xia, 2018b). Here I illustrate only the first two approaches.

7.4.1.4.1   Local Clock with Lineages Known A Priori to Evolve Differently

Suppose we have four lineages with very different evolutionary rates (Fig. 7.6a), with the lineages leading to OTU1 and OTU2 expected a priori to evolve at different rates from lineages leading to OTU3 and OTU4. Note that, although we labeled branch lengths (b_i) on the tree, in practice both branch lengths and pairwise distances are unknown and need to be estimated from the data. Thus, the input for the local-clock dating is a distance matrix, a topology, and a specification of which lineages have different rates.

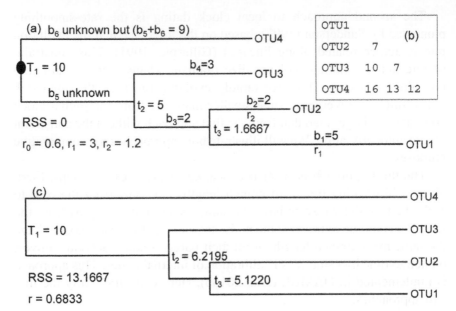

FIGURE 7.6 A 4-OTU tree with lineage-specific evolutionary rates (a). The branch lengths are indicated on the branch, together with the patristic distance matrix (c). T_1 is the calibration point, and t_2 and t_3 are dated with either (a) a local clock model with three rates (r_0, r_1, and r_2), or (c) a global clock model with a single rate (r).

Let us designate evolutionary rate from t_3 to OTU1 as r_1 and from t_3 to OTU2 as r_2. The rest of the lineages are assumed to evolve at the rate r_0. Given the evolutionary distances (Fig. 7.6b) and calibration time T_1 (Fig. 7.6a), we can obtain r_0, r_1, and r_2, as well as t_2 and t_3, by minimizing the following RSS

$$
\begin{aligned}
RSS = \ & (d_{12} - r_1 t_3 - r_2 t_3)^2 + (d_{13} - r_1 t_3 - r_0(t_2 - t_3) - r_0 t_2)^2 \\
& + (d_{14} - r_1 t_3 - r_0(t_2 - t_3) - r_0(T_1 - t_2) - r_0 T_1)^2 + (d_{23} - r_2 t_3 - r_0(t_2 - t_3) - r_0 t_2)^2 \\
& + (d_{24} - r_2 t_3 - r_0(t_2 - t_3) - r_0(T_1 - t_2) - r_0 T_1)^2 + (d_{34} - r_0 t_2 - r_0(T_1 - t_2) - r_0 T_1)^2
\end{aligned}
\tag{7.44}
$$

Note that the local-clock model specified in Eq. (7.44) is reduced to the global-clock model specified in Eq. (7.29) when $r_0 = r_1 = r_2$.

Taking partial derivatives of RSS in Eq. (7.44) with respect to r_0, r_1, r_2, t_2, and t_3, setting the derivatives to 0 and solving the resulting simultaneous equations, we obtain

$$r_0 = \frac{d_{34}}{2T_1}$$

$$r_1 = \frac{(2d_{12} + d_{13} + d_{14} - d_{23} - d_{24})d_{34}}{A}$$

$$r_2 = \frac{(2d_{12} + d_{23} + d_{24} - d_{13} - d_{14})d_{34}}{A}$$

$$t_2 = \frac{(d_{13} + 2d_{34} + d_{23} - d_{14} - d_{24})T_1}{2d_{34}} \qquad (7.45)$$

$$t_3 = \frac{(d_{12} + 2d_{34} - d_{14} - d_{24})T_1}{d_{34}}$$

$$A = 4(d_{12} + 2d_{34} - d_{14} - d_{24})T_1$$

With the actual d_{ij} values in Figure 7.6b, we have $r_0 = 0.6$, $r_1 = 3$, $r_2 = 1.2$, $t_2 = 5$, and $t_3 = 1.6667$. Because the d_{ij} values we used are the actual path lengths from the branch lengths shown in Figure 7.6a, i.e., d_{ij} values are accurate, the resulting RSS is 0, i.e., the fit of the distance matrix to the tree is perfect.

In contrast, if we assume a single evolutionary rate (i.e., a global clock), then we will have $r = 0.6833$, $t_2 = 6.2195$, $t_3 = 5.2122$, and RSS = 13.1667 (Fig. 7.6c). In other words, the increased evolutionary rates along lineages leading to OTU1 and OTU2 resulted in a poor fit of the distance matrix to the tree (i.e., a larger RSS) and the inflated estimates of t_2 and t_3 (especially t_3 due to the much faster evolutionary rate along the lineage leading to OTU1). Whether the two parameters in the local-clock model (i.e., r_1 and r_2) justify the decrease in RSS can be tested in the framework of model selection based on differences in RSS and the number of parameters (Xia, 2009), given that the rate differences are expected *a priori*.

7.4.1.4.2 The Rate-smoothing Approach for Local Clock Dating

The rate-smoothing approach (Sanderson, 1997) involves two steps. The first is to evaluate the tree to obtain the branch lengths, which can be done either by distance-based or ML methods. The second is to use the estimated branches to estimate divergence time with the constraint of rate autocorrelation.

With the distance matrix in Figure 7.6b, the branch lengths (b_i) can be evaluated by either NJ or FastME and are shown in Figure 7.6a. Branch lengths b_5 and b_6 cannot be separately evaluated by the distance-based methods without assuming a molecular clock and consequently only their summation, designated by b_{5+6} ($= b_5 + b_6$), is shown.

The second step in the rate-smoothing approach is to estimate local rates, which are r_1 ($= b_1/t_3$), r_2 ($= b_2/t_3$), r_3 [$= b_3/(t_2-t_3)$], and so on (Fig. 7.7). The method of rate-smoothing is to obtain t_2 and t_3 (with T_1 as the calibration time) as well as b_5 that minimize the following sum of squares:

$$RSS = (r_1 - r_3)^2 + (r_2 - r_3)^2 + (r_3 - r_5)^2 + (r_4 - r_5)^2 + (r_5 - r_0)^2 + (r_6 - r_0)^2$$

where   (7.46)

$$r_0 = \frac{b_{5+6}}{2T_1 - t_2}; t_2 < T_1; t_3 < t_2$$

The minimization results in t_3=5.4742, t_2=8.5016, and b_5=0.8992 (which leads to $b_6 = b_{5+6}-b_5 = 8.1008$), with minimized RSS equal to 0.2500. All local rates were shown in Figure 7.7. Note that RSS in Eq. (7.46) is not comparable to RSS in other equations.

The rate-smoothing approach implies that the evolutionary rate of the ancestral lineage will always be between the evolutionary rates of the child lineages, which reminds us of the dating approaches assuming a Brownian motion model. Theoretically, there is no strong reason to believe that the two-child lineage cannot both evolve faster than the ancestral lineage. However, with no external information available, the best guess of the evolutionary rate of the ancestral lineage should be some sort of average of the evolutionary rates of child lineages.

The application of Eq. (7.46) requires T_1 to be fixed because if T_1 is bounded with a minimum and maximum, then RSS will always be the smallest when T_1 equals the maximum. Specifically, when T_1 is increased n times, RSS will decrease by n^2 times. This suggests that a modified version of Eq. (7.46), i.e., $RSS_m = RSS*T_1^2$, might allow T_1 to be bounded. Unfortunately, such a modification only makes the model unidentifiable because RSS_m can be identical for any T_1, i.e., if we obtain RSS_m and rates r_i with $T_1 = T$, we can obtain the same RSS_m (but rates r_i/n) with $T_1 = n \cdot T$, where n is any positive real number.

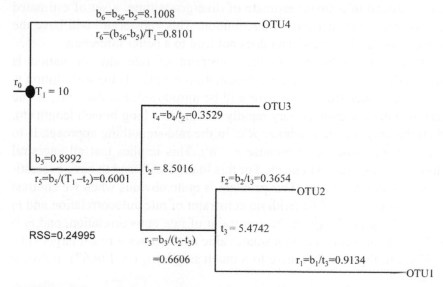

FIGURE 7.7   The estimated rates and divergence times from the rate-smoothing approach for local clock dating. T_1 is the calibration point.

It has been proposed that the rate-smoothing approach can incorporate fossil uncertainty by using the fossil date as a minimum age (Sanderson, 1997). For the reason in the previous paragraph, this proposed approach is impossible. Molecular sequences can be used to estimate branch lengths but not time and rate separately. If we increase the calibration time 10 times, then all estimated node times will be 10 times greater, and the resulting rates will simply be 10 times smaller. This is the problem shared by all dating approaches, including the likelihood and the Bayesian (Yang, 2006). Multiplying the calibration time by n and simultaneously dividing rate by n will not change the likelihood (or RSS_m in the LS approach). This invariance of likelihood with respect to calibration time due to the confounding of time and rate also causes problems in Bayesian inference.

With the LS approach we can also replace the calibration time T by a distribution (the equivalent of a Bayesian prior), e.g., a normal or exponential distribution with mean T and repeatedly sample from this distribution to obtain a set of estimated divergence times so that each internal node will have, instead of a single estimate of divergence time, a set of estimated divergence times that form a distribution. This "posterior" will have the same shape as the "prior" and does not lead to a better inference.

One main problem with the constraint of rate autocorrelation is whether the rate autocorrelation assumption is valid. If the assumption is false, then much estimation error will be introduced. For example, if one terminal lineage evolves very rapidly leading to a long branch length (b), then the only way to minimize RSS in the rate-smoothing approach is to increase the associated t because $r = b/t$. This implies that all ancestral nodes (parent, grandparent, etc.) of this lineage will tend to have overestimated divergence times. This problem is quite obvious when we contrast estimates in Figure 7.6a (with no constraint of rate autocorrelation and r_1 = 3) and Figure 7.7 (with the constraint of rate autocorrelation, and r_1 = 0.9134). Constraining r_1 to a small value necessitates a much larger t_3 (= 5.4742) in Figure 7.7 relative to a much smaller t_3 (= 1.6667) in Figure 7.6a.

7.4.1.5   NOTES ON DATING GENE DUPLICATION EVENTS

Gene duplication and subsequent subfunctionalization (i.e., the function of the parental gene is divided between the duplicated genes) and neofunctionalization (i.e., the duplicated gene acquires a new function) are important evolutionary events (Vlasschaert et al., 2015). Phylogenetic relationship and timing of gene duplication can help understand how duplicated genes evolve under which constraints (Vlasschaert et al., 2017). I wish to outline here a few caveats in dating gene duplication events as well as some special relationships among duplicated lineages that we can take advantage of in following evolutionary trajectories of duplicated genes.

Suppose we have 12 species (labeled *S1–S12*) related by the phylogeny in Figure 7.8A with gene A present in each species. A gene duplication event occurred at time T_0 (Fig. 7.8), giving rise to paralogous gene B represented in species *S1–S6* (Fig. 7.8A). While estimating T_0 is important, we will leave it aside momentarily and focus on another research problem. That is, which of the paralogous lineages (A lineage or B lineage) evolve faster. We can estimate $T_1–T_5$ by using gene B sequences in species *S1–S6* and T_1' to T_5' by using gene A sequences in species $S1$ and $S6$. As depicted in Figure 7.8B, we expect $T_i = T_i'$. Deviation from this expectation may be associated with differential mutation rates or functional constraints in these two gene lineages.

Now come back to T_0 in Figure 7.8. We can estimate T_0 if (1) all duplicated gene lineages are preserved and (2) the duplicated genes have evolved in conformation to the molecular clock hypothesis. If these two assumptions are met, then we just need to obtain gene sequences from S1A to S12A and S1B to S6B, build a tree and then date T_0 (Fig. 7.8B). Unfortunately, duplicated genes typically do not evolve in a clocklike manner, so we cannot use these gene sequences to date the duplication events. However, if we use a single-copy gene for dating, we can date only T_1 in Figure 7.8 but not T_0.

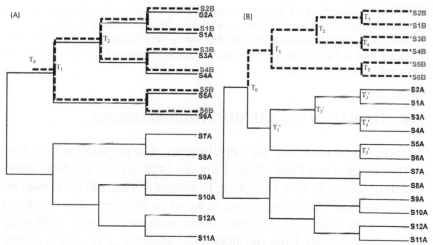

FIGURE 7.8   A gene duplication event occurred at time T_0 (A) with an alternative view in (B). We now have two copies (labeled A and B) for genes $S1$–$S6$.

What could be worse is when some paralogous lineages become lost during evolution (e.g., S5B and S6B in Fig. 7.9). This will mislead us to think that the gene duplication event occurred more recently than reality. Differential loss of paralogous genes in different lineages is long known to affect not only dating accuracy but also phylogenetic accuracy in general (Hudson, 1992).

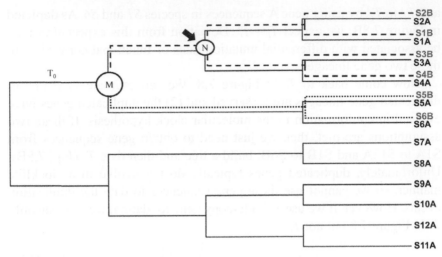

FIGURE 7.9 Illustration of lineage sorting (differential loss of paralogous genes in different lineages). The loss of paralogous gene B in lineages leading to species S5 and *S6* would result in underestimation of gene duplication time. Rather than identifying gene duplication time at T_0, we may think that gene duplication occurred somewhere along the branch connection nodes M and *N*.

7.4.2 TIP-DATING FOR RAPIDLY EVOLVING VIRUSES

The rationale of tip-dating for viral lineages was proposed a long time ago (Buonagurio and Fitch, 1986; Li et al., 1988; Saitou and Nei, 1986). Tip-dating (Drummond et al., 2003a; Drummond et al., 2003b) is used for rapidly evolving viral lineages and is based on different sampling times for calibration (Fig. 7.10). Distance-based methods for dating with serial samples have already been developed (Drummond et al., 2001; Drummond and Rodrigo, 2000; O'Brien et al., 2008; Yang et al., 2007). Given the phylogeny in Figure 7.10, we can easily write down the *RSS* for OLS method:

$$RSS = \left(\frac{d_{12}}{r} + 15 - 2t_1\right)^2 + \left(\frac{d_{13}}{r} + 10 - 2t_3\right)^2 + ... + \left(\frac{d_{56}}{r} + 30 + 25 - 2t_4\right)^2 \quad (7.47)$$

where d_{ij}/r is the time needed to generate a sequence divergence corresponding to d_{ij}. Note that, as I have shown before with the conventional internal-node calibrated dating, we can also write *RSS* as squared differences between the observed distance (d_{ij}) and the expected distance:

$$RSS = (d_{12} + 15r - 2rt_1)^2 + (d_{13} + 10r - 2rt_3)^2 + ... + (d_{56} + 30r + 25r - 2rt_4)^2 \quad (7.48)$$

To obtain r and t_i values, we take partial derivatives of RSS with respect to r and t_i, set the 6 partial derivatives to zero and solve the equation. The most recent sampling time (i.e., 1990) is taken at "present" and the estimated t_i values are the number of years from the respective internal node to the present. These t_i values are shown as italicized number next to their respective internal node in Figure 7.10, together with the actual year.

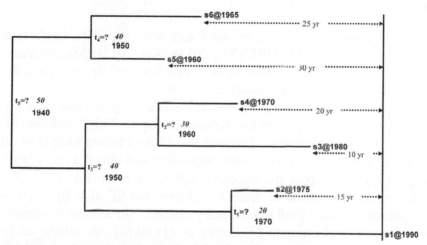

FIGURE 7.10 A viral sequence tree with sampling time embedded in sequence name (which is represented as species@samping_time). The estimated t_i values are in italics, with converted year under each t_i value.

7.4.3 OBTAINING CONFIDENCE INTERVALS BY USING BOOTSTRAPPING OR JACKKNIFING

While some dating results are published occasionally without an estimate of the variability of the estimated divergence time, such results are generally difficult to interpret with any confidence. A simple method to estimate the standard error of the time estimates is to use a resampling method, such as the bootstrap or jackknife, which has been used widely in molecular phylogenetics (see Felsenstein, 2004 for an extensive review). The method is applicable not only to aligned sequence data but also to other genetic data, such as allele frequency data with multiple loci.

For each resampled data set i and a fixed topology with N_n internal nodes, one evaluates branch lengths and obtains a set of estimated divergence time (T_{ij}, where $j = 1, 2, ..., N_n$). One can then obtain the standard error (SE) of T_j (designated by s_{Tj}) as the standard deviation of the resampled estimates:

$$s_{T_j} = \sqrt{\frac{\sum_{i=1}^{N}\left(T_{ij} - \bar{T}_j\right)^2}{N-1}}; \bar{T}_j = \frac{\sum_{i=1}^{N} T_{ij}}{N} \tag{7.49}$$

where N is the number of resampled data sets. The 95% confidence interval is $\bar{T}_j \pm 1.96 s_{T_j}$. DAMBE (Xia, 2013b; Xia, 2017a; Xia and Yang, 2011) uses this method to obtain SE of T_i values in both tip-dating and the conventional dating with calibrated internal nodes.

One might be wondering why we treat s_{Tj} as SE, given that s_{Tj} in Eq. (7.49) looks like an equation for standard deviation. This is because SE is "standard error of means." Suppose you take a random sample of 10 students from the first-year student population and obtain a mean body height ($\bar{x}_1$). You repeat the sampling 100 times to obtain $\bar{x}_1, \bar{x}_2, ... \bar{x}_{100}$. The standard deviation of these $\bar{x}_j$ values is the SE of x. In practice, we typically cannot afford to take many samples. We assume the central limit theorem and estimate SE simply by (1) taking one sample of 10 individuals, (2) compute the standard deviation (sd) from these values, and (3) obtain SE of x as sd/sqrt(10). When we take 100 bootstrapping samples to obtain $T_{i,1}$, $T_{i,2}$, ..., $T_{i,100}$, these $T_{i,j}$ values are equivalent to $\bar{x}_1, \bar{x}_2, ... \bar{x}_{100}$. So, the standard deviation of these means is SE. You may resample 100 times or 1000 times, s_{Tj} will be roughly the same.

As we have emphasized in Eq. (7.39), there are two sources of random error in dating, one from limited sequence data and one from limited fossil data. If the amount of sequence data is infinite, then the resampled distance matrices will be identical, leading to no variation in the estimated divergence time (Thorne and Kishino, 2005). This would give us false confidence in the estimated time with SE approaching 0. It is, therefore, important to keep in mind that the SE from resampling method estimates only uncertainty of sequence data without any consideration of uncertainty in fossil data. Therefore, an SE = 0 from resampling does not mean that the time estimates are precise. The confidence here pertains specifically to ε_{data} in Eq. (7.39). No amount of sequence data (or other data used to estimate branch lengths) can reduce the uncertainty associated with fossil dates, i.e., ε_{fossil} in Eq. (7.39) which can be estimated only from additional dated fossil data.

7.4.4   APPLICATION OF THE DATING METHODS

7.4.4.1   DATING THE DIVERGENCE TIME OF THE GREAT APES

The set of aligned mitochondrial sequences for seven ape species contains 9993 sites from 12 protein-coding genes (Cao et al., 1998). I chose this set of data to illustrate the LS-based dating method for comparison with results from a previous study based on Bayesian inference with the Markov chain Monte Carlo method (Rannala and Yang, 2007). I also performed dating with BEAST (Drummond and Rambaut, 2007) on the same data set. The same topology (Fig. 7.11) as in Rannala and Yang (2007) is used. Two fossil calibration points are indicated on the topology by $T_2 = 14$ million years (Myr) and $T_4 = 7$ Myr (Fig. 7.11), so we need to estimate only t_1, t_3, t_5, t_6, and the substitution rate (r). However, T_2 and T_4 can be further refined by using the least-square criterion.

The first and second codon positions are highly conserved in this set of sequences, with most of the substitutions observed at the third codon position. In the first part of the application, I will first use the 3331 third codon positions to illustrate the LS method with a single distance matrix. Choosing the third codon position is mainly because the third codon position is expected to evolve more in a clock-like manner than the first and second codon positions that are subject to strong purifying selection (Xia, 1998b; Xia et al., 1996). Although the third codon position is also under selection pressure mediated by differential abundance of tRNA species (Carullo and Xia, 2008; Xia, 2005, 2008), such selection is generally weak (Higgs and Ran, 2008) and expected to be much weaker than the purifying selection at the first and second codon positions.

The second part of the application illustrates the combined analysis involving more than one distance matrix. The combined analysis is performed on two distance matrices, one from codon positions 1 and 2 and the other from the third codon positions.

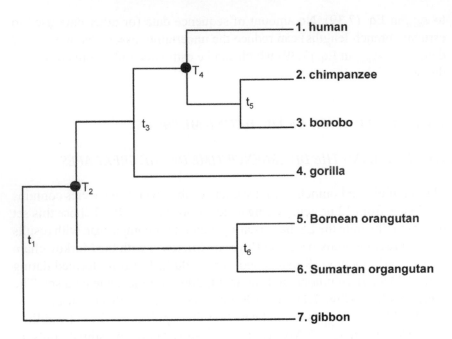

FIGURE 7.11   Topology for seven ape species. T_2 and T_4 are calibration points, and t_1, t_3, t_5, t_6, and substitution rate r are to be estimated. OTUs are numbered so that d_{ij} in the text refers to the evolutionary distance between OTUs i and j, e.g., d_{25} is the distance between chimpanzee and Bornean orangutan.

The evolutionary distance (d_{ij}, where i and j correspond to the taxon numbering in Figure 7.11, i.e., d_{12} is the distance between human and chimpanzee) is computed by using the simultaneous estimation method (Tamura et al., 2004) implemented in DAMBE (Xia, 2013b; Xia, 2017a) for the F84 substitution model which was used in Rannala and Yang (2007). Distances from codon positions 1 and 2 are in the upper triangle in Table 7.4 and those from the third codon positions are in the lower triangle in Table 7.4.

TABLE 7.4 Distance Matrix for the Seven Ape Species. Values in the lower triangle are from the third codon position and those in the upper triangle are from the first and second codon positions.

Species							
Human		0.03377	0.03298	0.04369	0.08152	0.07789	0.07964
chimpanzee	0.35614		0.01504	0.04288	0.07899	0.07589	0.07468
Bonobo	0.34434	0.11419		0.04207	0.07845	0.07604	0.07483
Gorilla	0.49710	0.46341	0.44526		0.07895	0.07840	0.07707
OrangutanB[1]	0.95933	0.94465	0.93699	0.99102		0.03050	0.08896
OrangutanS[2]	0.93121	0.94003	0.94296	0.98467	0.20216		0.08806
gibbon	1.33905	1.34517	1.31364	1.37386	1.42659	1.38938	

(1) Bornean orangutan.

(2) Sumatran orangutan.

7.4.4.1.1 Dating with a Single Distance Matrix

With the tree topology (Fig. 7.11) and the two calibration points (T_2 and T_4) indicated on the topology, the LS solution of the substitution rate (r) and the divergence time (t_1, t_3, t_5, and t_6) is

$$r = \frac{A}{4B}$$

$$t_1 = \frac{(d_{17} + d_{27} + d_{37} + d_{47} + d_{57} + d_{67})B}{3A} = \frac{(d_{17} + d_{27} + d_{37} + d_{47} + d_{57} + d_{67})}{12r}$$

$$t_3 = \frac{2(d_{14} + d_{24} + d_{34})B}{3A} = \frac{(d_{14} + d_{24} + d_{34})}{6r}$$

$$t_5 = \frac{2d_{23}B}{A} = \frac{d_{23}}{2r} \tag{7.50}$$

$$t_6 = \frac{2d_{56}B}{A} = \frac{d_{56}}{2r}$$

$$A = T_4(d_{12} + d_{13}) + T_2(d_{15} + d_{16} + d_{25} + d_{26} + d_{35} + d_{36} + d_{45} + d_{46})$$

$$B = 4T_2^2 + T_4^2$$

These LS-estimates are appropriate when the fossil dates are accurate, i.e., T_2 and T_4 (equal to 14 and 7 million years, respectively) are true divergence times of their respective nodes. The RSS is 0.04339 when the calibration points T_1 and T_2 are fixed, with r and t_i values estimated by using Eq. (7.50). The divergence times estimated, together with the standard error of the estimates, are shown in Figure 7.12a, with the evolutionary rate (r) equal to 0.0326 per million year, or 3.26 per 100 million years which is the unit in Rannala and Yang (2007).

When T_1 and T_2 are allowed to change to minimize RSS, RSS is reduced from 0.04339 to 0.0149 with the estimate of r equal to 3.105 per 100 million years which is similar to that in Rannala and Yang (2007) where they obtained $r = 3.11$ when a global clock is imposed and with soft-bounding of the divergence time. The dating details, together with the bootstrap-estimated standard error of the estimates, are shown in Figure 7.12b. These time estimates are similar to those from Rannala and Yang (2007) using the Bayes MCMC method (Fig. 7.13). For comparison, I have also estimated the divergence time by using BEAST (Drummond and Rambaut, 2007), which is now a leading method for estimating evolutionary rates and divergence times. Setting options with the HKY85 model, with no rate heterogeneity over site, with the clock model being "Relaxed clock: uncorrelated lognormal," with tree prior set to "Speciation: Yule process," with T_2 set to have a mean of 14 million years and standard error of 1.3 million years in a normal distribution, T_2 set to have a mean of 7 million years and standard error of 1.3 million years in a normal distribution, chain length equal to 1,000,000 and pre-burn-in of 10,000, we obtained time estimates very close to those from the LS method (Fig. 7.13).

7.4.4.1.2   Dating with Multiple Distance Matrices

Here we use two distance matrices to illustrate combined analysis with multiple distance matrices. The first distance matrix is from codon positions 1 and 2 of the ape mitochondrial sequences and the second distance matrix is from codon position 3 (upper and lower triangular matrices in Table 7.4, respectively). Because the distances from the third codon position are much greater than those from codon positions 1 and 2, we used both unscaled and scaled analyses for comparison. We should mention at the very beginning that it is not a good idea to combine highly heterogeneous genes or site partitions. So, it is not a good approach to combine the third codon position with first and second codon positions. We used the two matrices only to illustrate the method.

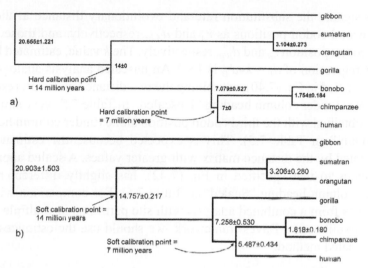

FIGURE 7.12 Dating the divergence of the great apes with the LS-based method with fixed (hard) calibration points (a) and soft calibration points (b). Each node is labeled by the mean±SE (standard error) estimated from 100 bootstrap samples. Two soft calibration points shown in the figure were used in dating.

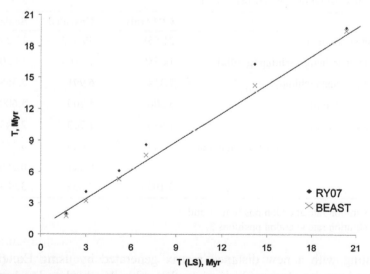

FIGURE 7.13 Comparing the LS-based dating (horizontal axis) and the dating based on Bayesian inference with Markov chain Monte Carlo (BI-MCMC) from Rannala and Yang (2007) and from BEAST (Vertical axis), all assuming a global clock.

Designate the substitution rate and evolutionary distance at the first and second codon positions as r_A and $d_{A.ij}$, respectively, and those at the third codon position r_B and $d_{B.ij}$, respectively. The k value, estimated by the linear regression of $d_B = k \bullet d_A$, is 13.9. An unscaled analysis analogous to that specified in Eq. (7.40), combining the two distance matrices, results in estimates (under column heading "Unscaled" in Table 7.5) very similar to those obtained with the third codon position alone (under column heading "CP3Only" in Table 7.5). This is expected because the estimation is dominated by the distance matrix with greater values. A scaled approach, analogous to that specified in Eq. (7.42), has slightly different results (under column heading "Scaled" in Table 7.5). For comparison with the estimates from a combined analysis with site partitions or multiple genes in the likelihood or Bayes framework, we should use the estimates from the unscaled method.

TABLE 7.5   Dating results for data at codon position 3 (CP3Only), for combined analysis of two matrices (one from codon positions 1 and 2 and the other from codon position 3) using unscaled approach (Unscaled) and scaled approach (Scaled). Initial values for T2 and T4 are 14 and 7 million years, respectively. Substitution rate r is measured by the expected number of substitutions per site per 100 Myr.

Time	CP3 Only	Unscaled	Scaled
t1 (gibbon-hominid)	21.558	20.312	17.239
T2 (orangutan-human+chimp+gorilla)	14.750	14.200	14.200
t3 (gorilla-human+chimp)	7.314	6.991	7.388
T4 (human-chimp)	5.500	5.200	5.600
t5 (chimp-bonobo)	1.830	1.709	2.243
t6 (Bornean orangutan-Sumatran orangutan)	3.244	3.029	4.345
$r_{12}^{(1)}$		0.241	0.259
$r_3^{(2)}$	3.105	3.356	3.603

(1) Substitution rate at codon positions 1 and 2.
(2) Substitution rate at codon positions 3.

Dating with a new distance matrix generated by using Eq. (7.43) produced results almost identical to that with the third codon position alone. This is understandable because the new d_{ij} is almost identical to d_{ij} based on the third codon position alone.

We have also performed dating and bootstrapping with the three site partitions (i.e., the three codon positions) as follows. Each site partition was bootstrapped separately, so each resampled data set will lead to three separate distance matrices for first, second and third codon positions, respectively. The three matrices are then combined into one matrix according to Eq. (7.43). The new matrix is then used for dating. This is repeated 100 times and the mean divergence time and the associated standard error are estimated in the same way as in Eq. (7.49). The results are similar to those in Figure 7.12, but the standard error is slightly larger, which is understandable because the second codon position violates the molecular clock hypothesis (likelihood ratio test. With the F84 model, lnL is -6381.9048 and -6388.4284, respectively, for a tree without a clock and with a global clock, $2\Delta lnL = 13.0471$, DF $= 5$, $p = 0.0229$). Combining third codon positions from different mitochondrial protein-coding genes invariably leads to reduced standard error.

7.4.4.2   DATING THE DIVERGENCE TIME OF THE MOUSE LEMURS

Here I compare the dating results between the LS method and BEAST (Drummond and Rambaut, 2007) by using the mouse lemur data set (Yang and Yoder, 2003). The data set consists of two mitochondrial genes (*COX2* and *Cyt-B*) from 35 mammalian species of which 26 are primate species. I used only the 604 third codon positions of the primate species because the third codon position evolves in a more clock-like manner than the other two codon positions (Yang and Yoder, 2003).

Three calibration points for primates and four calibration points for nonprimates were used in Yang and Yoder (2003). However, the calibration points for nonprimate species are somewhat doubtful as expressed in the original publications cited in Yang and Yoder (2003). So, I used only the three calibration points for the primates. I used BEAST with the settings identical to those for analyzing the great ape data except that the calibration points which are 77 million years for the root of primates, 35 million years for monkey/ape divergence, and 10 million years for human/gorilla divergence, i.e., the same as those used in Yang and Yoder (2003).

I first performed dating with BEAST and the LS-based method by using only the primate species. The dating results from the LS-based method (Fig. 7.14) are shown with each node labeled with the mean divergence time and the standard error estimated by 100 bootstrap samples. The results are nearly identical to those from BEAST (Fig. 7.15) where each node is labeled with a 95% high posterior density interval of the estimated divergence time. The mean divergence time from the LS-based method consistently falls right in the middle of the time interval from BEAST (Fig. 7.14 and Fig. 7.15).

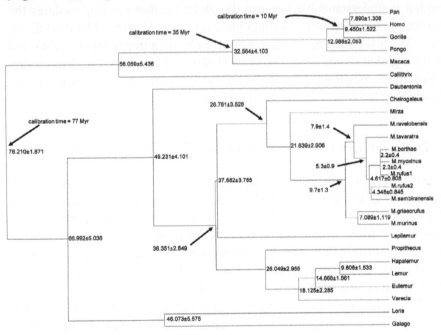

FIGURE 7.14 Dating the divergence of primates with the LS-based method. Each node is labeled with the mean divergence time and standard error (mean±s) estimated from 100 bootstrap samples. A global clock and the F84 substitution model were used. Three calibration points used are shown.

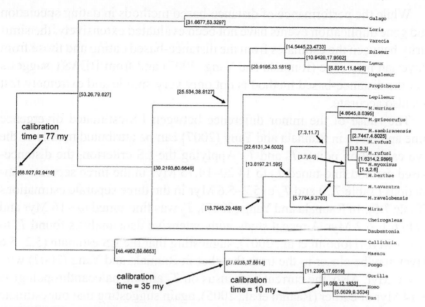

FIGURE 7.15 Dating the divergence of primates with BEAST. Each node is labeled with a 95% highest posterior density (HPD) interval of the estimated divergence time. A global clock and the HKY85 substitution model were used. Three calibration points used are shown.

To check whether there might be discordance with deep or shallow divergence times, I have plotted all corresponding divergence times from BEAST and from the LS-based method. The points effectively fall on a straight line (Fig. 7.16).

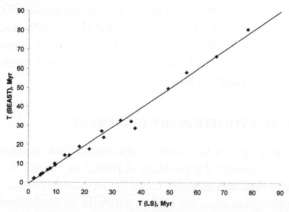

FIGURE 7.16 Concordance in dating results between the LS-based method, designated as T (LS) and BEAST, designated as T (BEAST). Results are from 26 primate species.

While the performance of distance-based methods in dating speciation and gene duplication events have not been evaluated extensively, the similarity between the estimates from the distance-based dating and those from Bayesian inference (Rannala and Yang, 2007) and from BEAST suggests that the distance-based method is not only very simple and extremely fast but also accurate.

The cause of the minor difference between LS-estimated divergence time and those in Rannala and Yang (2007) can be attributed mainly to the two calibration points T_2 and T_4. Applying the LS criterion, the distance-based method fine-tuned T_2 to 14.20–14.75 Myr in the three separate estimations (Table 7.5) and T_4 to 5.2–5.6 Myr in the three separate estimations (Table 7.5). In Rannala and Yang (2007), T_2 was fine-tuned to ~16 Myr and T_4 to 6.1–6.2 Myr. A recent study with extensive data analysis found T_4 to be 4.1 Myr (Hobolth et al., 2007), suggesting that the LS estimate (5.2–5.6 Myr) may be closer to the truth that that in Rannala and Yang (2007) with $T_4 > 6$ Myr. Also, the current consensus on T_2 among paleoanthropologists is 14 Myr or earlier (Raaum et al., 2005), again suggesting that our estimate here (14.20–14.75 Myr) may be closer to the truth that in Rannala and Yang (2007) with T_4 ranging from 15.8 to 16.3 with different clock models.

The dating method presented here should be useful for many new genome-based distances proposed in recent years. These include genome BLAST distances (Auch et al., 2006; Deng et al., 2006; Henz et al., 2005), breakpoint distances based on genome rearrangement (Gramm and Niedermeier, 2002; Herniou et al., 2001), distances based on the relative information between unaligned/unalignable sequences (Otu and Sayood, 2003), distances based on the sharing of oligopeptides (Gao and Qi, 2007), the composite vector distance (Xu and Hao, 2009) and composite distances incorporating several whole-genome similarity measures (Lin et al., 2009). However, how well these distances conform to the molecular clock has not been evaluated thoroughly.

7.5   IMPUTING EVOLUTIONARY DISTANCES

When we compile genes to create a supermatrix for constructing large trees, we may encounter the problem depicted in Figure 7.17 with Sp4 missing Gene A and Sp3 missing Gene B. Because Sp3 and Sp4 do not share any homologous sites, we cannot estimate an evolutionary distance between them. If we have to build a tree from these five species in Figure

7.17, we have to impute the missing distance D_{34}. Sometimes we may even have several D_{ij} missing and will need to impute them.

```
                Gene A                              Gene B
Sp1  CCGTTA...ACGGCTTTGCCGACGAC    ATCAGACGATGCG...AUGACGACTCACGATA
Sp2  CCGTCA...ACGACTTTGCCGACGAC    ACCAGACGATGCA...ACGACAACTTACGATA
Sp3  CCATTA...ACGGCTTTGCCGACGAC    ???????????????????????????????
Sp4  ???????????????????????????  ATCGGGCGACGCG...ACGACGACTCACGATA
Sp5  CTGTTA...ACGGCTTTGCCGACGAC    ATCAGACGATGCG...ACGGCGACTTACGATA
```

FIGURE 7.17 A sequence data set from concatenating Gene A and Gene B sequences. A distance cannot be computed between Sp3 and Sp4 because they share no homologous sites.

The LS method that was previously used to evaluate branch lengths given a topology is also frequently used for imputing missing distances. The general conceptual framework is to estimate the missing distances given different trees and then choose the best tree and the best estimates of missing distances that minimize the *RSS*.

7.5.1 A SPECIAL CASE

Before I illustrate the LS approach, I will present a special case that may seem to have an exact solution for missing values. Suppose we have four species (*S1–S4* in Fig. 7.18) with $D_{12} = 2, D_{14} = 5, D_{23} = 3, D_{24} = 5, D_{34} = 4$ but with D_{13} missing.

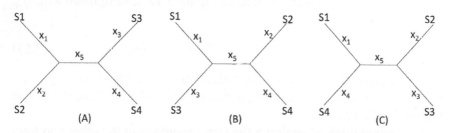

FIGURE 7.18 Topologies for Illustrating the Method of Imputing Missing Distances.

With the five known D_{ij} and five unknown xi values, we may take a wrong approach by thinking that, in this particular case, we have five unknowns and five equations and can solve for D_{13} exactly. For example, given a topology in Figure 7.18A, we can write the expected D_{ij} values, i.e., $E(D_{ij})$, as:

$$E(D_{12}) = x_1 + x_2$$
$$E(D_{14}) = x_1 + x_5 + x_4$$
$$E(D_{23}) = x_2 + x_5 + x_3 \qquad (7.51)$$
$$E(D_{24}) = x_2 + x_5 + x_4$$
$$E(D_{34}) = x_3 + x_4$$

These $E(D_{ij})$ values are termed patristic distances in phylogenetics. If we replace $E(D_{ij})$ by the observed D_{ij} values, we can solve the simultaneous equations in Eq. (7.51), which give the solution as

$$x_1 = \frac{D_{12}}{2} + \frac{D_{14}}{2} - \frac{D_{24}}{2}$$
$$x_2 = \frac{D_{12}}{2} + \frac{D_{24}}{2} - \frac{D_{14}}{2}$$
$$x_3 = \frac{D_{23}}{2} + \frac{D_{34}}{2} - \frac{D_{24}}{2} \qquad (7.52)$$
$$x_4 = \frac{D_{34}}{2} + \frac{D_{24}}{2} - \frac{D_{23}}{2}$$
$$x_5 = \frac{D_{14}}{2} + \frac{D_{23}}{2} - \frac{D_{12}}{2} - \frac{D_{34}}{2}$$

The missing D_{13} given the tree in Figure 7.18A, designated as $D_{13.A}$, can therefore be inferred as:

$$D_{13.A} = x_1 + x_5 + x_3 = D_{14} + D_{23} - D_{24} \qquad (7.53)$$

Thus, given the five known D_{ij} values above, we obtain $x_1 = x_2 = x_3 = x_5 = 1$, $x_4 = 3$, $D_{13.A} = 3$. The TL, defined as $TL = \Sigma x_i$, is 7 for the tree in Figure 7.18A, i.e., $TL_A = 7$.

One might think of applying the same approach to the other two trees in Figure 7.18B and 7.18C to obtain $D_{13.B}$ and $D_{13.C}$ as well as TL_B and TL_C, and choose as the best D_{13} and the best tree by using the ME criterion (Rzhetsky and Nei, 1992, 1994a), i.e., the tree with the shortest TL.

This approach has two problems. First, the approach fails with the tree in Figure 7.18B where the missing distance, D_{13}, involves two sister species. One can still write down five simultaneous equations but will find no solutions for x_i, given the five known D_{ij} values above, because the determinant of the coefficient matrix is 0. For the tree in Figure 7.18C, the solution will have $x_5 = -1$. A negative branch length is biologically undesirable and defeats the ME criterion for choosing the best tree and the associated estimate of D_{13}. Second, in most practical cases where missing distances are imputed there are more equations than unknowns, e.g., if we have five or more species with one missing distance.

7.5.2 THE LEAST-SQUARES APPROACH

Take $E(D_{ij})$ specifications in Eq. (7.51) for the tree in Figure 7.18A, the LS approach finds D_{13} and the best tree that minimize the RSS between the observed D_{ij} and the expected $E(D_{ij})$:

$$RSS = \sum \frac{\left[D_{ij} - E\left(D_{ij}\right)\right]^2}{D_{ij}^m} \qquad (7.54)$$

where m is typically 0 (OLS), 1, or 2. In the illustration below, we will take the OLS approach with $m = 0$. It has been shown before that OLS actually exhibits less topological bias than alternatives with m equal to 1 or 2 (Xia, 2006)

Given the three tree topologies, the results from the LS estimation are summarized in Table 7.6. Note that, for the tree in Figure 7.18B, there are multiple sets of solutions of x_i that can achieve the same minimum RSS of 1.

TABLE 7.6 Estimation results from minimizing RSS, with Trees A, B, and C as in Figure 7.18 and with the constraint of no negative branch lengths.

Site	Tree A	Tree B	Tree C
x_1	1	0	1
x_2	1	1.5	1.5
x_3	1	0	1
x_4	3	3.5	3.5
x_5	1	1	0
D_{13}	3	0	2
TL	7	6	7
RSS	0	1	1

We see a conflict between the LS criterion and the ME criterion in choosing the best tree and the best estimate of D_{13}. The ME criterion would have chosen Tree B with $TL_B = 6$ and $D_{13} = 0$ because TL_B is the smallest of the three TL values. In contrast, the LS criterion would have chosen Tree A with $RSS = 0$ and $D_{13} = 3$. The ME criterion is clearly inappropriate here for missing distance imputation because it tends to underestimate the missing distances to achieve the minimum tree length. For example, the missing distance involving two sister taxa would become 0 with ME criterion. I recommend the LS criterion for the simultaneous imputing of missing distances and inferring phylogenetic trees.

An earlier version of DAMBE implemented the LS approach above by using an iterative approach similar to the EM (expectation-maximization) algorithm as follows. For a given distance matrix with missing values, we simply fill in the missing D_{ij} values by guestimates, e.g., the average of the observed distances. These initial D_{ij} guestimates will be designated as $D_{ij,m0}$ where the subscript "$m0$" indicates missing distances at step 0. We now build a tree from the distance matrix that minimizes RSS in Eq. (7.54). From the resulting tree, we obtain the patristic distances $E(D_{ij})$ from the tree and replace $D_{ij.m0}$ by the corresponding $E(D_{ij})$ values which are now designated as $D_{ij.m1}$. We now again build a tree, obtain the corresponding $E(D_{ij})$ to replace $D_{ij.m1}$ so now we have $D_{ij.m2}$. We repeat this process until RSS does not decrease any further. This process can quickly arrive at a local minimum. Unfortunately, different topologies have different minimums and this approach is too often locked in a local minimum with a tree that does not achieve a global minimum RSS.

New version of DAMBE (since version 7) uses a downhill simplex method in multidimensions (Press et al., 1992, pp 408–412) when there are multiple missing values. This is repeated multiple times with different initial values for the points in the simplex to increase the chance of finding the global RSS associated with the missing distances and the tree. When there is a single missing distance, then the Brent's method (Press et al., 1992, pp 402–408) is used. Figure 7.19 shows an illustrative example. The distance matrix in Figure 7.19a is computed from aligned sequence data used before (Xia and Yang, 2011). Figure 7.19b is the phylogenetic tree built from this distance matrix. Suppose $D_{gibbon,orangutan}$ and $D_{gorrila.chimpazee}$ are missing (shaded in Fig. 7.19a) and need to be imputed. DAMBE yields $D_{gibbon,orangutan} = 1.3776$ and $D_{gorrila.chimpazee} = 0.4600$, which are close to the observed values (Fig. 7.19a). The final tree built from the distance matrix with the two missing distances is identical to Figure 7.19b except for a negligible difference in branch lengths.

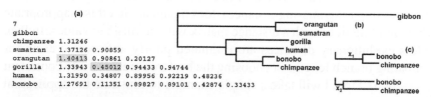

FIGURE 7.19 An example data set for imputing missing distances. (a) A real distance matrix computed from aligned sequences, but we pretend that the two shaded distances are missing. (b) A phylogenetic tree from the distance matrix. (c) A special case illustrating the problem of the estimation.

One can access the function in DAMBE (Xia, 2013b; Xia, 2017a) by clicking "File|Open other molecular data|Distance matrix file with missing value," and open a distance file in the format in Figure 7.19a with missing distances represented by "." (a period without quotation marks). The method in DAMBE has an advantage over a previous method (Kettleborough et al., 2015) that assumes a rooted tree and a molecular clock for building a tree and for inferring missing distances. Such assumptions are not needed and are too restrictive in practice.

There are cases where missing distances cannot be uniquely determined. For example, when the missing distance is for two sister taxa (e.g., the two chimpanzee species, designated bonobo and chimpanzee in Figure 7.19b), we can find a minimum *RSS* but the solution for the missing distance $D_{bonobo,chimpanzee}$ is not unique. That is, multiple $D_{bonobo,chimpanzee}$ values can generate the same *RSS*. Note that the patristic distances $E(D_{bonobo.i})$ and $E(D_{chimpanzee.i})$, where i stands for other species, do not depend on the branch length leading to the common ancestor from bonobo and chimpanzee. This branch can be as short as x_2 or as long as x_1 (Fig. 7.19c) but *RSS* in Eq. (7.54) will remain the same. Thus, in this particular case, a missing $D_{bonobo,chimpanzee}$ cannot be determined uniquely by LS methods. The only way to eliminate this problem is to have a more closely related species to break up the sister relationship so that the missing D_{ij} is not between two sister taxa.

7.6   DIFFERENT CRITERIA ARE GENERALLY CONSISTENT WITH EACH OTHER

The suggestion in the previous section that the ME criterion is inappropriate for imputing missing distances does not mean that it is inappropriate when building trees with a distance matrix with no missing values. In fact, unless evolutionary distances are estimated poorly, different criteria for evaluating branch lengths or choosing the best tree are generally consistent (Xia, 2006). Here I will take a simple example to illustrate the application of these different criteria.

Suppose we have the distance matrix in Figure 7.20A and the three possible topologies for four OTUs (*S1– S4*, Fig. 7.20B–D). We will use two ways to evaluate branch length, with $m = 0$ and $m = 1$, respectively, in Eq. (7.11). The branch lengths differ slightly with the two methods (Table 7.7), so do the tree length and *RSS*. However, using either the ME criterion (i.e., the tree with the shortest tree length is the best tree) or the least-square criterion (i.e., the tree with the smallest *RSS* is the best tree), lead to the conclusion that the two trees in Figure 7.20B and Figure 7.20D are equally good but the tree in Figure 7.20C is worse.

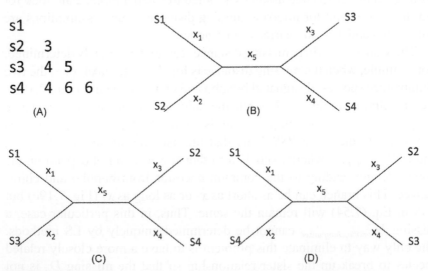

FIGURE 7.20   A distance matrix for four OTUs (*S1* to *S4*) and three topologies.

TABLE 7.7 Results of evaluating branch lengths by ordinary least-square with $m = 0$ in Eq. (7.11) and weighted least square with $m = 1$ in Eq. (7.11), with no negative branch length allowed. letters under column heading 'Tree' correspond to those in Figure 7.20.

M	Tree	$x1$	$x2$	$x3$	$x4$	$x5$	TreeLen	RSS
0	B	0.75	2.25	2.75	3.25	0.25	9.25	0.25
	C	0.833333	2.333333	2.833333	3.333333	0	9.333333	0.333333
	D	0.75	2.25	2.75	3.25	0.25	9.25	0.25
1	B	0.763159	2.23684	2.78947	3.210522	0.236845	9.236835	0.052632
	C	0.827586	2.275862	2.896552	3.310345	0	9.310344	0.068966
	D	0.736842	2.184207	2.815786	3.263154	0.236847	9.236835	0.052632

KEYWORDS

- minimum evolution criterion
- least-squares criterion
- simultaneously estimated distance
- substitution models
- fossil-based dating
- calibration
- tip-dating

CHAPTER 8

Maximum Likelihood Methods in Phylogenetics

ABSTRACT

I first present the fundamental conceptual framework of likelihood methods and likelihood ratio test, and then address the main topics in this chapter with a detailed illustration of the pruning algorithm used to evaluate log-likelihood (*lnL*) of a topology given a set of aligned sequences and a substitution model, with or without assuming a molecular clock. This is followed by likelihood ratio test for molecular clock, handling of missing data with the pruning algorithm and statistical tests of alternative topologies. The chapter concludes with a presentation of the starless bias and confounding effect between topology and parameter estimation with a warning that the rate heterogeneity over sites, as characterized by the shape parameter of gamma distribution, generally should not be taken as a sequence feature when topology is uncertain. With the same set of aligned sequences, one may observe no rate heterogeneity with one topology but high rate heterogeneity with another topology.

8.1 INTRODUCTION

The likelihood-based phylogenetic method was championed by Joe Felsenstein and popularized by his DNAML program in the PHYLIP package (Felsenstein, 2014). There is some similarity between the maximum parsimony (MP) and the maximum likelihood (ML) method. Both operate on a set of aligned sequences typically represented as an $N \times L$ character matrix, where N is the number of sequences and L is the aligned sequence length. If one learns how to evaluate one site, one knows how to evaluate all sites. The core algorithms of the two methods take the alignment and a topology as input, assign a value to each of the L sites and sum up the values as a criterion for choosing the best topology. The site-specific value is the substitution cost (c_i) in MP and log-likelihood (lnL_i) in ML. The best topology is one with the smallest Σc_i in MP or the largest ΣlnL_i in ML, where $i = 1, 2, \ldots, L$. While there are many books written about ML phylogenetic methods, perhaps the most comprehensive one is by Felsenstein (2004).

Likelihood-based phylogenetic methods are model-based, involving two categories of models: (1) A substitution model with continuous rate ratio parameters and (2) tree models with discrete topology and continuous branch length parameters for a given topology. It is conceivable that all tree models could be wrong. For example, with four species, we have a star tree and three unrooted trees. If a gene evolves along the star tree and another three genes each evolve along each of the three unrooted trees and if we concatenate all these four gene sequences together, then no single topology can possibly be correct. Likelihood methods behave in strange ways in such a scenario, which will be illustrated after we have gained the conceptual framework of the likelihood method in phylogenetics.

The key algorithm for the ML method is the pruning algorithm (Felsenstein, 1973, 1981; 2004, pp 253–255) for computing the likelihood based on equilibrium frequencies and transition probabilities in phylogenetic reconstruction. The pruning algorithm not only speeds up computation but also offers a natural and statistically valid way to handle missing data.

This chapter deals only with tree reconstruction by the ML method based on sequence data. For the ML method for computing pairwise evolutionary distances, please review the chapter on substitution models and the chapter on distance-based phylogenetic methods. For comparative methods using the likelihood approach based on Brownian motion model, with a post hoc modification for characterizing directional changes, please read the chapter on comparative methods.

We will first present simple examples of likelihood-based estimation to illustrate the rationale of the ML approach and likelihood ratio test (LRT). This is followed by a detailed illustration of the likelihood calculation given a topology and a set of aligned sequences. Both a brute-force approach and the pruning algorithm are explained, with and without imposing a molecular clock. The basic knowledge needed for this chapter is tree traversal and transition probabilities derived from substitution models. Readers who do not know transition probabilities should review a previous chapter on substitution models. We will illustrate the likelihood method with the simplest scenario with four sequences labeled *S1* to *S4* and three possible unrooted trees. We need to compute the log-likelihood (*lnL*) for each tree and choose the tree with the maximum likelihood as the ML tree. The last section makes an important point that topology and substitution models are confounded, leading to some unexpected aspects of ML methods (Xia, 2014).

8.1.1   THE RATIONALE OF MAXIMUM LIKELIHOOD APPROACH

ML is a criterion for both parameter estimation and model selection, i.e, the best set of parameter values or the best model should be those that maximize the likelihood. Recall that we always need to have a criterion whenever we need to choose one from several alternatives. The MP criterion states that the best tree is one with the fewest changes. The minimum evolution criterion in distance-based methods states that the best tree is one with the shortest tree length. In the chapters on substitution models and distance-based phylogenetic methods, we have used the least-squares criterion (both the ordinary and the weighted least-squares). A set of branch lengths is the best if they minimize the residual sum of squares. Maximum likelihood is just one of these criteria for making a choice among alternatives.

Let us illustrate the ML approach with a few examples. Suppose we wish to estimate the proportion of males (*p*) of a fish population in a large lake. A random sample of N fish contains M males. With the binomial distribution, the likelihood, which is the probability mass function for discrete variables, is

$$L = \frac{N!}{M!(N-M)!} p^M (1-p)^{N-M} . \tag{8.1}$$

The maximum likelihood criterion states that the best p should maximize the likelihood value given the observation. This maximization process is simplified by maximizing the natural logarithm of L instead:

$$\ln L = A + M \ln(p) + (N-M)\ln(1-p)$$

$$\frac{\partial \ln L}{\partial p} = \frac{M}{p} - \frac{N-M}{1-p} = 0 \tag{8.2}$$

$$p = \frac{M}{N} .$$

The likelihood estimate of the variance of p is the negative reciprocal of the second derivative,

$$Var(p) = -\frac{1}{\dfrac{\partial^2 \ln(L)}{\partial p^2}} = -\frac{1}{-\dfrac{M}{p^2} - \dfrac{N-M}{(1-p)^2}} = \frac{p(1-p)}{N} \,. \tag{8.3}$$

Note that the likelihood method needs a model (binomial distribution in our example) to formulate the likelihood function, which is in Eq. (8.1) for our example. For this reason, the likelihood method is always model-based.

8.1.2   LIKELIHOOD RATIO TEST AND INFORMATION-THEORETIC INDICES

The likelihood ratio test is for model selection involving nested models, that is, a general model and special model which is a special case of the general model. Suppose we wish to know whether body height differs between male and female students. We randomly sampled seven male and six female students and measured body height (shown in the first two columns in Table 8.1). We consider three hypotheses (or models). The first (M1) assumes that male and female students do not differ in body height and all 13 values represent sample values from the same normal distribution specified by mean μ and standard deviation σ. The likelihood for continuous variables is the probability density function. For example, the likelihood for a body height of 170:

$$L(170 \mid M1) = \frac{1}{\sigma\sqrt{2\pi}} e^{-\frac{1}{2}\left(\frac{170-\mu}{\sigma}\right)^2} \tag{8.4}$$

The log-likelihood function for the 13 sample values is

$$\ln L_{M1} = \ln[L(170 \mid M1)] + \ln[L(175 \mid M1)] + \dots + \ln[L(160 \mid M1)] \tag{8.5}$$

which is a function of two unknowns (μ and σ). The likelihood criterion states that the best μ and σ should maximize lnL. We thus take partial derivatives of lnL_{M1} with respect to μ and σ, set the partial derivatives to zero and solve the two simultaneous equations. This gives us $\mu = 173.0769$ and $\sigma = 6.719239$, and $lnL_{M1} = -43.21084$. lnL for individual observations are shown in Table 8.1, in the two columns under the heading of M1. This M1 is equivalent to the null hypothesis of no difference in body height between male and female students.

Suppose we now have a second hypothesis (M2) that sample values from males and females belong to two different normal distributions, with the male population specified by μ_M and σ_M, and the female population specified by μ_F and σ_F. Now the same sample value (e.g., 170) for a male and a female student will have different likelihoods, denoted $L_{M.170}$ and $L_{F.170}$ below

$$L(170, male \mid M2) = \frac{1}{\sigma_M \sqrt{2\pi}} e^{-\frac{1}{2}\left(\frac{170-\mu_M}{\sigma_M}\right)^2} ; L(170, female \mid M2) \frac{1}{\sigma_F \sqrt{2\pi}} e^{-\frac{1}{2}\left(\frac{170-\mu_F}{\sigma_F}\right)^2} \quad (8.6)$$

TABLE 8.1 Body height (in cm) measured from seven male (M) and six female (F) students. Three models (M1, M2, and M3) are evaluated, assuming normal distribution. M1: male and female students do not differ in body height and all 13 values represent sample values from the same population; M2: the seven male and six female sample values are from two populations differing in both mean and standard deviation; M3: the seven male and six female sample values are from two populations differing in mean but having the same standard deviation.

Height		M1 (μ, σ)		M2 $(\mu_M, \sigma_M, \mu_F, \sigma_F)$		M3 (μ_M, μ_F, σ)	
M	F	lnL_M	lnL_F	$lnLM$	$lnLF$	$lnLM$	$lnLF$
170	170	−2.92876	−2.92876	−3.92540	−2.49898	−3.92540	−2.58489
175	165	−2.86487	−3.54639	−2.63108	−2.49893	−2.63108	−2.58485
175	172	−2.86487	−2.83676	−2.63108	−2.93880	−2.63108	−2.92317
180	170	−3.35471	−2.92876	−2.54483	−2.49898	−2.54483	−2.58489
181	168	−3.51913	−3.10936	−2.67254	−2.31048	−2.67254	−2.43991
179	160	−3.21244	−4.71774	−2.46543	−4.06956	−2.46543	−3.79288
185		−4.39828		−3.66665		−3.66665	

Designate male and female height as *MH* and *FH*, respectively, the log-likelihood (*lnL*) for the seven male and six female sample values is

$$\ln L_{M2} = \sum_{i=1}^{7} \ln L(MH_i \mid M2) + \sum_{i=1}^{6} \ln L(FH_i \mid M2) \quad (8.7)$$

Now the function lnL_{M2} has four parameters. The maximum likelihood estimates of these parameters (i.e., the parameters that maximize lnL_{M2}) are $\mu_M = 177.8570$, $\sigma_M = 4.5491$, $\mu_F = 167.4998$, and $\sigma_F = 3.9896$, with the resulting $lnL_{M2} = -37.3527$. The log-likelihood of the 13 individual sample values are shown in Table 8.1 in the two columns under M2.

Which model (M1 or M2) is the more preferable? M1 is simpler, with only two parameters, but is it too simple to describe nature adequately? What criterion should we use to discriminate between these two models? We cannot use lnL as a criterion because it will always be greater for the more complicated model, just like R^2 in linear models. R^2 is a measure of how well a model fits the data in a least-squares context, and lnL is a measure of how well a model fits the data in a likelihood context. If we use R^2 or lnL as a criterion for model selection, then complicated models will always be favored against simple models.

A series of models are termed nested models if the simpler model is a special case of the more complicated model. For example, the following are nested models because the second can be reduced to the first if $b = 0$, and the third can be reduced to the second if $b_2 = 0$:

$$y = a$$
$$y = a + bx \quad\quad\quad (8.8)$$
$$y = a + b_1 x + b_2 x^2$$

In our case, M1 and M2 are nested models because M2 is reduced to M1 if $\mu_M = \mu_F = \mu$ and $\sigma_M = \sigma_F = \sigma$.

Nested models can be tested by the likelihood ratio test (LRT). Any statistical significance test will have two essential quantities: a statistic that measures the difference between the two models (two hypotheses) and a known distribution of the statistic. The statistic in LRT is $2\Delta lnL$ (twice the difference in lnL between the two nested models, which is often referred to as the likelihood-ratio chi-square) which follows approximately the χ^2 distribution with the degree of freedom being ΔP (the difference in the number of parameters between the two nested models). In our example, $\Delta P = 4-2 = 2$, and $2\Delta lnL = 2*(lnL_{M2}-lnL_{M1}) = 11.7162$. With two degrees of freedom, $p = 0.0029$. Note that the null hypothesis being tested in LRT is that M1 and M2 are equally good, and this null hypothesis is rejected at $p = 0.0029$, so we adopt M2 and conclude that male and female students differ highly significantly in μ or σ or both.

Now suppose we have a third hypothesis (M3) stating that the male and female populations differ in μ but not in σ, i.e., $\mu_M \neq \mu_F$ but $\sigma_M = \sigma_F = \sigma$. Is this M3 as good as M2? We can do the same calculation to obtain μ_M = 177.8570, μ_F = 167.4998, and σ = 4.5491 with lnL_{M3} = −37.4476. The lnL for individual sample values are also shown in Table 8.1 in the two columns under M3. The likelihood ratio chi-square $2\Delta lnL$ = 0.1897. With one degree of freedom, p = 0.6631, so we cannot reject the null hypothesis that M3 and M2 are equally good. The principle of parsimony therefore dictates that M3 is the best model.

An alternative to likelihood-ratio test is the information-theoretic indices such as AIC (Akaike, 1973, 1974) and BIC (Schwarz, 1978) defined as

$$AIC = -2\ln L + 2p \qquad (8.9)$$

$$BIC = -2\ln L + p\ln(n) \qquad (8.10)$$

where p is the number of parameters and n is the sample size. AIC and BIC differ only in the second term, with BIC penalizes parameter-rich models more than AIC. The best model is the one with the smallest AIC or BIC value. For our example, AIC is 90.4210 for M1, 82.7054 for M2, and 80.8952 for M3. So M3 strikes the best balance between simplicity and sufficiency. Similarly, BIC is 91.5509 for M1, 84.9652 for M2, and 82.5900 for M3. So M3 is also the best model based on the BIC criterion.

8.2 LIKELIHOOD METHOD IN PHYLOGENETIC RECONSTRUCTION

Likelihood methods in phylogenetics differ fundamentally from the conventional likelihood methods illustrated above. Likelihood methods are consistent for continuous variables. Similarly, model selection involving nested models by LRT is well-accepted. However, using the ML criterion for model selection involving models that are not nested is controversial. This is perhaps best illustrated by a fictitious example. Suppose four species with three unrooted resolved trees, as well as a star tree. Also, suppose four genes each evolving along one of the four trees (star tree and three resolved trees). If we now concatenate the four gene sequences together, then none of the four trees is correct for the data. Application of the ML criterion when all tree models are wrong can lead to very bizarre results including outlandish branch estimates.

While I will illustrate some problems involving the likelihood method at the end of the chapter, our focus here is to gain a detailed understanding of the likelihood method in phylogenetics, with particular emphasis on tree traversal and the pruning algorithm used to compute likelihood. It would be very helpful if readers can review (1) the material on substitution models, especial those model-specific transition probabilities which are required for computing likelihood and (2) tree traversal that we encountered in the chapter on MP method.

8.2.1   THE BRUTE-FORCE APPROACH

The ML method, like the MP method we learned before, is site-oriented. Once we learned how to calculate the likelihood for one site, we know how to calculate for all sites. Given a site in a set of aligned sequences and a topology (Fig. 8.1A), we have two internal nodes numbered 5 and 6 with unknown states (Fig. 8.1B), leading to 16 possible nucleotide configurations with the same topology (Fig. 8.1C). At first sight, it seems that we need to sum up 16 terms to obtain the likelihood of each site. The likelihood for site 1 is

$$L_1 = \pi_A P_{AA}(b_1) P_{AA}(b_2) P_{AA}(b_5) P_{AG}(b_3) P_{AG}(b_4) + \pi_C P_{CA}(b_1) P_{CA}(b_2) P_{CA}(b_5) P_{AG}(b_3) P_{AG}(b_4)$$
$$+ \ \dots \ + \pi_T P_{TA}(b_1) P_{TA}(b_2) P_{TT}(b_5) P_{TG}(b_3) P_{TG}(b_4) \tag{8.11}$$

where π_A, π_C, π_G, and π_T are equilibrium nucleotide frequencies, b_1 to b_5 are branch lengths (Fig. 8.1B), and P_{AA}, P_{AG}, ..., P_{TT} are transition probabilities derived from a given substitution model. Because we do not know the state of the internal node, we assign the probability of each state according to nucleotide frequencies. One can express the likelihood for other sites in the same way. For example, the likelihood for site 5 is

$$L_5 = \pi_A P_{AA}(b_1) P_{AA}(b_2) P_{AA}(b_5) P_{AA}(b_3) P_{AA}(b_4)$$
$$+ \pi_C P_{CA}(b_1) P_{CA}(b_2) P_{CA}(b_5) P_{AA}(b_3) P_{AA}(b_4) \tag{8.12}$$
$$+ \ \dots \ + \pi_T P_{TA}(b_1) P_{TA}(b_2) P_{TT}(b_5) P_{TA}(b_3) P_{TA}(b_4)$$

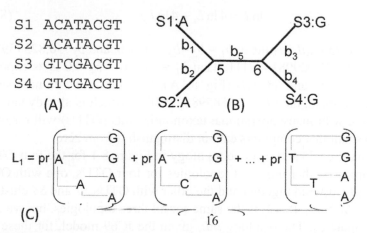

S1 ACATACGT
S2 ACATACGT
S3 GTCGACGT
S4 GTCGACGT

(A)

(B)

(C)

FIGURE 8.1 Computing likelihood with a brute-force approach involving one site (site 1) in a set of four aligned sequences (A). Nodes 5 and 6 have unknown states that could be A, C, G, or T (B), generating 16 different combinations (C). We need to compute likelihood for each site designated L_1 to L_{16}. The log-likelihood of a tree is $lnL = \sum ln(L_i)$, and the maximum likelihood tree is the one with the highest lnL among all possible topologies.

For illustration, we may take equal nucleotide frequencies and the simplest JC69 model with only two distinct transition probabilities:

$$P_{ii}(b) = \frac{1}{4} + \frac{3}{4}e^{-4b/3}, P_{ij}(b) = \frac{1}{4} - \frac{1}{4}e^{-4b/3} \tag{8.13}$$

where b is branch length between neighboring nodes.

Because the JC69 model assumes that the four nucleotides replace each other with equal rate, the four sequences in Figure 8.1A have only two site patterns, one shared among sites 1–4 and the other shared among sites 5–8. Sites sharing the same site pattern for a given substitution model means that these sites have the same likelihood, so we do not need to calculate them individually. Given this, the 16 terms for the first site pattern in Eq. (8.11) can be reduced to seven terms because many terms are identical. For example, seven terms are identical and equal to $P_{ij}(b_1)*P_{ij}(b_2)*$ $P_{ij}(b_3)* P_{ij}(b_4)* P_{ij}(b_5)*0.25$ when internal nodes 5 and 6 are occupied by nucleotide pairs (C, A), (C, T), (G, A), (G, C), (G, T), (T, A), (T, C), where the first nucleotide in each pair is at node 5 and second at node 6. Similarly, the 16 terms for the second pattern in Eq. (8.12) can be reduced to five terms. The tree lnL given the four sequences in Figure 8.1A is

$$\ln L = 4\ln L_1 + 4\ln L_5 \qquad\qquad (8.14)$$

Maximizing lnL results in $b_1 = b_2 = b_3 = b_4 = 0$, and $b_5 = 0.823959217$, with $lnL = -21.029981488111$. That $b_1 = b_2 = b_3 = b_4 = 0$ is as expected because $S1 = S2$ and $S3 = S4$ (Fig. 8.1A). Note that if we do not use lnL but use L instead, then $L = 7.358598123*10^{-10}$, which is already small. A larger tree with many operational taxonomic units (OTUs) will results in an L so small that computers cannot distinguish it from zero.

We have evaluated just one topology in Figure 8.1 for the four OTUs. There are two other unrooted topologies for four OTUs, one with OTUs $S1$ and $S3$ clustered together and the other with OTUs $S1$ and $S4$ clustered together. L_5 in Eq. (8.12) is the same for all three topologies, but we need to recompute L_1. The resulting lnL, given the JC69 model, for these two topologies are the same and equal to -30.96960809. Thus, the topology in Figure 8.1B, with $S1$ and $S2$ clustered together and $b_1 = b_2 = b_3 = b_4 = 0$, and $b_5 = 0.823959217$, is the best tree of the three, because it has the largest lnL ($= -21.029981488111$). Recall that all three phylogenetic methods we have covered so far, the MP, the distance-based and the likelihood methods, have an explicit criterion for choosing the best tree. The MP chooses the tree with the smallest substitution cost as the best tree, distance-based methods choose the tree with the shortest tree length (minimum evolution criterion) or with the smallest residual sum of squares (least-squares criterion) as the best tree and the maximum likelihood method choose the tree with the highest lnL as the best tree.

8.2.2 THE PRUNING ALGORITHM

The brute-force approach for computing lnL is unnecessary and is not used in practice other than classroom or textbook illustration. The pruning algorithm (Felsenstein, 1973, 1981; 2004, pp 253–255), illustrated below, economizes the computation substantially.

As in the MP method, we only need to illustrate the application of the pruning algorithm for a single site because all sites are computed the same way. For any given topology, e.g., the four-species topology in Figure 8.1B, we first define a likelihood vector (L_j) for each of the nodes including the leaf nodes. The vector contains four elements for nucleotide sequences, 20 for amino acid sequences or the number of sense codons for codon sequences with codon-based models. We will use nucleotide sequences for illustration but the computation is the same for amino acid or codon sequences.

We have four sequences with the first site being A, G, C, and T for species 1, 2, 3, and 4, respectively (Fig. 8.2). Our task is to compute the lnL_1 for this first site with the pruning algorithm. The computation is the same for all other sites.

For a leaf node j with a nucleotide s (where s is either A, C, G, or T), $L_j(s) = 1$, and $L_j(\bar{s}) = 0$ (Fig. 8.2). For example, for the first sequence with nucleotide A, $L_1(A) = 1$, and $L_1(C) = L_1(G) = L_1(T) = 0$. For an internal node j with two offspring (o_1 and o_2), L_j is recursively defined as

$$L_j(s) = \left[\sum_{k=0}^{3} P_{sk}(b_{j,o_1})L_{o_1}(k)\right]\left[\sum_{k=0}^{3} P_{sk}(b_{j,o_2})L_{o_2}(k)\right] \qquad (8.15)$$

where s is either A, C, G, or T, k takes value of 0, 1, 2, 3 corresponding to nucleotides A, C, G, T, $b_{j,o1}$ is the branch length between internal node j and its offspring o_1 and P_{sk} is the transition probability from state s to state k (where s and k are A, C, G, or T for nucleotide sequences). Transition probabilities P_{sk} and its derivation from various substitution models have been detailed in the chapter on substitution models. You may view the two terms in Eq. (8.15) as two ways for the internal node j to reach the two offspring.

The application of Eq. (8.15) is straightforward. Take for example internal node 5 with its two offspring nodes 1 and 2,

$$L_5(A) = \left[\sum_{k=0}^{3} P_{Ak}(b_1)L_1(k)\right]\left[\sum_{k=0}^{3} P_{Ak}(b_2)L_2(k)\right] \qquad (8.16)$$

Because $L_1(A) = 1, L_1(C) = L_1(G) = L_1(T) = 0, L_2(G) = 1, L_2(A) = L_2(C) = L_2(T) = 0, L_5(A)$ becomes

$$L_5(A) = P_{AA}(b_1)P_{AG}(b_2) \qquad (8.17)$$

The other three elements, as well as L_j vectors for other internal nodes, are listed in Figure 8.2.

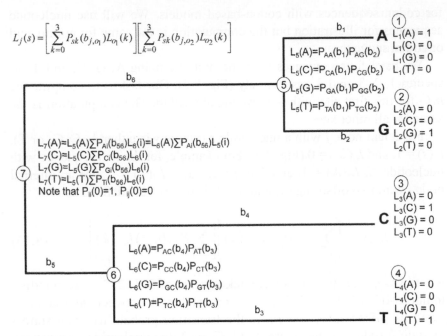

$$L_j(s) = \left[\sum_{k=0}^{3} P_{sk}(b_{j,o_1})L_{o_1}(k) \right] \left[\sum_{k=0}^{3} P_{sk}(b_{j,o_2})L_{o_2}(k) \right]$$

FIGURE 8.2 Likelihood computation with the pruning algorithm on a four-species tree. Node j is represented by a vector (L_j) of four elements for nucleotide sequences or 20 for amino acid sequences. L_j is computed according to Eq. (8.15) shown on the upper-left. b_5 and b_6 cannot be estimated separately without assuming a molecular clock, only their summation (b_{56}) is used in likelihood calculation.

Internal Node 7 is special in that we cannot estimate b_5 and b_6 separately because the substitution model is time-reversible and the resulting tree is consequently unrooted. We simply move Node 7 to the location of Node 6 (or Node 5), so that either b_5 or b_6 is 0 and the other is then equal to (b_5+b_6) represented as b_{56} in L_7 in Figure 8.2. If b_5 is 0, then $P_{ii}(b_5) = 1$ and $P_{ij}(b_5) = 0$, i.e., no time for anything to change. This leads to the simplified equations for computing $L_7(i)$ in Figure 8.2. The final likelihood for the tree is

$$L = \sum_{i=0}^{3} \pi_i L_7(i) \tag{8.18}$$

where π_i is the equilibrium frequency of nucleotide i, and reflects the assumption that sufficient time has elapsed for the frequencies to reach equilibrium. Note that, for the JC69 model, $\pi_i = 1/4$.

The application of the pruning algorithm to the aligned sequences and the topology in Figure 8.1 with the JC69 model will also result in $b_1 = b_2 = b_3 = b_4 = 0$, and $b_5 = 0.823959217$, with $lnL = -21.029981488111$, just as we have obtained with the brute-force approach. The benefit of the pruning algorithm is the reduction of repeated calculation.

8.2.3 SEARCHING TREE SPACE AND CHOOSING THE BEST TREE

Likelihood-based methods are slow. We have 16 combinations with only two internal nodes in Figure 8.1 for nucleotide sequences and would have 400 terms with two internal nodes for amino acid sequences. If you have a large number of OTUs with many internal nodes, then the amount of computation increases very rapidly. Although the pruning algorithm reduces the amount of computation involved, it does not change the fact that likelihood methods for phylogenetic reconstruction are very slow. It has been criticized before that many published ML trees are not authentic ML trees because the computer programs implementing likelihood phylo-genetic reconstruction checked only a small subset of possible trees (Xia, 2007b).

Some implementations will first use an uphill search by starting with a 3-OTU tree with an internal node and three branches. The 4th OTU can be added to one of the three branches, leading to three alternative 4-OTU trees that are evaluated to produce an lnL value for each tree. Only the best of the three trees (i.e., with the largest lnL) is kept. To this 4-OTU tree with five branches is added the 5th OTU to generate five alternative topologies. They are evaluated to generate five lnL values. The one with the highest lnL is used to continue the addition of the 6th OTU and so on. Once all OTUs have been added, the topology is modified locally in various ways and re-evaluated to see if any modification leads to a higher lnL value than the original. This continues until further modification does not lead to higher lnL. fastDNAML (Olsen et al., 1994) takes this approach to speed up the computation. The most frequent local modification is nearest-neighbor interchanging, subtree pruning and regrafting, tree bisection and reconnection. Note that these tree modification and re-evaluation is used not only for likelihood-based phylogenetic reconstruction but also for the MP method such as PAUP (Swofford, 1993), and distance-based method such as FastME (Desper and Gascuel, 2002, 2004). In TreeBase, there are phylogenetic studies using both MP and ML methods, sometimes the MP tree, when used to compute the *lnL*, actually has greater *lnL* than the reported ML tree. This implies that the ML method used has never had a chance to encounter the reported MP tree.

8.3 LIKELIHOOD METHOD AND MOLECULAR CLOCK

Recall that molecular phylogenetics has two main objectives: (1) resolving the branching pattern and (2) dating evolutionary events such as specia-tion events or gene duplication events. We have learned how to use the likelihood method for phylogenetic reconstruction. However, to perform dating, one needs to test for the validity of the molecular clock hypothesis and use the clock for dating. The actual dating is now typically done in the Bayesian framework popularized by BEAST (Drummond and Rambaut, 2007) partly because the ML approach does not permit a natural way of incorporating uncertainty on the fossil dates. However, the likelihood ratio test is still used widely to test the molecular clock hypothesis.

To test the molecular clock hypothesis, we compare two models, with one imposing a clock and one without imposing a molecular clock. The model with a clock is a special case of the model without a clock, so the two are nested and can be tested by the likelihood ratio test. We need to compute *lnL* for both models. The null hypothesis is that the two models are equally good in fitting the data. If we have long sequence alignment (i.e., good power to detect differences between models) but the molecular clock hypothesis is not rejected, then we can calibrate the clocked tree to perform dating.

8.3.1 PRUNING ALGORITHM AND MOLECULAR CLOCK

This section illustrates the calculation of likelihood given the sequence alignment and topology in Figure 8.3. The pruning algorithm is the same as before except that we constrain $b_1 = b_2$, $b_3 = b_4$, and $(b_1 + b_5) = (b_3 + b_6)$. For simplicity, we will again use the JC69 model, which allows us to reduce the eight aligned sites (Fig. 8.3) to three site patterns: Pattern 1 for sites 1–2, pattern 2 for sites 3–4 and pattern 3 for sites 5–8. Thus, we only need to compute the likelihood for sites 1, 3, and 5.

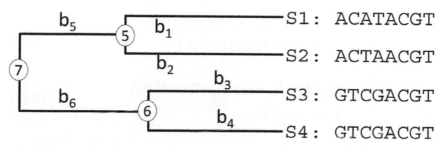

FIGURE 8.3 Sequence alignment and topology for illustrating likelihood calculation with a molecular clock. Imposing a molecular clock implies $b_1 = b_2$, $b_3 = b_4$, and $(b_1 + b_5)$ $= (b_3 + b_6)$. So there are only three branch lengths to estimate. Without a clock we would need to estimate five branch lengths: b_1, b_2, b_3, b_4, and b_{56}.

For site 1 (site pattern 1), the likelihood vector L for the internal nodes 5, 6, and 7 are

$$L_{5.1}(A) = P_{AA}(b_1)P_{AA}(b_2) = P_{ii}^2(b_1)$$
$$L_{5.1}(C) = P_{CA}(b_1)P_{CA}(b_2) = P_{ij}^2(b_1) = L_{5.1}(G) = L_{5.1}(T) \qquad (8.19)$$

where $L_{5.1}$ denotes the L vector for internal node 5 with site pattern 1.

$$L_{6.1}(A) = P_{AG}(b_3)P_{AG}(b_4) = P_{ij}^2(b_3) = L_{6.1}(C) = L_{6.1}(T)$$
$$L_{6.1}(G) = P_{GG}(b_3)P_{GG}(b_4) = P_{ii}^2(b_3) \qquad (8.20)$$

$$L_{7.1}(A) = \left[\sum_{k=0}^{3} P_{Ak}(b_5)L_{5.1}(k)\right]\left[\sum_{k=0}^{3} P_{Ak}(b_6)L_{6.1}(k)\right]$$
$$L_{7.1}(C) = \left[\sum_{k=0}^{3} P_{Ck}(b_5)L_{5.1}(k)\right]\left[\sum_{k=0}^{3} P_{Ck}(b_6)L_{6.1}(k)\right]$$
$$L_{7.1}(G) = \left[\sum_{k=0}^{3} P_{Gk}(b_5)L_{5.1}(k)\right]\left[\sum_{k=0}^{3} P_{Gk}(b_6)L_{6.1}(k)\right] \qquad (8.21)$$
$$L_{7.1}(T) = \left[\sum_{k=0}^{3} P_{Tk}(b_5)L_{5.1}(k)\right]\left[\sum_{k=0}^{3} P_{Tk}(b_6)L_{6.1}(k)\right]$$

For site 3 (site pattern 2), the L vectors for internal nodes 5 and 6 are specified below, and $L_{7.1}$ is specified the way as that in Eq. (8.21) except that $L_{5.1}$ and $L_{6.1}$ are, respectively, replaced by $L_{5.2}$ and $L_{6.2}$ specified below:

$$L_{5.2}(A) = L_{5.2}(T) = P_{ii}(b_1)P_{ij}(b_1)$$
$$L_{5.2}(C) = L_{5.2}(G) = P_{ij}^2(b_1)$$

(8.22)

$$L_{6.2}(A) = L_{6.2}(G) = L_{6.2}(T) = P_{ij}^2(b_3)$$
$$L_{6.2}(C) = P_{ii}^2(b_3)$$

(8.23)

For site 5 (site pattern 3), the L vectors for internal nodes 5 and 6 are shown below and L_7 is specified the way as that in Eq. (8.21) except that $L_{5.1}$ and $L_{6.1}$ are, respectively, replaced by $L_{5.3}$ and $L_{6.3}$ specified below:

$$L_{5.3}(A) = P_{ii}^2(b_1)$$
$$L_{5.3}(C) = L_{5.3}(G) = L_{5.3}(T) = P_{ij}^2(b_1)$$

(8.24)

$$L_{6.3}(A) = P_{ii}^2(b_3)$$
$$L_{6.3}(C) = L_{6.3}(G) = L_{6.3}(T) = P_{ij}^2(b_3)$$

(8.25)

The likelihood for the three site patterns, designated as L_1, L_2, and L_3, are

$$L_1 = \frac{1}{4}\sum_{i=0}^{3} L_{7.1}(i); \quad L_2 = \frac{1}{4}\sum_{i=0}^{3} L_{7.2}(i); \quad L_3 = \frac{1}{4}\sum_{i=0}^{3} L_{7.3}(i);$$

(8.26)

where 1/4 is the equilibrium frequencies (π_i) for the JC69 model. The log-likelihood (lnL) given the topology and the sequence alignment in Figure 8.3 is

$$\ln L = 2\ln(L_1) + 2\ln(L_2) + 4\ln(L_3)$$

(8.27)

which has three unknown branch lengths (b_1, b_3, and b_5). The b_1, b_3, and b_5 values that maximize lnL, subject to the constraints that branch lengths cannot be negative, are $b_1 = 0.1597105$, $b_3 = 0$, and $b_5 = 0.3011361$. Given the clock constraint that $(b_1 + b_5) = (b_3 + b_6)$, we have $b_6 = b_1 + b_5 - b_3 =$

0.460846. The L-BFGS-B algorithm (Zhu et al., 1997) is often used for constrained optimization, e.g., with the lower bounds for branch lengths set to zero. The resulting $lnL = -27.63046$, with $L_1 = 0.02970894$, $L_2 = 0.003665145$, and $L_3 = 0.09584556$. Note that variable sites, in general, will have a smaller likelihood than conserved sites.

8.3.2 TESTING MOLECULAR CLOCK WITH LRT

Before one calibrates the clocked tree with dated fossils, it is customary to test the clock hypothesis by LRT. Note that a tree without a clock is more general than a tree with a clock. With the former, we need to estimate (N-2) more branch lengths than with the latter, where N is the number of OTUs. With four OTUs, a tree without a clock will have five branch lengths to estimate, in contrast to only three in a tree with a clock. The procedure of LRT is to estimate lnL for the tree with and without the clock, designated lnL_{clock} and $lnL_{no.clock}$, respectively. The likelihood ratio chi-square is $2(lnL_{no.clock}-lnL_{clock})$ with (N-2) degrees of freedom. To discriminate between the two models, one typically needs to have much longer sequences than those in Figure 8.3, for two reasons. First, there would be little statistical power to reject the null hypothesis if we have little data, even if the null hypothesis is false. Second, the likelihood ratio chi-square may not follow chi-square distribution when there is little data, so that the resulting p value will not be accurate.

The sequences in Figure 8.3 cannot be used to illustrate the test of molecular clock because *S3* and *S4* are identical and *S1* and *S2* diverge equally from *S3/S4*, so we know a priori that the sequences conform to the clock hypothesis. In other words, the clock model and the nonclock model will have the same lnL. If we change the third site of *S3* from C to T, then, again applying the JC69 model and the pruning algorithm as illustrated before for the clock and no-clock hypotheses, we will find lnL equal to -31.2924 with clock and -30.4874 without clock. This gives us the likelihood ratio chi-square of $2\Delta lnL$ equal 1.6099. With two degrees of freedom, $p = 0.4471$ so we do not reject the molecular clock hypothesis. Keep in mind that this illustration has two problems because of the short sequences (sequence length of 8). First, there is little power to reject the null hypothesis. Second, approximate of $2\Delta lnL$ distribution by χ^2 distribution may not be accurate with small samples. Fortunately, we always have more data in real research.

8.4 POTENTIAL BIAS IN HANDLING OF MISSING DATA WITH THE PRUNING ALGORITHM

The pruning algorithm facilitates the handling of missing data. The key requirement for handling missing data is that what is missing will not contribute anything to the choice of the best tree. The maximum likelihood method, when implemented properly, is not biased with missing data. However, phylogenetic bias may be induced by missing data in conjunction with rate heterogeneity over sites. I will illustrate the handling of missing data by the pruning algorithm and the potential phylogenetic bias based on a previous publication (Xia, 2014).

Suppose we have data in Figure 8.4a and need to evaluate the three possible unrooted trees (T_1, T_2, and T_3 in Fig. 8.4). It is obvious that the only information we have for the data set is the distance between $S1$ and $S2$, so we should not be able to discriminate among the three topologies. We also note that, given the JC69 model, the sequences in Figure 8.4a have two site patterns, with the first four sites sharing one site pattern (i.e., with the same site-specific likelihood) and the last four sites sharing the other site pattern. We, therefore, need to compute the log-likelihood for only the first site (lnL_1) and the fifth site (lnL_5) and multiply them by 4 to get lnL for the entire alignment.

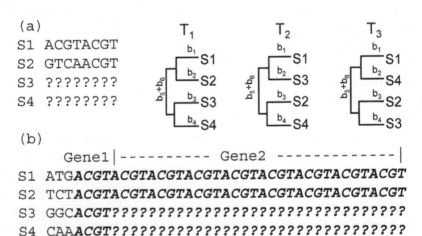

(a)
```
S1  ACGTACGT
S2  GTCAACGT
S3  ????????
S4  ????????
```

(b)
```
         Gene1 | - - - - - - - - - Gene2  - - - - - - - - - - - - |
S1  ATGACGTACGTACGTACGTACGTACGTACGTACGTACGT
S2  TCTACGTACGTACGTACGTACGTACGTACGTACGTACGT
S3  GGCACGT????????????????????????????????
S4  CAAACGT????????????????????????????????
```

FIGURE 8.4 Aligned sequences with missing data for illustrating missing data handling by the likelihood method and the potential bias induced by missing information in conjunction with rate heterogeneity.

The computation of lnL_1, given Topology T_1, is illustrated in Figure 8.5. For an unknown or missing nucleotide, we simply set $L_j(A) = L_j(C) = L_j(G) = L_j(T) = 1$. The likelihood calculation then proceeds exactly as before. The log-likelihood (lnL) for all eight sites, given topology T_1 in Figure 8.4, is

$$\ln L = 4\ln L_1 + 4\ln L_5 \tag{8.28}$$

which, upon maximization, leads to $b_1 + b_2 = 0.8239592165$ and $lnL = -21.02998149$. Terms containing b_3, b_4, and b_5+b_6 all cancel out, i.e., the sequences in Figure 8.4a have no information for estimating b_3, b_4, and b_5+b_6, which again is what we would have expected. The resulting distance between $S1$ and $S2$ $(=b_1 + b_2)$ is the same if we just use the distance formula for two sequences. Thus, adding two sequences with all information missing does not distort our estimate of the distance between $S1$ and $S2$.

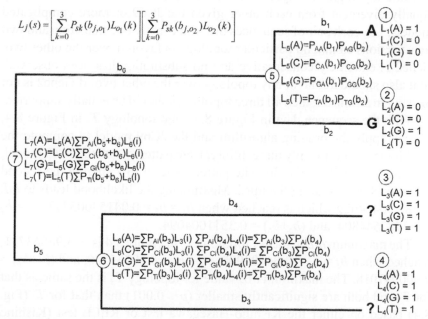

FIGURE 8.5 Likelihood computation with the pruning algorithm and missing data.

If we perform the computation again with topology T_2 in Figure 8.4, we will have exactly the same lnL, but b_5+b_6 will be 0 and $b_1+b_3=0.8239592165$ (i.e., the distance between OTUs $S1$ and $S2$ is 0.8239592165 as before). This again is perfectly consistent with our common sense. Topology T_3 in Figure 8.4 will lead to the same lnL and the same conclusion with distance between $S1$ and $S2$ being 0.8239592165.

Our happy feeling with the likelihood method, however, does not last forever. Suppose now we have sequence data in Figure 8.4b, with Gene1 being variable but Gene2, which is missing in $S3$ and $S4$, is so conservative as to be invariant. In practice, Gene1 and Gene2 could be different segments within the same gene, e.g., the conserved and variable domains in ribosomal RNAs with no clear boundary between them. Note that the three variable sites at the 5'-end could be scattered over different sites in the data instead of clumping together to be as easily recognizable as in Figure 8.4b.

The sequences are intentionally made not to favor any one of the three possible topologies in Figure 8.4. For Gene1, the four OTUs are exactly equally divergent from each other given the JC69 or more complicated models, i.e., each pair of sequences differ in exactly one transition and two transversions so that no particular topology is favored over the other two. Gene2 is extremely conservative and no substitution has been observed, so it also should not favor any topology over the other two. If Gene2 is not missing in $S3$ and $S4$, then all three topologies should be equally supported.

With the sequence data in Figure 8.4b and topology T_1 in Figure 8.4, we can apply the pruning algorithm and the JC69 model to compute the likelihood. There are only three different site patterns with the JC69 model, i.e., sites 1 to 3 share the first site pattern, sites 4 to 7 sharing the second and sites 8 to 39 sharing the third. Maximizing the likelihood leads to lnL = −83.56464029 which is reached when $b_1 = b_2 = 0.04153005797$, $b_3 = b_4$ = 0.3787544804, and $(b_5+b_6) = 0.3511004094$.

The maximum lnL value for topology T_2 in Figure 8.4 is −83.96663731, reached when $b_1 = b_3 = 0.04184900$, $b_2 = b_4 = 0.60765526$, and (b_5+b_6) = 0.000947018. The maximum lnL value for topology T_3 is the same as that for T_2 and both are significantly smaller ($p < 0.001$) than that for T_1 (Fig. 8.4) based on either the Kishino-Hasegawa test or RELL test (Kishino and Hasegawa, 1989) or Shimodaira & Hasegawa test (Shimodaira and Hasegawa, 1999).

We have previously mentioned that the most fundamental criterion for missing data handling methods is that the missing data should not contribute phylogenetically relevant information. The demonstration above shows clearly that missing data do contribute such information, even with the likelihood approach. If the data are not missing, then the three topologies will be equally supported. So, the bias in favor of Topology T_1 in the presence of missing data can only be attributed to the presence of missing data.

While the phylogenetic bias in the sequence configuration in Figure 8.4b favors the grouping S_1 and S_2 together, one can easily envision scenarios in which S_1 and S_2 would repulse each other, e.g., when the last 32 sites in Figure 8.4b are far more variable than the first seven sites. Thus, the direction of the bias cannot be predicted before data analysis.

8.5 STATISTICAL TEST OF ALTERNATIVE PHYLOGENETIC HYPOTHESES

Phylogeneticists often encounter problems in which different morphological or paleontological data support different trees. One can use molecular data to evaluate these alternative hypotheses in a likelihood framework (Xia, 2000). Such tests are often termed phylogenetic incongruence tests.

Phylogenetic incongruence test is frequently used in testing alternative phylogenetic hypotheses and, in particular, in detecting lateral gene transfer (LGT) events. Among closely related enterobacterial species, some have genes coding proteins for lactose metabolism (e.g., *Escherichia coli* and *Klebsiella pneumoniae*) and some do not (e.g., *Shigella flaxneri, Salmonella enterica, Serratia marcescens, Yersinia pestis*). *E. coli* and *Sh. Flaxneri* are the most closely related phylogenetically, yet they differ in lactose utilization. This leads to at least two possible evolutionary scenarios. First, a lactose-metabolizing function may be absent in the enterobacterial ancestor but gained independently along lineages leading to *E. coli* and *K. pneumoniae* (e.g., by LGT). Second, the function is present in the ancestor but lost in all species except for lineages *E. coli* and *K. pneumoniae*. If lactose-metabolizing genes are never involved in LGT, then the first scenario, where lineages E and H gained lactose-metabolizing function independently, would be highly implausible. In contrast, if lactose-metabolizing genes are frequently involved in LGT, then this scenario cannot be excluded.

How would we know if a gene is frequently involved in LGT? Lack of LGT in a gene implies that the gene tree should approximate a species tree. A gene frequently involved in LGT tends to have a gene tree incompatible with the species tree. A species tree is typically approximated by a tree built from two types of genes (Rivera et al., 1998): (1) Informational genes encoding the machinery for transcription, translation, DNA replication, and (2) operational genes ("housekeeping genes") for cellular metabolic processes, such as biosynthesis of amino acids, fatty acids, nucleotides, cell envelope proteins. A gene tree incompatible with a species tree is an indication of LGT. Such tests have led to the discovery of the rampant occurrence of LGT, prompting the suggestion that the cenancestor is neither a single cell nor a single genome but is instead an entangle bank of heterogeneous genomes with relatively free flow of genetic information. Out of this entangled bank of frolicking genomes arose probably many evolutionary lineages with a gradually reduced rate of horizontal gene transfer confined mainly within individual lineages (Xia and Yang, 2013). Only three (Archaea, Eubacteria, and Eukarya) of these early lineages have representatives survived to this day.

LGT events distort phylogenetic signals in the gene. Such genes are poor phylogenetic markers. The late Ernst Mayr, once in an argument against using parasites as markers to infer phylogeny in a conference, stated that two birds can exchange parasites but never exchange their heads or wings or legs (Paterson et al., 1995). The point is that we should use characters such as heads, wings, and tails that are ancestrally inherited instead of parasites that could be laterally transferred to build phylogenetic relationships. Laterally transferred genes are equivalent to laterally trans- ferred parasites in terms of recovering phylogenetic relationships.

Suppose we have the sequence data (Fig. 8.6) from housekeeping genes, a species tree (T_1) and a lactose operon gene tree (T_2). We wish to test whether T_1 is significantly better than T_2 given the housekeeping gene sequences with the null hypothesis being that T_2 is just as good as T_1. MP, ML, and distance-based methods have all been used for such significance tests but here we illustrate with only MP and ML methods.

For the ML method, we compute the log-likelihood (lnL) for each of the nine sites (Fig. 8.6) given T_1 and T_2, respectively (lnL_1 and lnL_2 for T_1 and T_2, respectively, Table 8.2). We have already learned how to obtain site-specific likelihood in the chapter on ML method using the pruning algorithms. A paired-sample t-test can then be applied to test whether mean lnL_1 is significantly different from mean lnL_2. For our data in Table 8.2, $t = 4.107$, DF = 8, $p = 0.0034$, two-tailed test). So we reject the null hypothesis and conclude that the lactose operon gene tree (T_2) is significantly worse than the species tree (T_1). A natural explanation for the phylogenetic incongruence is LGT, although there are other processes that can distort phylogenetic signals and generate gene trees significantly different from a species tree.

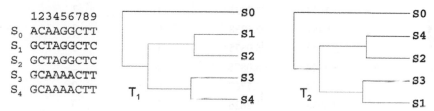

              123456789
S_0 ACAAGGCTT
S_1 GCTAGGCTC
S_2 GCTAGGCTC
S_3 GCAAAACTT
S_4 GCAAAACTT

FIGURE 8.6   DNA sequence data for significance tests of two alternative topologies.

For the MP method, we compute the minimum number of changes (NC) for each site given T_1 and T_2 (Fig. 8.6), respectively (NC_1 and NC_2 Table 8.2). We have already learned how to obtain site-specific NC in the chapter on MP method using either the Fitch algorithm or the Sankoff algorithm. We can then perform a paired-sample t-test as before to test whether mean NC_1 is significantly smaller than NC_2, in one of three ways. The first is to use the entire nine pairs of data, which yields $t = -2.5298$, DF = 8, $p = 0.0353$, and a decision to reject the null hypothesis that T_1 and T_2 are equally good at the 0.05 significance level. In other words, we adopt the alternative hypothesis that T_1 is significantly better than T_2. Second, we may use only the five polymorphic sites in the paired-sample t-test, which would yield $t = -4$, DF = 4, and $p = 0.0161$. This leads to the same conclusion with greater confidence. The third is to use only the four informative sites if Fitch algorithm is used to compute NC. We have four NC_1 values all equal to 1 and four NC_2 values all equal to 2. With no within-group variation, p value is then 0, also leading to rejection of the null hypothesis. In the chapter on MP, we have mentioned mixed models in which "Tree" is the fixed effect and "Site" is taken as a random effect. The mixed model can also be used in discriminating between alternative phylogenetic trees with site-specific lnL in Table 8.2.

TABLE 8.2 Phylogenetic incongruence tests with maximum likelihood (ML) and maximum parsimony (MP) methods. lnL_1 and lnL_2 are site-specific log-likelihood values based on the F84 Model and T_1 and T_2 (Fig. 8.6), respectively, and NC_1 and NC_2 are the minimum number of changes required for each site given T_1 and T_2, respectively.

	ML		MP	
Site	lnL_1	lnL_2	NC_1	NC_2
1	−4.0975	−4.0990	1	1
2	−2.0634	−2.7767	0	0
3	−5.1147	−7.7335	1	2
4	−1.9481	−2.6238	0	0
5	−3.2142	−5.0875	1	2
6	−3.2142	−5.0875	1	2
7	−2.0634	−2.7767	0	0
8	−2.3938	−3.2626	0	0
9	−3.1090	−3.8572	1	2

When the phylogenetic incongruence test is applied to real lactose operon data, it was found that the lactose operon gene tree is somewhat compatible to the species tree, and the case for LGT is therefore not strong (Stoebel, 2005). This suggests the possibility that the lactose operon was present in the ancestor but has been lost in a number of descendent lineages. In contrast, the urease gene cluster, which is important for long-term cytoplasmic pH homeostasis in the bacterial gastric pathogen, *Helicobacter pylori* (Sachs et al., 2003; Xia, 2018a, Chapter 17; Xia and Palidwor, 2005), generate gene trees significantly different from the species tree (unpublished result). This suggests that the urease gene cluster is involved in LGT and has implications in emerging pathogens. For example, many bacterial species pass through our digestive system daily and it is conceivable that some of them may gain the urease gene cluster and become acid-resistant with the consequence of one additional pathogen for our stomach.

One may note that significant incongruence between the gene tree and species tree does not imply LGT because events, such as gene duplication and lineage-specific gene loss (lineage sorting), can also lead to phylogenetic incongruence (Page, 2003). This is illustrated in Figure 8.7 with five species labeled Sp1 to Sp5. A gene duplication event occurred at node N in Figure 8.7a, leading to paralogous genes A and B in all subsequent lineages. Differential gene losses occurred subsequently (Fig. 8.7b), leading to the loss of A1, B2, and A3, which would mislead us to think that gene duplication has never occurred and that the gene has always been in a single-copy state. Using these five gene sequences, B1, B3, A2, *A4,* and A5, we would arrive at the wrong tree (Fig. 8.7c) that is different from the true tree in Figure 8.7a. Thus, the phylogenetic incongruence test can only be used to identify poor phylogenetic markers. Genes involved in LGT are typically poor phylogenetic markers but a poor phylogenetic marker may not necessarily be an LGT gene.

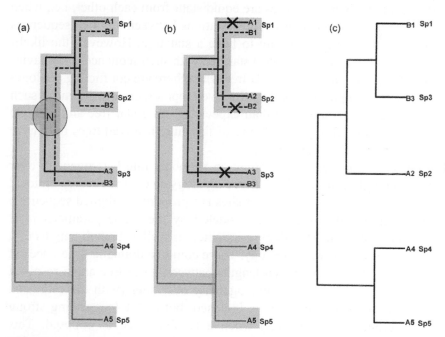

FIGURE 8.7 Phylogenetic incongruence can result from gene duplication and lineage-specific gene loss. (a) A gene duplication event occurred at Node N. (b) Genes A1, B2 and B3 were lost in evolution. (c) Phylogenetic tree resulting from the remaining 5 gene sequences is different from the true tree (shaded).

The illustration above shows that claiming LGT of gene A by showing a significant discrepancy between the gene A tree and species tree is another example of conclusion through a backdoor. That is, we do not have direct evidence of LGT, but claimed LGT because we are at a loss to explain the discrepancy between the gene A tree and species. We have previously mentioned that the CODEML approach of detecting positive selection is also an example of conclusion through a backdoor. One does not have any direct evidence of positive selection but claimed positive selection because a particular neutral model does not seem sufficient to fit the data.

8.6   STARLESS PROPENSITY AND PARAMETER ESTIMATION BIAS

There are two peculiarities associated with the likelihood methods (Xia, 2019a). First, when sequences are equidistant from each other, i.e., when the number of various types of substitutions between any two sequences is exactly the same, we desire to have a star tree. However, the likelihood method may not generate a star tree with such sequences, a behavior dubbed starless bias. In a 4-OTU tree when there are conflicting phylogenetic signals supporting the three resolved topologies equally, and if such conflicting signals are more than expected from a star tree and a single substitution model, e.g., JC69, any of the three resolved trees may have tree *lnL* greater than the star tree.

Second, fitting gamma distribution to model rate heterogeneity over sites is strongly confounded with tree topology, in contrast to conventional belief that rate heterogeneity over sites is a property of aligned sequences. Rate heterogeneity over site is modeled by the shape parameter α of gamma distribution. This shape parameter, as well as branch lengths of a tree, is confounded with topology. There could be dramatic differences in the estimated α and in branch lengths between a star tree and a resolved tree. One may find no rate heterogeneity over sites (with the estimated $\alpha > 10,000$) when a star tree is imposed, but $\alpha < 1$ (suggesting strong rate heterogeneity over sites) when a resolved tree is imposed. This highlights the point that "rate heterogeneity" is not a sequence-specific feature independent of tree topology. One should not interpret a small α to mean that some sites are under strong purifying selection and others not. I substantiate these observations here with numerical illustrations published in a previous study based on the JC69 model (Xia, 2019a).

While the dependence of parameter estimation on tree topology seems obvious, it might still benefit from an analogous example in statistics (Fig. 8.8A) where two different combinations of models and parameter estimates can both explain perfectly the variation in the y variable. If we know for sure that Model 1 (Fig. 8.8A) is correct, then there is little controversy to report the two slopes (1 and 2, respectively, for x_1 and x_2) which provide us with meaningful information. However, these two slope parameters would make little sense if Model 2 (Fig. 8.8A) is in fact correct and vice versa.

The three variables in Fig. 8.8A are equivalent to aligned sequences, the two models are equivalent to alternative topologies (both model and topology being discrete variables), the model parameters (e.g., coefficients 1 for x_1 and 2 for x_2 in Model 1) given the model are equivalent to branch lengths and substitution model parameters given the topology. The branch lengths and substitution model parameters are meaningful only if the topology is correct, just as the slope parameters for Model 1 and Model 2 (Fig. 8.8A) are meaningful only if the model is correct. This is particularly relevant to dating speciation and gene duplication events. If the topology is incorrect, then the branch length estimates could be meaningless. Consequently, inferred speciation dates or gene duplication dates could potentially be meaningless as well. Similarly, choosing substitution models when the true topology is unknown could also be potentially meaningless. As will be shown later, a set of sequences will appear to have no rate heterogeneity over sites with a star tree but high rate heterogeneity over sites with a resolved tree.

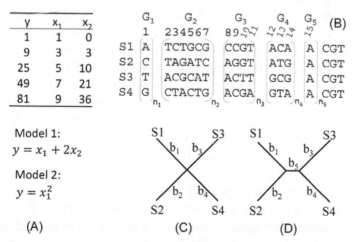

FIGURE 8.8 Models and parameters in statistical estimation. (A) Three variables and two models. (B) Representative site patterns for four species. A total of 256 possible site patterns with four sequences, classed into 15 site pattern classes relevant to the JC69 model and further boxed into five site pattern groups (G_1 to G_5). Sites within each group jointly support equally the three alternative resolved trees. (C) A star tree. (D) One of three resolved trees with $b_5 > 0$.

8.6.1   SITE PATTERNS CLASSIFICATION AND SEQUENCE REPRESENTATION

With four aligned sequences, there are 256 possible site patterns which can be collapsed into 15 site patterns for the JC69 model (Fig. 8.8A). Different combinations of these 256 site patterns support different substitution models and different topologies. The transition probabilities needed for likelihood calculation for the JC69 and other substitution models have been derived in the chapter on nucleotide-based substitution models.

Sites in G_1 have all four OTUs (*S1–S4*) with different nucleotides, with 24 unique site patterns represented as a single G_1 site in Figure 8.8A (because JC69 sees these 24 site patterns as equivalent, i.e., with the same site likelihood). Sites in G_2 each have three different nucleotides, with a total of 144 unique site patterns. Only six sites are used to represent them in Figure 8.8A because JC69 sees these 144 unique sites in this group as equivalent to one of the six representative sites. Sites in G_3 feature two nucleotides, with three OTUs having the same nucleotide and a total of 48 unique sites represented by four sites in Figure 8.8A. Sites in G_4 also feature two nucleotides, with two OTUs sharing one nucleotide and the other two OTUs sharing the other (i.e., they are the traditional informative sites in Fitch parsimony). There are 36 unique G_4 sites represented by three sites in Figure 8.8A. G_5 sites are monomorphic, with four unique site patterns represented by site 15 in Figure 8.8A. The five groups of sites (G_1–G_5 in Fig. 8.8A) support the three unrooted topologies equally. This is obvious for G_1 and G_5 sites. The six sites in G_2, shown in Figure 8.8A, jointly also support the three topologies equally, so do the four sites in G_3 and three sites in G_4. This site pattern classification (Xia 2019a) was included for your convenience (so you don' t need to search for the original reference).

Note that, with a star tree and JC69, we cannot have G_1, G_2, and G_4 sites without having G_3 sites first. With low sequence divergence along a star tree, almost all polymorphic site patterns should be G_3 sites. The star tree bias occurs when there is a surplus of G_4 sites relative to the expectation from a strict JC69 model. Note that the three sites in G_4 each support an alternative resolved topology.

Subscripts n_1 to n_5 in Figure 8.8A mean multiples of the enclosed sites, e.g., an n_2 of 10 means that the six G_2 sites in Figure 8.8A are repeated 10 times (for a total of 60 sites). A site combination of $(n_1, n_2, n_3, n_4, n_5)$, where n_i corresponds to those in Figure 8.8A, means a set of aligned sequences containing n_1 G_1 sites, n_2 G_2 sites (i.e., n_2*6 sites), n_3 G_3 sites (for a total of n_3*4 sites), and so on (Fig. 8.8A). A set of four sequences of length 256 containing all 256 possible site patterns is specified as (24, 24, 12, 12, 4). Such a set of sequences will naturally have equal nucleotide frequencies and twice as many transversions as transitions, i.e., the equilibrium ratio of substitution saturation. A set of sequences with any combinations of (n_1, n_2, n_3, n_4, n_5) are equidistant from each other from a JC69 perspective and we would desire to have a star tree (Fig. 8.8B) instead of one of the three resolved trees (Fig. 8.8C). A set of four aligned sequences equidistant from each other can be simply specified by (n_1, n_2, n_3, n_4, n_5).

Not all (n_1, n_2, n_3, n_4, n_5) combinations are equally likely under the JC69 model with a star tree. For example, the site pattern combination (24, 24, 12, 96, 32) has a near-zero chance to occur with a star tree and a strict JC69 model because given a star tree with $x_5 = 0$, G_4 sites can only emerge through independent substitutions along each of the four branches (i.e., all G_4 sites result from convergent substitutions). This means that we cannot have G_4 sites in a star tree without first having G_3 sites, so G_4 sites should not be more frequent than G_3 sites given a star tree and JC69. However, when different genes evolving under JC69 models with different rates (and potentially with different evolutionary histories and conflicting phylogenetic signals) are concatenated, strange site pattern combinations, such as (24, 24, 12, 96, 32), may occur and cannot be dismissed as unreal.

8.6.2 THE STAR TREE BIAS

The site pattern combination (24, 24, 12, 96, 32) implies that the four sequences will remain equidistant from each other but the likelihood method will not favor a star tree in spite of equidistance among sequences. As I mentioned before, G_3 sites are the first site pattern to appear in sequence evolution along a star tree. In contrast, a G_4 site requires a minimum of two substitutions when $x_5 = 0$ (Fig. 8.9C), but only a minimum of one with a resolved tree from a parsimony perspective (Fig. 8.9D). Thus, if aligned sequences have few G_3 and many G_4 site patterns, then these G_4 sites will have a low likelihood for a star tree because they all require two independent substitutions which is likely only when there are many G_3 sites. In contrast, any of the three resolved tree will have 1/3 of G_4 sites requiring only one substitution (and consequently a high likelihood) and 2/3 of the G_4 sites requiring two independent substitutions. In short, when there are too many G_4 sites relative to G_3 sites, tree lnL will tend to be greater with $x_5 > 0$ (i.e., a resolved tree) than with $x_5 = 0$ (a star tree).

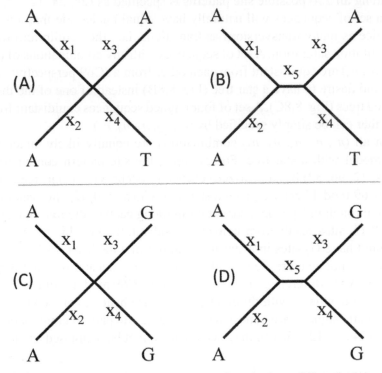

FIGURE 8.9 G_3 and G_4 sites support star tree and resolved tree differently. (A) and (B) a G_3 site mapped to a star tree and a resolved tree, respectively. (C) and (D) a G_4 site mapped to a star tree and a resolved tree, respectively.

It might help to illustrate this with a numerical example. Suppose we have a set of four aligned sequences characterized by site pattern combination (24, 24, 12, 96, 32). We can evaluate tree lnL by using either the R script files (New2.R and NewGamma3.R at http://dambe.bio.uottawa.ca/Include/software.aspx) or alternative likelihood methods. Assuming no rate heterogeneity over sites, tree lnL is -2947.793 with a star tree (with x_5 in Fig. 8.9 set to 0), but is greater ($lnL = -2943.148$) with x_5 allowed to be greater than 0. Thus, although the sequences are equidistant, a star tree is not favored by the likelihood method. If we model rate heterogeneity over sites by gamma-distributed rate, then lnL for the star tree is still -2947.793 but lnL for any of the three resolved tree is much greater

(lnL = −2918.782, obtained when the shape parameter α = 0.745). A likelihood ratio test will conclusively reject the star tree (which has one fewer branch than any of the three resolved tree).

8.6.3 RATE HETEROGENEITY OVER SITES IS CONFOUNDED BY TREE TOPOLOGY

It is quite easy to see tree topology and the estimate of rate heterogeneity over sites confounding each other. Let us focus on G_4 site patterns. With a star tree in Figure 8.9C, all G_4 sites require exactly the same number of changes (a minimum of two substitutions per site from a parsimony perspective). In other words, there is no rate heterogeneity among G_4 sites with a star tree. However, for a resolved tree in Figure 8.9D, 1/3 of the G_4 sites (with identical nucleotides between sister groups as in Fig. 8.9D) would require only one substitution from the parsimony perspective. The other 2/3 of the G_4 sites (with different nucleotides between sister groups) would require a minimum of two substitutions. Thus, from a parsimony perspective, 1/3 of the G_4 sites evolve at a rate half as fast as the other 2/3 of the sites. Likewise with the likelihood perspective when multiple substitutions are corrected, 2/3 of the G_4 sites will have a substitution rate at least twice as large as 1/3 of the G_4 sites, giving rise to rate heterogeneity among G_4 sites. This rate heterogeneity over G_4 sites is not present with a star tree. Thus, the relative numbers of G_4 and G_3 sites (denoted n_4 and n_3, respectively, Fig. 8.8A) affect not only the tendency to reject the star tree but also the estimation of the rate heterogeneity over sites.

Table 8.3 shows the results of phylogenetic analysis of site pattern combination (24, 24, 12, 96, 32), computed by the two R scripts (Xia, 2019a) as well as by PhyML. Both R scripts implement the likelihood method with the JC69 model (Jukes and Cantor, 1969) with four OTUs. New2.R assumes a constant rate over sites and estimates branch lengths for the star tree (with four branches) and a resolved tree (with five branches). NewGamma3.R does the same but with a continuous gamma-distributed rate over sites. They are plain text files that can be copied and pasted into an R window to generate results presented in the paper.

When a constant rate is assumed the tree lnL is −2943.148 for a resolved tree in contrast to −2947.793 for a star tree (Table 8.3). A likelihood ratio test would lead to $2\Delta lnL$ = 9.29, DF = 1, p = 0.0023 and a rejection of the star tree in favor of a resolved tree. The star tree has equal branch lengths (Table 8.3) and the resolved tree has one zero-length terminal branch ($b_4 = 0$, Table 8.3).

TABLE 8.3 Evaluate two alternative topologies and their branch lengths (b_i) in Figure 8.8C (with b_5 set to 0 and not evaluated) and Figure 8.8D, based on site pattern combination (24, 24, 12, 96, 32).

Method[1]	b_1	b_2	b_3	b_4	b_5[2]	α[3]	*lnL*
New2.R	0.849814	0.849814	1.693866	0	0.850	N/A	−2943.148
	1.020276	1.020276	1.020276	1.020276	N/A	N/A	−2947.793
PhyML	0.849942	0.849764	1.694148	0.000015	0.850	N/A	−2943.148
NewΓ3	2.783640	1.133961	1.575337	2.343977	10	1	−2930.116
	3.359848	1.413517	1.886961	2.886549	30	0.843	−2921.743
	3.767304	1.850750	2.302868	3.315211	50	0.745	−2918.782
	1.020429	1.020429	1.020429	1.020429	N/A	10000	−2947.797
PhyML	2.213152	1.976554	2.206997	1.968304	10	0.814	−2927.806

(1) software used to evaluate topology
(2) N/A indicates star tree (b5 not estimated)
(3) N/A indicates constant rate over sites (α not estimated)

The phylogenetic result with JC69+Γ rejects the star tree more strongly. The maximum lnL for the resolved tree (with α = 0.745, Table 8.3) is −2918.782. Comparing this with the star tree, $2\Delta lnL = 58.03$, DF = 1, $p = 2.58*10^{-14}$. The branch lengths of the resolved tree are odd, with a very long internal branch (b_5) relative to the four terminal branches (Table 8.3).

One point we wish to highlight involves branch length estimates when gamma distribution is used to model rate heterogeneity over sites. With the JC69 model, it is reasonable to set the maximum branch length to 10 in maximizing tree *lnL* because longer branch leads to transition probabilities of JC69 effectively equal to 1/4. This is not so with gamma distribution. We may intuitively appreciate this by contrasting between transition probability p_{ij} for the constant-rate JC69 model and the average p_{ij} for the JC69+Γ model:

$$P_{ij.constant} = \frac{1}{4} - \frac{1}{4}e^{\left(-\frac{4b}{3}\right)}; P_{ij.gamma} = \frac{1}{4} - \frac{1}{4}\left(1 + \frac{4b}{3\alpha}\right)^{-\alpha} \tag{8.29}$$

If $\alpha = 10000$ (no rate heterogeneity over sites), then $b = 10$ would result in both p_{ij}, with or without gamma distribution, to be effectively 0.25. That is, the sequences have experienced full substitution saturation. Increasing b beyond 10 would have little effect on tree lnL. However, if $\alpha \leq 1$ (strong rate heterogeneity over sites), then the same $b = 10$ will result in $p_{ij.gamma}$ = 0.232558. It takes a much larger b value ($b > 100$) for $p_{ij.gamma}$ to get close to 0.25. Table 8.3 shows that, when b_5 is increased from 10 to 30 and 50 with gamma-distributed rates, the tree lnL change substantially. This implies that setting the maximum branch length to 10 in PhyML may not be a good idea.

The estimated parameter values in Table 8.3 confirm a point we have made before. First, when the star tree is imposed, there is no rate heterogeneity over sites, with the shape parameter α in the order of 10000 (Table 8.3). However, the estimated α becomes 0.745 when b_5 (x_5 in Fig. 8.1D) is allowed to be greater than 0, indicating strong rate heterogeneity over sites. This highlights that the α parameter is much confounded by tree topology and cautions against interpreting it as strictly a sequence feature. A small α is often interpreted to mean strong purifying selection constraining certain sites but not others. However, the α parameter clearly depends on both sequences and the tree topology.

I hope that these illustrations will be sufficient to convince the reader that the shape parameter α, as estimated in phylogenetic analysis, is conditional on topology. It may be considered as a sequence feature only when the topology is known.

KEYWORDS

- **maximum likelihood**
- **pruning algorithm**
- **phylogenetic incongruence test**
- **likelihood ratio test**
- **rate heterogeneity over sites**
- **molecular clock hypothesis**
- **missing data**

CHAPTER 9

Phylogeny-Based Comparative Methods

ABSTRACT

Are genes functionally related so that they are often present or absent jointly in different evolutionary lineages? Does a phenotypic character evolve in response to an environmental factor? Are two phenotypic characters evolve jointly over time? All these questions involve the relationship between one variable (or a set of variables) and another variable (or another set of variables). Conventional statistical methods without taking phylogeny into consideration are inappropriate for quantifying the relationships because of coancestry. This chapter introduces the phylogeny-based comparative methods that are crucial for quantifying and understanding the relationship among genes, between genotype and phenotype, and between phenotype and environmental factors. The independent contrast methods for continuous variables, in both least-squares and likelihood framework, were illustrated in great detail, together with various modifications. This is followed by numerical illustration of the pruning algorithm and the likelihood ratio test used to model association between discrete variables.

9.1 INTRODUCTION

Comparative methods are pioneered by Felsenstein (1985b) and popularized by Harvey and Pagel (1991). They represent a broad category of phylogeny-based statistical inferential methods and should be extremely useful in characterizing the relationship between continuous and discrete variables to understand the relationship between genes, between phenotypes and genotypes, and how environmental changes affect genes, genomes, and phenotypes. This chapter covers the fundamentals of phylogeny-based comparative methods, and is an expanded version of Xia (2013a, Chapter 2).

Large-scale comparative genomics involves the type of framework (Xia 2013a, pp. 21–23) aimed to understand functional association among genes and among phenotypes as well as between genes and phenotypic traits and between genotype/phenotype and the environmental variables (Fig. 9.1). G_{ij} refers to Gene j in species i and the same subscript notations apply to a phenotypic trait (P_{ij}) and environmental factor E_{ij}. The most straightforward genetic variables (G_{ij}) are the presence/absence of genes, so the G_{ij} variables will be binary. The loss/gain of one gene may affect the loss/gain of another gene. For example, the presence of a type II restriction enzyme in bacteria that cuts DNA at a specific restriction site dictates the presence of a methyltransferase that modifies the same recognition site in the host genome to protect it from being digested by the restriction enzyme. The two genes are, therefore, strongly associated, with the presence of the type II restriction enzyme always associated with the methyltransferase. Similarly, phenotypic traits can also be associated. For example, uncertainty in genetic relatedness can select against parental care or other altruistic behavior (Xia, 1992, 1993, 1995a).

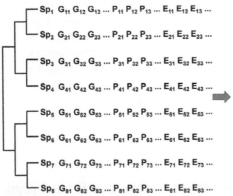

• $G_{.i}$ is associated with $G_{.j}$: functional dependence between $G_{.i}$ and $G_{.j}$, e.g., type II ENase needs methyltransferase
• $P_{.i}$ is associated with $P_{.j}$: functional dependence of phenotypic traits, e.g., flight is associated with light bone.
• $G_{.i}$ is associated with $P_{.j}$: genotype/phenotype association, e.g., urease gene cluster confers acid-resistance in bacteria.
• $P_{.i}$ is associated with $E_{.j}$: adaptation of certain phenotype to certain environmental factors, e.g., codon usage in bacteria phage and host tRNA pool

FIGURE 9.1 Data framework for detecting the association between genes (G), between phenotypic variables (P) and environmental variables (E). Redrawn with modification from Fig. 2.1 in Xia (2013a)

Similarly, a change in $G_{.j}$ may have a phenotypic effect. G_{ij} could be associated with one or more of the phenotypic variables (P_{ij}). For example, a change in G_{ij} may result in drug resistance (P_{ij}) in a bacterial species or genetic disease in human (P_{ij}). Evolutionary biologists are particularly interested in whether certain changes in the G variables and P variables are in response to the environmental variables (E_{ij}), such as temperature and genome size (Xia 1995). For example, gaining a urease gene cluster as well as efficient regulation of urease activity in response to acidic environment facilitates the adaptation of bacterial pathogen, *Helicobacter pylori,* to the acidic environment of the mammalian stomach (Xia, 2018a; Xia and Palidwor, 2005). The comparative genomic data illustrated in Figure 9.1 allows us to characterize millions of pairwise relationships simultaneously and to build gene interaction networks.

9.2   THE NECESSITY OF PHYLOGENY-BASED COMPARATIVE METHOD

One might wonder why we need to use phylogeny-based comparative methods to study the relationship among the G, P, and E sets of variables. Can't we just erase the tree in Figure 9.1 and happily analyze the remaining data matrix with a variety of multivariate statistical methods? The problem is that each row of data in Figure 9.1 is not independent of the data in other rows. Two rows of data corresponding to two closely related species are expected to be similar, especially for the G set of variables, than two rows of data corresponding to two distantly-related species. This violates the assumption of conventional statistics where independence of sampling points is assumed.

This problem is graphically illustrated in Figure 9.2 for two variables X and Y. One may mistakenly conclude a positive relationship between X and Y when the 16 data points are taken as independent (when the tree in Figure 9.2 is ignored). A phylogenetic tree superimposed on the points allows us to see immediately that the data points are not independent. All eight points on the left side of Figure 9.2 share one common ancestor, so do the eight points on the right side. So, the superficial association between X and Y could be due to a single coincidental change in X and Y in one of the two common ancestors. One needs to use the phylogeny-based method, such as independent contrasts (Felsenstein, 1985b; 2004, pp 432–459) or the generalized least-square method (Martins and Hansen, 1997; Pagel, 1997, 1999) when assessing the relationship between quantitative variables.

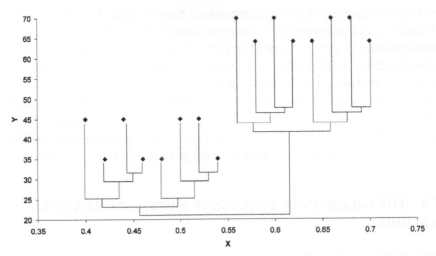

FIGURE 9.2 Phylogeny-based comparison is important for evolutionary studies. The data points, when wrongly taken as independent, would result in a significant positive but spurious relationship between Y and X (which represent any two continuous variables, e.g., $GC\%$ and OGT).

In what follows, I will numerically illustrate the comparative methods (Barker and Pagel, 2005; Felsenstein, 1985b; Harvey and Pagel, 1991; Pagel, 1994; Schluter et al., 1997) for characterizing the association between any two columns of data shown in Figure 9.1. The simplest data set in Figure 9.1 would have only two columns of data, and that is the type of data I will use to illustrate the comparative method for the continuous and discrete variables. I have taken this minimum but sufficient approach throughout the book.

Note that N columns of data would imply $N*(N-1)/2$ pairwise associations, so large-scale comparative genomic studies almost always lead to multiple comparisons. Suppose we take two samples of six individuals from the same population and test the difference in body height between the two samples. Because the two samples are from the same population, we expect no significant differences in body height. However, if we sample repeatedly, eventually we may have one sample of individuals that happen to be mostly short ones and the other sample of individuals that happen to be mostly tall ones. If we reject the null hypothesis of equal body height (which is true given that we are sampling from the same population), then we would have committed a type I error. We, therefore, need a protocol to reduce the chance of committing this type I error. Both the conventional Bonferroni and the more recent false discovery rate (FDR) methods are for this purpose, and both necessarily would elevate the chance of committing a type II error (falsely accepting the null hypothesis when it is false) which is also undesirable. FDR represents a key development in recent studies of statistical significance tests and achieves a better compromise than the conventional Bonferroni method (Benjamini and Hochberg, 1995; Benjamini and Yekutieli, 2001; Ge et al., 2008). These methods were illustrated numerically in detail in Xia (2018, pp. 85–87)

9.3 THE COMPARATIVE METHOD FOR CONTINUOUS CHARACTERS

There are two phylogeny-based approaches to characterize the relationship between the two continuous variables, one by the least-squares (LS) approach (Martins and Hansen, 1997; Pagel, 1997, 1999) and the other based on the random-walk Brownian motion model (Felsenstein, 1985b; 2004, pp 432–459) and the more general Ornstein-Uhlenbeck model. The LS approach is descriptive, i.e., not based on a mechanistic model of character evolution, in contrast to the Brownian motion model (BMM) which is mechanistic. A strict BMM does not accommodate directional changes, with the consequence that the ancestral states of the variables lie somewhere between those of descendent lineages. The LS approach has various ways of accommodating directional changes.

Directional changes do happen often in evolution. For example, various mammalian lineages have in general increased their body size from their humble beginning of tiny insectivores. The ancestral state of the body size, estimated with the assumption of the random-walk Brownian motion model, would be substantially greater than the true ancestral state. This shortcoming can be accommodated by the generalized least-square method (Martins and Hansen, 1997; Pagel, 1997, 1999). The generalized least-square method has an implicit assumption that, if a variable has exhibited directional change, then longer branches should be associated with greater changes. Many traits at the molecular level do conform to this assumption. For example, GC-biased mutation leads to directional changes in genomic $GC\%$, so longer time (i.e., greater divergence) would imply longer branches and greater changes in genomic $GC\%$. Similarly, differences in codon usage is also expected to be small between closely related species but mutations and consequent differences in tRNA pool would lead to divergence in codon usage pattern. That is, greater divergence time tends to be associated with longer branches which, in turn, is associated with greater differences in codon usage among different lineages. In contrast, if the tree is built from gene sequences, but the trait is morphological or physiological, then the differences in trait may not be correlated with divergence time or branch lengths. For example, body size change in different mammalian lineages may not be related well to branch lengths on a tree built from aligned sequences. In this case, the assumed association between branch length and trait values may be weak or nonexistent. In addition, the assumption also leads to the restriction that the method for assessing directional change cannot be used with ultrametric trees, i.e., trees with leaves having equal distance to the root, such as trees built with a molecular clock. I present an LS approach that does not require this assumption, but with one or more ancestral states known or estimated. For example, the ancestral body size of mammals is roughly the size of a rat.

9.3.1 PHYLOGENY-BASED INDEPENDENT CONTRASTS FOR CONTINUOUS TRAITS

Here I illustrate the method of phylogeny-based independent contrasts with two continuous variables: genomic $GC\%$ and its optimal growth temperature (OGT) in different bacterial species. Genomic $GC\%$ represents a genomic feature and OGT an environmental variable (a G variable and an E variable in Fig. 9.1). Wide variation in genomic $GC\%$ is observed in bacterial species. A popular selectionist hypothesis is that bacterial species living in high temperature should have high genomic $GC\%$ for two reasons. First, an increased GC usage, with more hydrogen bonds between the two DNA strands, would stabilize the physical structure of the genome (Kushiro et al., 1987; Saenger, 1984). Second, the high temperature would need more thermostable amino acids (Argos et al., 1979) which are typically encoded by GC-rich codons. Such a hypothesis predicts that genomic $GC\%$ should increase with OGT in bacterial species.

The prediction above, however, is not supported by experimental evolution (Xia et al., 2002). A bacterial species, *Pasteurella multocida*, was cultured under increasing temperatures for more than 14,400 generations. $GC\%$ was estimated for the ancestral and derived strains by probing both with many AT-rich and GC-rich RAPD primers. If the derived strain has increased genomic $GC\%$ during this period of adaptation to increased culture temperature, one would expect to observe more amplification of the GC-rich primers and less amplification of AT-rich primers in the derived strain than in the ancestral strain. However, the opposite was observed (Xia et al., 2002). A comparative sequence analysis (Galtier and Lobry, 1997) also does not support the prediction.

Surprisingly, it has been found that $GC\%$ of rRNA genes is highly correlated with OGT (Dalgaard and Garrett, 1993, p 535; Galtier and Lobry, 1997; Hurst and Merchant, 2001; Nakashima et al., 2003; Wang et al. 2006). In particular, when the loop and stem regions of rRNA are studied separately, it was found that the hyperthermophilic bacterial species not only have a higher proportion of GC in the stems but also longer stems (Wang et al., 2006). In contrast, the $GC\%$ in the loop region correlates only weakly with OGT. Because stems function to stabilize the RNA secondary structure which is functionally important, these results are consistent with the hypothesized selection for RNA structural stability in high ambient temperatures.

Here we will not bother ourselves with biological details. We just want to learn how to perform a phylogeny-based comparative study on the relationship between genomic $GC\%$ and OGT. Suppose eight bacterial species $(s_1 - s_8)$ whose OGT and $GC\%$ of rRNA genes have been measured and plotted in Figure 9.3. A phylogeny of the eight species, with branch lengths designated as v_1 to v_{14}, are also plotted in Figure 9.3. Note that the branch lengths in Figure 9.3 are not scaled to v_1-v_{14}. Are OGT and $GC\%$ positively correlated as we have hypothesized? If we ignore the phylogeny and simply do a linear regression of $GC\%$ on OGT based on the eight points, we get a slope of 0.1726 ($p = 0.1317$). However, as we have mentioned before, such a regression is not appropriate because the eight points are not independent.

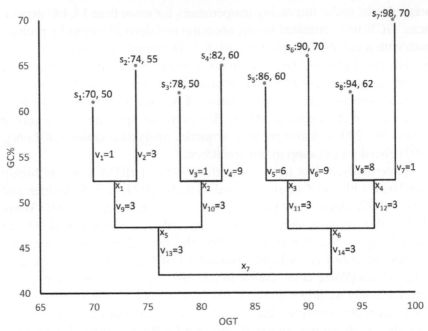

FIGURE 9.3   A phylogeny of eight bacterial species (s_1 to s_8) each labeled with optimal growth temperature (OGT) and $GC\%$ of the stem region of rRNA genes in the format of "OGT, $GC\%$." The branch lengths (v_1–v_{14}) are next to the branches and not scaled, e.g., v_7 (= 1) looks longer than v_8 (= 8). Ancestral nodes are designated by x_1 to x_7.

The conceptual rationale of independent contrasts is that, although the eight points are not independent, it is valid to contrasts the two sister taxa. For example, we can contrast between s_1 and s_2, between s_3 and s_4 as well as between x_1 and x_2, between x_3 and x_4, and so on. This requires the reconstruction of the ancestral states at x_1 to x_7 either by using the LS method or by the method based on the Brownian motion model. We can then compute independent contrasts, and finally characterize the relationship between the independent contrasts. The difference between the LS method and the method on the Brownian motion model illustrated below is in the reconstruction of the ancestral states. The LS method does not guarantee that all contrasts are independent because it does not ensure that the covariance between (s_1–s_2) and x_1, or covariance between (s_3–s_4) and x_2, is 0. In other words, contrasts such as (s_1–s_2), (s_3–s_4), and (x_1–x_2) may not be independent of each other. For this reason, I name the contrasts as quasi-independent below. In contrast, the method explicitly based on the Brownian motion model does lead to independent contrasts.

9.3.2 THE LS METHOD FOR QUASI-INDEPENDENT CONTRASTS

The LS method outlined here is designated quasi-independent contrasts because there is no guarantee that all contrasts are independent of each other. Without an explicit mechanistic model, the bare-bone LS approach will infer the ancestral states at x_1 to x_7 by minimizing the following residual sum of squares (RSS):

$$RSS = \sum_{i=1}^{n-1} \left[\frac{(O_{i1} - P_i)^2}{W_{i1}^m} + \frac{(O_{i2} - P_i)^2}{W_{i2}^m} \right] \tag{9.1}$$

where $n-1$ is the number of internal nodes for a rooted tree with n leaves, P_i is the value of the internal node i, O_{i1}, and O_{i2} are the values of the two offspring of P_i, W_{i1}, and W_{i2} are the two associated weighting factors which could be the branch lengths leading to the two offspring or the variance of the branch lengths and m is a constant typically taking the value of 0, 1, or 2. Taking OGT in Figure 9.3 for example, with branch lengths (v) as the weight factor and $m = 1$, we have

$$RSS = \sum_{i=1}^{n-1} \left[\frac{(O_{i1} - P_i)^2}{v_{i1}} + \frac{(O_{i2} - P_i)^2}{v_{i2}} \right]$$

$$= \sum_{i=1}^{n-1} \left[\frac{(70 - x_1)^2}{1} + \frac{(74 - x_1)^2}{3} + \frac{(78 - x_2)^2}{1} + \ldots + \frac{(x_5 - x_7)^2}{3} + \frac{(x_6 - x_7)^2}{3} \right] \tag{9.2}$$

We now have a function of RSS with seven parameters (x_1 to x_7). To find the values for x_1 to x_7 that minimize RSS, we take partial derivatives of RSS with respect to x_i, setting the seven partial derivatives to 0 and solve for x_i. The resulting OGT values for x_1 to x_7 are shown in Table 9.1a, with the minimized RSS equal to 48.89225. We can obtain the genomic $GC\%$ values for x_1 to x_7 in the same way and the resulting values are shown in Table 9.1a as well, with minimized $RSS = 53.9290$.

TABLE 9.1   Estimated ancestral states of optimal growth temperature (OGT) and genomic $GC\%$ by the least-squares method (a), together with quasi-independent contrasts (b).

(a)	OGT	$GC\%$	(b)	C_{OGT}	$C_{GC\%}$
x_1	72.4355	62.2193	s_1-s_2	−4	−4
x_2	78.3487	62.4838	s_3-s_4	−4	−3
x_3	88.5382	65.2229	s_5-s_6	−4	−3
x_4	95.6732	68.4172	s_7-s_8	4	8
x_5	78.1777	63.0963	x_1-x_2	−5.9132	−0.2645
x_6	89.3201	66.0753	x_3-x_4	−7.1349	−3.1943
x_7	83.7489	64.5858	x_5-x_6	−11.1424	−2.9790

Now we can compute the quasi-independent contrasts (designated by C) as the difference between the two offspring sharing the same ancestor, e.g., between s_1 and s_2, s_3 and s_4, x_1 and x_2, and so on. With eight species, we have seven ($= n-1$, where n is the number of species) quasi-independent contrasts (Table 9.1b). The quasi-independent contrasts between s_1 and s_2 and between x_1 and x_2 for OGT are illustrated below:

$$C_{s_1-s_2.OGT} = OGT_{s_1} - OGT_{s_2} = 70 - 74 = -4$$
$$C_{x_1-x_2.OGT} = OGT_{x_1} - OGT_{x_2} = 72.4355 - 78.3487 = -5.9132$$

(9.3)

The final step in performing quasi-independent contrasts is to assess the relationship between C_{OGT} and $C_{GC\%}$, specifically whether an increase in OGT will result in an increase in $GC\%$. That is, whether the two variables are positively correlated as hypothesized. There are three ways to assess the relationship. The first is parametric by performing a linear regression of $C_{GC\%}$ on C_{OGT}, forcing the intercept equal to 0. The resulting slope is 0.4728. The regression accounts for 52.28% of the variation in $C_{GC\%}$. The square root of 52.28%, equal to 0.7231, is the correlation coefficient between the two. This relationship between C_{OGT} and $C_{GC\%}$ is significant ($p = 0.0252$, one-tailed test). The reason for the one-tailed test is because of our directional hypothesis of a positive relationship between the two variables. One may also do a regression of C_{OGT} on $C_{GC\%}$, which will result in a slope of 1.1059. The correlation coefficient and the p value would be the same.

In short, with the phylogenetic control, we see a clear association between OGT and $GC\%$ that would have been missed without a phylogeny. The phylogeny-based comparative method approximates the control-treatment experiment. The ancestral population is the "test organism" that nature has separated into two groups, one "treated" with low ambient temperature (reflected in low OGT) and the other with high ambient temperature (reflected in high OGT). We check if the group treated with higher temperature have high $GC\%$ than the group treated with low temperature. This phylogeny-based inference may recover a relationship not obvious without a phylogeny (Fig. 9.3). Similarly, it may reveal a spurious relationship that seems superficially strong (Fig. 9.2).

An alternative to the parametric test above is to use binomial distribution. For example, given the null hypothesis of no relationship between the two variables, we expect half of the (C_{OGT}, $C_{GC\%}$) pairs to have the same sign (i.e., both positive or both negative) and the other half to have different signs. Thus, for a binomial distribution, we have $p = q = 0.5$. We observe all seven pairs to have the same sign (Table 9.1b). The probability of observing seven pairs to have the same sign is $0.5^7 = 0.0078$, which is the p value for the one-tailed test of our null hypothesis. So, we reject the null hypothesis and conclude that there is indeed a positive relationship between OGT and $GC\%$.

One may also assess the relationship between C_{OGT} and $C_{GC\%}$ by using χ^2-test. With seven contrasts, we expect 3.5 pairs to have the same sign and another 3.5 to have different signs. Although the rule of thumb for χ^2-test is that the expected values should be generally equal or greater than 5, we will carry out the test nevertheless. The observation of seven pairs to have the same sign and zero pair to have different signs (Table 9.1b) gives us

$$\chi^2 = \frac{(7-3.5)^2}{3.5} + \frac{(0-3.5)^2}{3.5} = 7 \tag{9.4}$$

with one degree of freedom, $p = 0.0082$.

Phylogeny-based comparison is easy to understand conceptually. If one finds organisms living in ephemeral environment always practicing the r-strategy, and those in stable environment always practicing the K-strategy, in many diverse evolutionary lineages, then we are more certain of the association between reproductive strategy and environment than observing the association in only two lineages.

It is simple to incorporate known ancestral values into the estimation in the LS framework. For example, if the ancestral states at x_7 are known with $OGT = 90$ and genomic $GC\% = 70$, then we simply replace x_7 in Eq. (9.2) with the known value and estimate x_1 to x_6. The estimated values, together with the quasi-independent contrasts, are shown in Table 9.2. Regressing $C_{GC\%}$ on C_{OGT} yields a slope of 0.4683, $p = 0.0259$ (one-tailed). Incorporating known ancestral states allows us to accommodate directional evolution such as the overall body size increase in mammalian species. The two nonparametric approaches mentioned previously will generate the same results as before because the two values in each of the seven pairs in Table 9.2b have the same sign.

TABLE 9.2 Estimated ancestral states (x_1 to x_6) of optimal growth temperature (OGT) and genomic $GC\%$ by the least-squares method (a), with OGT and $GC\%$ known to be 90 and 70, respectively, for x_7, together with quasi-independent contrasts (b).

(a)	OGT	GC%	(b)	C_{OGT}	$C_{GC\%}$
x_1	72.9221	62.6407	s_1-s_2	−4	−4
x_2	78.9102	62.9700	s_3-s_4	−4	−3
x_3	90.0700	66.5496	s_5-s_6	−4	−3
x_4	96.3150	68.9732	s_7-s_8	4	8
x_5	80.6108	65.2036	x_1-x_2	−5.9880	−0.3293
x_6	92.1283	68.5076	x_3-x_4	−6.2450	−2.4236
x_7	90	70	x_5-x_6	−11.5176	−3.3040

One can modify the basic LS approach outlined above to accommodate different scenarios (Martins and Hansen, 1997; Pagel, 1997, 1999). One may also scale the quasi-independent contrasts above with a weight factor. I explain the unweighted and weighted contrasts (WC) below in the context of independent contrasts based on Brownian motion model.

9.3.3 INDEPENDENT CONTRASTS BASED ON BROWNIAN MOTION MODEL

While the derivation and mathematical justification of the phylogeny-based comparative method is quite complicated, the most fundamental assumption is the Brownian motion model (Felsenstein, 2004, pp 391–414) which appears reasonable for neutrally evolving continuous characters (the null hypothesis). Here I illustrate the actual computation of independent contrasts with the same numerical example in Figure 9.3. I believe that one generally cannot interpret the results properly if one does not know how the results are obtained.

The computation is recursive and is exactly the same for any quantitative variable. So, we will only illustrate the computation involving OGT. One may repeat the computation involving $GC\%$ as an exercise.

The computation is of three steps. First, we recursively compute the ancestral values for internal (ancestral) nodes x_1 to x_6. The ancestral value for internal node x_7 can also be computed, but it does not have a sister taxon to contrast against. We treat these ancestors as if they were new taxa and compute the branch lengths leading to these ancestral nodes. Let us illustrate this with the two sister species s_1 and s_2. The OGT of their ancestor (x_1) is inferred from the OGT values of its two descendants. If we assume a molecular clock, then OGT for x_1 (OGT_{x1}) will simply be the average of OGT_{S1} and OGT_{S2}, or $OGT_{x1} = 0.5*OGT_{S1} + 0.5*OGT_{S2}$. With different branch lengths, we may write $OGT_{x1} = f*OGT_{S1} + (1-f)*OGT_{S2}$. The f value should be chosen in such a way that the covariance between $(OGT_{S1}-OGT_{S2})$ and OGT_{x1} is 0. This f value turns out to be $v_2/(v_1+v_2)$. The LS method in the previous section does not guarantee that the covariance is zero, hence the designation of "quasi-independent contrasts." In short, we have:

$$OGT_{x_1} = \frac{v_2}{v_1+v_2}OGT_{s_1} + \frac{v_1}{v_1+v_2}OGT_{s_2} = \frac{3\times70}{4} + \frac{1\times74}{4} = 71 \qquad (9.5)$$

The weighting scheme in Eq. (9.5) has two consequences. First, because f is within the range of $[0,1]$, OGT for an ancestor is always between the two OGT values for the two descendants. Second, the ancestral state is more similar to the state of the descendent node with a short branch than the other with a long branch. This makes intuitive sense as a descendent node diverged much from the ancestor should be less reliable for inferring the ancestral state than a descendent node diverged little from the ancestor. We now treat x_1 as if it is a new taxon and compute the branch lengths leading to it from its ancestor (x_5) as

$$v_{x_1} = \frac{v_1 v_2}{v_1+v_2} + v_9 = \frac{1\times3}{1+3} + 3 = 3.75 \qquad (9.6)$$

We do the same for x_2 to x_4, and the associated OGT_{xi} and v_{xi} values are listed in Table 9.3a. The computation of the ancestral states for x_5 and x_6 is similar to that in Eq. (9.5), e.g.,

$$OGT_{x_5} = \frac{v_{x_2} OGT_{x_1}}{v_{x_1} + v_{x_2}} + \frac{v_{x_1} OGT_{x_2}}{v_{x_1} + v_{x_2}} = \frac{3.9 \times 71}{7.65} + \frac{3.75 \times 78.4}{7.65} \approx 74.63 \qquad (9.7)$$

TABLE 9.3 Computed ancestral states (OGT_{xi} and GC_{xi}) and the branch lengths (v_{xi}) for the seven ancestral nodes (a), together with unweighted contrast (C_{OGT} and $C_{GC\%}$) in (b) and weighted contrasts (WC_{OGT} and $WC_{GC\%}$) in (c).

(a) OGT	$GC\%$	v_{xi}	(b) C_{OGT}		$C_{GC\%}$	$SumV$	(c) WC_{OGT}	$WC_{GC\%}$
x_1	71.0000	62.0000	3.7500	s_1-s_2	-4	-4	4	-2	-2
x_2	78.4000	62.3000	3.9000	s_3-s_4	-4	-3	10	-1.2649	-0.9487
x_3	87.6000	64.2000	6.6000	s_5-s_6	-4	-3	15	-1.0328	-0.7746
x_4	97.5556	69.1111	3.8889	s_7-s_8	4	8	9	1.3333	2.6667
x_5	74.6275	62.1471	4.9118	x_1-x_2	-7.4000	-0.3000	7.6500	-2.6755	-0.1085
x_6	93.8644	67.2903	5.4470	x_3-x_4	-9.9556	-4.9111	10.4889	-3.0740	-1.5164
x_7	83.7489	64.5858		x_5-x_6	-19.2370	-5.1432	10.3588	-5.9770	-1.5980

Now we can take the second step to compute the unweighted contrasts (designated by C) as well as the sum of branch lengths linking the two contrasted taxa. With eight species, we have seven ($= n-1$, where n is the number of species) contrasts (Table 9.3b). These unweighted contrasts, as well as the sum of branch lengths ($SumV$) associated with the contrasts, are illustrated below for those between s_1 and s_2 and between x_1 and x_2 for OGT in Eq. (9.8).

$$C_{s_1-s_2.OGT} = OGT_{s_1} - OGT_{s_2} = 70 - 74 = -4$$
$$SumV_{C_{s_1-s_2}} = v_1 + v_2 = 1 + 3 = 4$$
$$C_{x_1-x_2.OGT} = OGT_{x_1} - OGT_{x_2} = 71 - 78.4 = -7.4 \qquad (9.8)$$
$$SumV_{C_{x_1-x_2}} = v_{x_1} + v_{x_2} = 3.75 + 3.9 = 7.65$$

All the computed unweighted contrasts for both OGT and $GC\%$, as well as the associated $SumV$ values, are listed in Table 9.3b. We can now take the third step of obtaining independent WC by dividing each unweighted contrast by the square root of the associated $SumV$. For example,

$$WC_{s_1-s_2.OGT} = \frac{C_{s_1-s_2.OGT}}{\sqrt{SumV_{C_{s_1-s_2}}}} = \frac{-4}{\sqrt{4}} = -2$$

$$WC_{x_1-x_2.OGT} = \frac{C_{x_1-x_2.OGT}}{\sqrt{SumV_{C_{x_1-x_2}}}} = \frac{-7.4}{\sqrt{7.65}} = -2.6755$$

(9.9)

These independent contrasts for OGT thus computed, together with those for $GC\%$, are shown in Table 9.3c. Now we need to assess the relationship between WC_{OGT} and $WC_{GC\%}$, specifically whether an increase in OGT will result in an increase in $GC\%$. The tests used here are the same as those used in the LS framework in the previous section. The first test is parametric by performing a linear regression of $WC_{GC\%}$ on WC_{OGT}, forcing the intercept equal to 0. The resulting slope is 0.3959. The regression accounts for 54.50% of the variation in $WC_{GC\%}$. The square root of 54.50%, equal to 0.7382, is the correlation coefficient between the two. These slopes and the correlation coefficients, as well as the result of a significance test, are in the default output in the CONTRAST program in PHYLIP (Felsenstein, 2014) and DAMBE (Xia, 2017a, 2018b). The relationship between WC_{OGT} and $WC_{GC\%}$ in Table 9.3c has a $p = 0.0219$ (one-tailed test). You may use the other significance tests we outlined in the previous section. Because the two values in each pair have the same sign, the hypothesized positive relationship is consistently supported and the p values from the two nonparametric tests will be the same as those in the LS approach in the previous section.

One shortcoming of the method of independent contrasts is that the value of the ancestral state is always somewhere between the two values of the descendants. For example, the OGT and $GC\%$ values for the root x_7 are expected to be 82.8207 and 57.8610, respectively. This implies that it cannot detect directional changes over time. For example, if the ancestor is small in body size and all descendants have increased in body size over time, then the Brownian motion model assumed by the method of independent contrasts is no longer applicable.

However, if we actually know that the ancestral values of OGT and $GC\%$ at x_7 are 90 and 70, respectively, then these values obviously deviate much from the Brownian expectation. A well-known example is the body size of modern mammals which has in general increased substantially from that of the ancestral insectivores since the time of dinosaurs. The Brownian model would lead to the inference of an ancestral body size much larger than that of the insectivore ancestor. It is therefore essential for us to incorporate the known ancestral state to improve the inference.

Here, I present a simple post hoc LS approach to incorporate the ancestral information in the estimation of the values at nodes x_1 to x_6. The RSS for variable OGT (RSS_{OGT}) is specified below:

$$
RSS_{OGT} = \left[90 - \left(\frac{v_{x5} OGT_{x6}}{v_{x5} + v_{x6}} + \frac{v_{x6} OGT_{x5}}{v_{x5} + v_{x6}} \right) \right]^2 +
$$

$$
\left[OGT_{x6} - \left(\frac{v_{x3} OGT_{x4}}{v_{x3} + v_{x4}} + \frac{v_{x4} OGT_{x3}}{v_{x3} + v_{x4}} \right) \right]^2 + \left[OGT_{x5} - \left(\frac{v_{x1} OGT_{x2}}{v_{x1} + v_{x2}} + \frac{v_{x2} OGT_{x1}}{v_{x1} + v_{x2}} \right) \right]^2 +
$$

$$
\left[OGT_{x4} - \left(\frac{v_7 OGT_{s8}}{v_7 + v_8} + \frac{v_8 OGT_{s7}}{v_7 + v_8} \right) \right]^2 + \left[OGT_{x3} - \left(\frac{v_5 OGT_{s6}}{v_5 + v_6} + \frac{v_6 OGT_{s5}}{v_5 + v_6} \right) \right]^2 +
$$

$$
\left[OGT_{x2} - \left(\frac{v_3 OGT_{s4}}{v_3 + v_4} + \frac{v_4 OGT_{s3}}{v_3 + v_4} \right) \right]^2 + \left[OGT_{x1} - \left(\frac{v_1 OGT_{s2}}{v_1 + v_2} + \frac{v_2 OGT_{s1}}{v_1 + v_2} \right) \right]^2
$$

(9.10)

where 90 is the known ancestral value of OGT at the root, and the terms inside the parentheses are the expected OGT values as illustrated before, e.g., Eq. (9.5). To obtain the least-square estimates of OGT values at internal nodes x_1 to x_6, we take the partial derivatives of RSS_{OGT} with respect to OGT_{x1}, OGT_{x2}, ..., OGT_{x6}, set them to zero and solve the six resulting simultaneous equations. The new estimated values of OGT at x_1 to x_6 are 72.0763, 79.5959, 87.8990, 98.7664, 78.3063, and 98.1243, respectively. The new values suggest that the OGT values have decreased in most descendent lineages from the ancestral value of 90.

The least-square framework is not limited to one known ancestral value. For example, if OGT_{x5} is known, it can be substituted into Eq. (9.10) so that we will only need to estimate five unknown ancestral OGT values. The same computation can be done for $GC\%$ or any other variable with one or more known ancestral values. The independent contrasts can be computed the same way as before, except that the new ancestral values are then used.

9.4   THE COMPARATIVE METHODS FOR DISCRETE CHARACTERS

Discrete characters arise in many ways. The simplest discrete data are binary and include presence/absence of genes, pathogenic islands, etc. A genome typically encodes many genes. The presence or absence of certain genes, certain phenotypic traits, and environmental conditions jointly represent a major source of data that can be analyzed by comparative methods for discrete data. Genomic data have been increasing rapidly, with 11977 prokaryotic genomes on May 29, 2012, but 99081 on May 28, 2017. The availability of such annotated genomes, as well as the availability of powerful phylogenetic software packages such as MEGA (Kumar et al., 2016), PAUP* (Swofford, 2000), PHYLIP (Felsenstein, 2014), BEAST (Drummond and Rambaut, 2007), and DAMBE (Xia, 2001), greatly facilitates the compilation of data for comparative genomics illustrated in Figure 9.1.

9.4.1   STUDYING ASSOCIATION BETWEEN BINARY VARIABLES

Many genes work together and complement each other to accomplish a biological function. For example, Type II ENase (restriction endonuclease) in bacteria is always accompanied by the same type of MTase (methyltransferase) recognizing and modifying the same site. ENase cuts the DNA at specific sites and defends the bacterial host against invading DNA phages. MTase modifies (methylates) the same site in the bacterial genome to prevent ENase from cutting the bacterial genome. Obviously, ENase activity without MTase is suicidal, so MTase must accompany ENase. A bacterium cannot lose the MTase without first losing the ENase. Although rare, MTase can be present without the associated ENase. For example, *E. coli* possesses two unaccompanied MTases, Dam and Dcm. Some bacteriophages carry one or more MTases to modify their own genome so as to nullify the hostile action of the host ENases. Association between genes, such as that between genes encoding ENase and MTase, offers us a way to bioinformatically identify enzymes that are potential partners working in concert.

The functional complementation also explains why the activity of many ENases depends on S-adenosylmethionine (AdoMet) availability

(Sistla and Rao, 2004). AdoMet serves as the methyl donor for MTase. Without AdoMet, the restriction sites in the host genome will not be modified even in the presence of MTase because of the lack of the methyl donor, and ENase activity will then kill the host. So, it is selectively advantageous for ENase activity to depend on the availability of AdoMet.

Aside from association between genes, we are often interested in the association between gene function and environmental variables. For example, urease activity is often associated with an acidic environment in bacterial species, such as *Helicobacter pylori*, *Klebsiella pneumoniae*, and *Serratia marcescens*. *H. pylori* inhabits the acidic environment in mammalian stomach and the two other species can generate acids by fermentation leading to acidification of their environment. The presence of urease, which catalyzes urea to produce ammonia, can help maintain cytoplasmic pH homeostasis and allow the bacteria to tolerate environmental pH of 5 or even lower. Thus, characterizing such association between gene function and environment helps us understand evolution and adaptation to a specific environment.

Urease gene cluster serves as one of the two key acid-resistant mechanisms in the bacterial pathogen *Helicobacter pylori* in mammalian stomach, with the other mechanism being a positively charged cell membrane that alleviates the influx of protons into the cytoplasm. The latter mechanism is established by comparative genomics between *H. pylori* and its close relatives as an adaptation to the acidic environment in the mammalian stomach (Xia, 2018a, Chapter 17; Xia and Palidwor, 2005).

Association of variables goes beyond molecular data. For example, it has been hypothesized that insects on volcano islands in the ocean are associated the evolution of wing loss, partly because the winged form is more likely to get blown into the ocean waves and drowned. This involves the association between a habitat (volcano island) and a morphological trait (wing). Both variables can be coded in binary. Testing such association can also be carried out in the same likelihood framework described below.

Not only can association between genes or between genes and their function lead to biological insights, but the lack of certain expected association can also shed light on gene functions. For example, a set of *ERG* genes involved in de novo cholesterol biosynthesis are strongly conserved among various animal lineages. However, some of these genes are also strongly conserved in *Drosophila melanogaster* and *Caenorhabditis elegant* that are unable to synthesize cholesterol, i.e., a decoupling of the genes and their expected function. Comparative genomics studies suggest that the *ERG* homologs in *D. melanogaster* and *C. elegant* have evolved to acquire new functions (Vinci et al., 2008).

The identification of association either between two genes (e.g., between a type II ENase and a type II MTase) or between a gene and an environmental variable (e.g., between urease activity and acidic habitat) represents the same statistical problem. However, a statistician without biological background may misconstrue the problem and might use a 2×2 contingency table with values $N_{+/+}$, $N_{+/-}$, $N_{-/+}$, $N_{-/-}$ and Fisher's exact test to identify the association between two columns without taking the phylogeny into consideration. However, such an approach can lead to both false negatives and false positives. Figure 9.4 illustrates this potential problem. A phylogeny of 12 species (Fig. 9.4A) is shown with four genes (X1, X2, Y1, and Y2) whose presence and absence are encoded as 1 and 0, respectively (Fig. 9.4B). A statistician not well versed in evolutionary biology, if tasked to quantify association between genes X1 and X2, may ignore the phylogeny. He most likely will compile a contingency table shown in Figure 9.4C and perform a Fisher's exact test. This would result in a p value of 0.0183 from a likelihood ratio chi-square test and the statistician will conclude a significant association between genes X1 and X2, i.e., they tend to be either both present or both absent. The same analysis applied to studying the association between Y1 and Y2 will reach exactly the same conclusion with the same p value (because the four numbers in the contingency table will be the same as in Figure 9.4C.

The phylogeny in Figure 9.4A helps us to see that the 12 rows of data are not independent. The superficial association between X1 and X2 could be caused by a single gene-loss event in the common ancestor of Sp9–Sp12 if the common ancestor had both X1 and X2, or a single gene-gain event in the common ancestor of Sp1–Sp8 if the common ancestor did not have X1 and X2. All the four "0 0" entries or the eight "1 1" entries for X1 and X2 could simply be the consequence of shared ancestral characters. In contrast, the association between Y1 and Y2 are almost independent of the phylogeny.

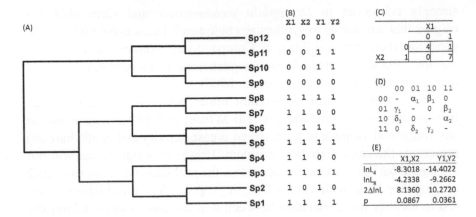

FIGURE 9.4 Comparative methods for discrete binary characters, given a known phylogeny (A). The presence and absence (designated by 1 and 0, respectively) of four genes are recorded for each species (B). The contingency table for the association between X1 and X2 without considering the phylogeny would generate a $p = 0.0183$ (likelihood ratio chi-square test) suggesting a significant association between X1 and X2. The instantaneous rate matrix (D), with notations following Felsenstein (2004), shows the relationship among the four character designations, i.e., 00 for both genes absent, 01 for the absence of gene 1 but presence of gene 2, 10 for the presence of gene 1 but absence of gene 2 and 11 for both genes present. The diagonals are constrained by each row sum equal to 0. (E) Summary statistics for a likelihood ratio test (see text for explanation).

We need a phylogeny-based method to assess the significance of such associations between two discrete variables. The rationale is shown in Figure 9.4D. Two genes, each with two states (presence/absence), have four possible joint states and eight rate parameters (α_1, α_2, β_1, β_2, δ_1, δ_2, γ_1, and γ_2) to be estimated from the data (Fig. 9.4). If gene loss/gain is independent between the two genes, then then the substitution rates between 00 and 01 (α_1), and between 10 and 11 (α_2) are expected to be the same. That is, the gain/loss of the second gene is independent of the presence/absence of the first gene. Similarly, we expect $\beta_1 = \beta_2$, $\gamma_1 = \gamma_2$, and $\delta_1 = \delta_2$. This would reduce the eight rate parameters to four parameters. We, therefore, can compute the log-likelihood for the eight-parameter model and the four-parameter model given the tree and the data, designated lnL_8 and lnL_4, respectively, and perform a likelihood ratio test with test statistic being $2(lnL_8 - lnL_4)$ and four degrees of freedom (Pagel et al., 2004). The result of the significance test (Fig. 9.4E) shows no significant association between X1 and X2 ($p = 0.0867$), but significant association between Y1 and Y2 ($p = 0.0361$).

Note that we assume in Figure 9.4D that multiple changes cannot occur, that is, state "00" and state "11" cannot change into each other, neither can state "01" and state "10." Such changes are filled with 0 in Figure 9.4D. In Markov chain parlance, states that can reach from each other are said to communicate. They belong to the same communicating classes. States "00" and "11" cannot communicate directly but can communicate via states "01" and "10"

The discovery of a significant association should be followed by searching for the cause of the association. A biologically significant association is a functional association, that is, the two genes mutually depend on each other in accomplishing a function. I have previously mentioned the association between type II restriction enzyme in bacteria and DNA methyltransferase genes. Type II restriction enzymes in bacteria cut DNA at a specific restriction site, which necessitates the presence of a methyltransferase that modify the same recognition site in the host genome to protect it from being digested by the restriction enzyme. The two genes are thus strongly associated, with the presence of the type II restriction enzyme always associated with the methyltransferase. Another example of functional association is between genes *IRE1* and *HAC1* in a number of fungal lineages, both being required for unfolded protein response (Xia, 2019b). However, the association between two genes identified by the likelihood ratio test above does not necessarily imply functional association because other mechanisms can also give rise to a significant association. For example, bacteriophages and plasmids can integrate their genomes into their host genomes, or contribute a segment of their genomes (e.g., a segment containing Gene1 and Gene2) to their host genomes. Such phage- or plasmid-contributed genes naturally would be associated because bacterial genomes will either have the linked Gene1 and Gene2 (the "1 1" configuration) when the bacterial host genome receives the segment bearing Gene1 and Gene2 or do not (the "0 0" configuration) when the host is not infected by phage or plasmid. However, in the study of gene presence/absence data, such linkage-mediated copresence or coabsence is assumed not to occur. Such cotransmitted genes should be considered as a single gene entity instead of two independently distributed genes. In fact, the substitution model that is used to calculate the likelihood for the 4-parameter and 8-parameter models assumes that state "00" and state "11" cannot change into each other (Fig. 9.4D).

9.4.2   THE PRUNING ALGORITHM AND THE LIKELIHOOD RATIO TEST

A phylogeny-based comparative analysis (Barker and Pagel, 2005; Pagel, 1994) characterizes the state transition by a Markov chain and uses a likelihood ratio test to detect the presence of the association between genes or between a gene function and an environmental condition. Two genes, each with two states (presence/absence), have four possible joint states and eight rate parameters (α_1, α_2, β_1, β_2, δ_1, δ_2, γ_1, and γ_2) to be estimated from the data (Fig. 9.4D). When the gain or loss of one gene is independent of the other gene, then $\alpha_1 = \alpha_2$, $\beta_1 = \beta_2$, $\delta_1 = \delta_2$, and $\gamma_1 = \gamma_2$, with only four rate parameters to be estimated. Thus, we compute the log-likelihood for the eight-parameter model and the four-parameter model given the tree and the data, designated lnL_8 and lnL_4, respectively, and perform a likelihood ratio test with test statistic being $2(lnL_8 - lnL_4)$ and four degrees of freedom (i.e., the difference in the number of parameters between the two models). It is the same pruning algorithm that we learned in the chapter on likelihood-based phylogenetic methods that we will use to compute lnL_8 and lnL_4.

I illustrate the computation of lnL_8 by using a simpler tree with only four operational taxonomic units or OTUs (Fig. 9.5). The joint states, represented by binary numbers 00, 01, 10, and 11, correspond to decimal numbers 0, 1, 2, and 3 which will be used to denote the four states in some equations below. The likelihood for the eight-parameter model is

$$L_8 = \sum_{z=0}^{3} \sum_{y=0}^{3} \sum_{x=0}^{3} \pi_z P_{zx}(b_6) P_{x0}(b_1) P_{x3}(b_2) P_{zy}(b_5) P_{y0}(b_3) P_{y3}(b_4) \qquad (9.11)$$

Note that the state of the internal node is unknown so we need to consider all four possible states.

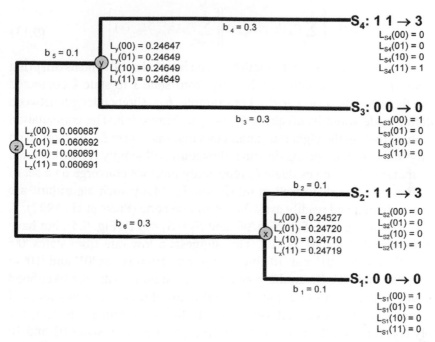

FIGURE 9.5 Four-OTU tree with branch lengths (b_1 to b_6) for illustrating likelihood computation by the pruning algorithm. The L vectors are computed recursively according to Eqs. (9.12)–(9.13).

Eq. (9.11) may seem to suggest that we need to sum up 4^3 terms. However, the amount of computation involved is greatly reduced by the pruning algorithm (Felsenstein, 1981). Although we have already illustrated the pruning algorithm in the chapter on maximum likelihood methods on phylogenetics, students appear to benefit from another application of the algorithm in a slightly different context. To implement this algorithm, we define a vector L with elements $L(0)$, $L(1)$, $L(2)$, and $L(3)$, corresponding to L(00), L(01), L(10) and L(11) in Fig. 9.5, for every node including the leaves. I will use L(0) and L(00), L(1) and L(01), L(2) and L(10), and L(3) and L(11) interchangeably. L for leaf i is defined as

$$L_i(s) = \begin{cases} 1, & \text{if } s = S_i \\ 0, \text{otherwise} \end{cases} \tag{9.12}$$

L for an internal node i (which is node x, y or z in Fig. 9.5) with two offspring (o_1 and o_2) is recursively defined as

$$L_i(s) = \left[\sum_{k=0}^{3} P_{sk}(b_{i,o_1})L_{o_1}(k) \right]\left[\sum_{k=0}^{3} P_{sk}(b_{i,o_2})L_{o_2}(k) \right]$$ (9.13)

where $b_{i,o1}$ means the branch length between internal node i and its offspring o_1, and P_{sk} is the transition probability from state s to state k computed from the rate matrix (Fig. 9.4b). For example, $b_{x,S1}$ (branch length between internal node x and its offspring S_1) is b_1 in Figure 9.5. The computation involves finding the eight rate parameters that maximize L_8. As there is no analytical solution, the maximizing algorithm will simply try various rate parameter values and evaluate L_8 repeatedly until we converge on a set of parameter values that result in maximum L_8. Many such algorithms are well explained and readily available in source code (Press et al., 1992).

Note that we have $S_1 = S_3 = $ '00' and $S_2 = S_4 = $ '11' (Fig. 9.5), but have not observed states '01' or '10'. This suggests a low rate from states '00' and '11' to states '01' and '10', but a high rate from states '01' and '10' to states '00' and '11'. Given the very limited amount of data, the likelihood surface is expected to be quite flat and many different combinations of the rate parameters can get very close to the maximum L_8. In fact, the only constraint on the rate parameters is high rates from states 01 and 10 to states 00 and 11 (i.e., large $\delta_1 + \gamma_1 + \alpha_2 + \beta_2$) and low rates from states 00 and 11 to states 01 and 10 (i.e., small $\delta_2 + \gamma_2 + \alpha_1 + \beta_1$). This should be obvious when we look at the four OTUs in the tree (Fig. 9.5), with only 00 and 11 being observed at the leaves. This implies that 01 and 10 should be transient states, quickly changing to 00 or 11, whereas 00 and 11 are relatively conservative stable states. One of the rate matrices that approaches the maximum L_8 is

$$Q = \begin{bmatrix} & 00 & 01 & 10 & 11 \\ 00 & -16.47 & 13.15 & 3.32 & 0 \\ 01 & 1.10 & -135653.97 & 0 & 135652.87 \\ 10 & 1816.49 & 0 & -20308.04 & 18491.54 \\ 11 & 0 & 18.30 & 207.21 & -225.52 \end{bmatrix}$$ (9.14)

The rate of transition from states 01 and 10 to states 00 and 11 is 644.5 times greater (the true rate should be infinitely greater) than the other way around, which implies that we will almost never observe 01 and 10 states. Note that the likelihood method is strictly data-based. If we do not observe states 01 and 10, then the probability of entering these states from other states will be effectively zero. We have previously mentioned that if we take a sample of three fish, all being males, from a lake, then the likelihood estimate of the proportion of males is 1 which is most likely wrong. However, the likelihood method will insist that the estimate is 1. Just as the observation of no female fish may be due to the sample being too small, the lack of observation of 01 and 10 states in our example most likely is also due to the small sample size. In such cases, Bayesian approach would offer a more reasonable description of data and models (Barker and Pagel, 2005; Pagel and Meade, 2006). However, this primer is strictly non-Bayesian.

The transition probability matrices with branch lengths of 0.1 and 0.3, which are computed as e^{Qt}, where t is the branch length, are, respectively,

$$P(0.1) = \begin{bmatrix} & 00 & 01 & 10 & 11 \\ 00 & 0.54616 & 0.00011 & 0.00467 & 0.44908 \\ 01 & 0.51459 & 0.00011 & 0.00499 & 0.48038 \\ 10 & 0.51738 & 0.00011 & 0.00496 & 0.47759 \\ 11 & 0.51458 & 0.00011 & 0.00499 & 0.48034 \end{bmatrix}$$

(9.15)

$$P(0.3) = \begin{bmatrix} & 00 & 01 & 10 & 11 \\ 00 & 0.53145 & 0.00011 & 0.00482 & 0.46377 \\ 01 & 0.53144 & 0.00011 & 0.00482 & 0.46382 \\ 10 & 0.53144 & 0.00011 & 0.00482 & 0.46382 \\ 11 & 0.53144 & 0.00011 & 0.00482 & 0.46382 \end{bmatrix}$$

We can now compute L_8 by using the pruning algorithm. First, L_{S1} to L_{S4} are straightforward from Eq. (9.12) and shown in Figure 9.5. L_x and L_y are computed according to Eq. (9.13). Because $L_{S1}(01) = L_{S1}(10) = L_{S1}(11) = 0$, and $L_{S2}(00) = L_{S2}(01) = L_{S2}(10) = 0$, so any multiplication involving these terms are also zero, $L_x(k)$ and $L_y(k)$ are much simpler than what is implied in the equation:

$$L_x(00) = P_{00,00}(0.1)P_{00,11}(0.1) = 0.54616 \times 0.44908 = 0.24527$$
$$L_x(01) = 0.51459 \times 0.48038 = 0.24720$$
$$L_x(10) = 0.51738 \times 0.47759 = 0.24710$$
$$L_x(11) = 0.51458 \times 0.48037 = 0.24719$$

(9.16)

Similarly, $L_y(00)$, $L_y(01)$, $L_y(10)$, and $L_y(11)$ are computed the same way and have values 0.24647, 0.24649, 0.24649, and 0.24649, respectively. L_z is also computed by applying Eq. (9.13), e.g.,

$$L_z(00) = AB = 0.246207 \times 0.246487 = 0.060687, \; where$$
$$A = [P_{00,00}(b_6)L_x(00) + P_{00,01}(b_6)L_x(01) + P_{00,10}(b_6)L_x(10) + P_{00,11}(b_6)L_x(11)]$$
$$= 0.246207 \tag{9.17}$$
$$B = [P_{00,00}(b_5)L_y(00) + P_{00,01}(b_5)L_y(01) + P_{00,10}(b_5)L_y(10) + P_{00,11}(b_5)L_y(11)]$$
$$= 0.246487$$

$L_z(01)$, $L_z(10)$, and $L_z(11)$ are 0.060692, 0.060691, and 0.060691, respectively. The final L_8 is

$$L_8 = \sum_{k=0}^{3} \pi_k L_z(k) = 0.060687 \times 0.5 + 0.060691 \times 0.5 = 0.060689 \tag{9.18}$$
$$\ln L_8 = \ln(L_8) = -2.802$$

where we used the empirical frequencies for π_k, although π_k could also be estimated as parameters of the model. Note that states 01 and 10 are not observed, and π_{01} and π_{10} are consequently assumed to be 0 in Eq. (9.18). Note that computer implementations of the algorithm often assign very small frequencies, e.g., 0.000001, to such states that have not been observed. This assignment is based on our belief that the zero frequencies of π_{01} and π_{10} are not real but are due to insufficient sampling. This also serves as an argument to take a Bayesian approach which is beyond the coverage of the book.

The computation of lnL_4 is simpler because only four rate parameters need to be estimated, and is equal to -5.545. If quite a large number of OTUs are involved, then twice the difference between lnL_8 and lnL_4, designated $2\Delta lnL$, follows approximately the χ^2 distribution with 4 degrees of freedom. For our fictitious example, $2\Delta lnL = 5.486$, which leads to $p = 0.241$, i.e., the eight-parameter model is not significantly better than the four-parameter model. Such a result is not surprising given the small number of OTUs with little statistical power to discriminate between alternative hypotheses. Figure 9.4E shows the significance test with more reasonable sample size.

Mapping genes and gene functions to a phylogeny have revealed the loss of a single-copy *Maelstrom* gene in fish. *Maelstrom* performs an essential function, and its loss suggests that the essential function has been fulfilled by a nonhomologous gene (Zhang et al., 2008). Thus, the same phenotype can have different genotypes. Such findings that a specific molecular function can be performed by evolutionarily unrelated genes suggest a fundamental flaw in research effort to identify the minimal genome by identifying shared orthologous genes (Mushegian and Koonin, 1996). The rationale for such an approach is this. Suppose a minimal organism needs to perform three essential functions designated {x, y, z}, and three different genes, designated {*A, B, C*}, encode products that perform these three functions. If we have a genome (*G1*) with five genes {*A, B, C, D, E*} and another genome (*G2*) with four genes {*A, B, C, F*}, with genes of the same letter being orthologous, then shared orthologous genes between *G1* and *G2* are {*A, B, C*} which would be a good approximation of the minimal genome. However, it is possible that *G1* = {*A, D, E*} for essential functions {x, y, z} and *G2* = {*A, C, F*} for the same set of essential functions {x, y, z}. Both are already minimal genomes by the definition above, but the intersection of *G1* and *G2* is only {*A*}, which is a severe underestimation of a minimal genome. Creating a cell with such a "minimal" genome is doomed to fail.

The comparative methods still need further development. For example, one difficulty with the comparative methods for the continuous and discrete characters is what branch lengths to use because different trees, or even the same topology with different branch lengths, can lead to different conclusions. One may need to explore all plausible trees to check the robustness of the conclusion.

Key steps in comparative genomics involve the compilation of data in the form of Figure 9.1, perform data analyses, such as measuring association and assessing statistical significance, and present biologically significant results. All these can be computationally automated with various software packages such as DAMBE (Xia, 2012b, 2013a). A recently developed XML-based rich data format, named NeXML (Vos et al., 2012), is particularly suitable for large-scale comparative genomics.

KEYWORDS

- **independent contrasts**
- **pruning algorithm**
- **likelihood method**
- **least-squares method**
- **continuous variables**
- **discrete variables**
- **phylogeny-based comparative methods**

Appendix

1.1 THE DELTA METHOD FOR DERIVING PARAMETER VARIANCE

Delta method has been used extensively in deriving variances of parameters (Kimura and Ohta, 1972; Waddell and Steel, 1997a; Xia, 2007a: pp 256–262). When a variable Y is a function of a variable X, that is, $Y = F(X)$, the delta method allows us to obtain approximate formulation of the variance of Y if (1) Y is differentiable with respect to X and (2) the variance of X is known. The same can be extended to more variables. Take for example the simplest case of $Y = F(X)$. Regardless of the functional relationship between Y and X, we always have

$$\Delta Y \approx \left(\frac{dY}{dX} \right) \Delta X \tag{1}$$

$$(\Delta Y)^2 \approx \left(\frac{dY}{dX} \right)^2 (\Delta X)^2. \tag{2}$$

where ΔY and ΔX are small changes in Y and X, respectively.

Note that the variance of Y is the expectation of the squared deviations of Y, that is,

$$V(Y) = E(\Delta Y)^2$$
$$V(X) = E(\Delta X)^2. \tag{3}$$

Replacing $(DY)^2$ and $(DX)^2$ in Eq. (2) with $V(Y)$ and $V(X)$, we have

$$V(Y) \approx \left(\frac{dY}{dX} \right)^2 V(X). \tag{4}$$

This relationship allows us to obtain an approximate formulation of the variance of either Y or X if we know either $V(X)$ or $V(Y)$.

1.1.1 VARIANCE OF ALLELE FREQUENCY FOR A RECESSIVE ALLELE

As students are always eager to have more illustrative examples, and because I myself belong to the lesser folks who cannot see the beauty of equations without rendering them to numbers, I will present another example, taken from a book on population genetics (Li, 1976), in which we know the variance of Y and want to estimate the variance of X.

Given a locus with one dominant allele (A) and one recessive allele (a), we have only two distinguishable phenotypes, dominants (AA, Aa) and recessives (aa). You might be interested to know that the severe human disease cystic fibrosis is determined by one locus with a dominant allele and a recessive allele. The disease is caused by homozygosity for the recessive allele. How to estimate the frequency of the recessive allele and its variance?

Let D and R be the observed numbers of dominants and recessives in a sample of N random individuals ($N = D + R$). Our estimate of the frequency of allele a, designated q, is

$$q^2 = R / N$$
$$q = \sqrt{R / N} \tag{5}$$

In the case of cystic fibrosis, suppose we found four patients out of 10,000 surveyed, so $q = 1/50$. Now we proceed to find the variance of q. From the binomial distribution, we know the variance of q^2 to be

$$V(q^2) = \frac{q^2(1-q^2)}{N} \tag{6}$$

In the framework of the delta method with $Y = F(X)$, we have $Y = q^2$, $X = q$, and $dY/dX = 2q$. We already know the variance of Y (i.e., q^2) in Eq. (6), and the variance of X can be obtained as follows

$$V(Y) = \frac{q^2(1-q^2)}{N} = \left(\frac{dY}{dq}\right)^2 V(q) = (2q)^2 V(q)$$

$$V(q) = \frac{V(Y)}{(2q)^2} = \frac{\frac{q^2(1-q^2)}{N}}{4q^2} = \frac{1-q^2}{4N} \tag{7}$$

You might have noticed that, $q^2 = R/N$ and $(1-q^2) = D/N$. So we have

$$V(q) = \frac{1-q^2}{4N} = \frac{D/N}{4N} = \frac{D}{4N^2} \tag{8}$$

In the case of cystic fibrosis with $N = 10,000$ and $R = 4$, $q = 1/50$, $V(q) = 0.000002499$.

1.1.2 VARIANCE OF JC69 DISTANCE

The delta method is not needed for deriving the variance of JC69 distance (D_{JC69}) because D_{JC69} does have a likelihood estimator of its variance, but we will apply the delta method just for illustrating the method. We note that D_{JC69} is a function of P_{diff} (the proportion of sites differing between two aligned sequences), and the variance of P_{diff} is known from the binomial distribution:

$$D_{JC69} = -\frac{3}{4}\ln\left(1 - \frac{4P_{diff}}{3}\right) \tag{9}$$

$$V(P_{diff}) = \frac{P_{diff}(1 - P_{diff})}{L} \tag{10}$$

where L is the length of the two aligned sequences. From the expression of D_{JC69} in Eq. (9), we have

$$\frac{\partial D_{JC69}}{\partial P_{diff}} = \frac{1}{1 - \frac{4P_{diff}}{3}}$$

$$V(D_{JC69}) = \left(\frac{\partial D_{JC69}}{\partial P_{diff}}\right)^2 V(P_{diff}) = \frac{P_{diff}(1 - P_{diff})}{L\left(1 - \frac{4P_{diff}}{3}\right)^2}. \tag{11}$$

which is the same as the likelihood estimator.

1.1.3 THE VARIANCE OF K80 DISTANCE

The distance for the K80 model is

$$D_{K80} = 2\alpha t + 4\beta t = \frac{1}{2}\ln(a) + \frac{1}{4}\ln(b), \text{ where}$$

$$a = \frac{1}{1 - 2P - Q} \text{ and } b = \frac{1}{1 - 2Q}. \tag{12}$$

The variance of D_{K80} can be derived by the delta method as before:

$$dD_{K80} = \left(\frac{\partial D_{K80}}{\partial P}\right)dP + \left(\frac{\partial D_{K80}}{\partial Q}\right)dQ = d_1 \bullet dP + d_2 \bullet dQ \tag{13}$$

$$V(D_{K80}) = (dD_{K80})^2 = [d_1 \bullet dP + d_2 \bullet dQ]^2$$
$$= d_1^2 dP^2 + 2d_1 d_2 dPdQ + d_2^2 dQ^2$$
$$= d_1^2 V(P) + 2d_1 d_2 Cov(P,Q) + d_2^2 V(Q) \tag{14}$$
$$= [d_1 \quad d_2] \begin{bmatrix} V(P) & Cov(P,Q) \\ Cov(P,Q) & V(Q) \end{bmatrix} \begin{bmatrix} d_1 \\ d_2 \end{bmatrix}.$$

Recall that P stands for the proportion of sites that differ by a transitional change and Q stands for the proportion of sites that differ by a transversional change. Designate R as the proportion of identical sites ($R = 1 - P - Q$). From the trinomial distribution of $(R + P + Q)^L$, we have:

$$V(P) = \frac{P(1-P)}{L}$$
$$V(Q) = \frac{Q(1-Q)}{L} \tag{15}$$
$$Cov(P,Q) = -\frac{PQ}{L}.$$

Substituting these into Eq. (14), we have the variance of D_{K80}:

$$V(D_{K80}) = (dD_{K80})^2 = \frac{a^2 P + c^2 Q - (aP + cQ)^2}{L} \tag{16}$$

where $c = (a + b)/2$, with a and b defined in Eq. (12).

Note that Eq. (14) is a general equation for computing the variance by the delta method. For any function $Y = F(X_1, X_2, ..., X_n)$, the variance of Y is obtained by the variance-covariance matrix of X_i multiplied left and right by the vector of partial derivatives of Y with respect to X_i.

1.2 ILLUSTRATION OF EXPECTATION–MAXIMIZATION (EM) ALGORITHM

EM algorithm is used often in bioinformatics. Here is a numerical illustration (the simplest possible, I believe) of the EM algorithm to estimate q (the frequency of the recessive allele a). Note that in this particular case we do not need to use the EM algorithm to estimate q because q is already given in Eq. (5). However, gaining some familiarity with the EM algorithm may be useful in other situations.

There are three genotypes involving the cystic fibrosis locus, AA, Aa, and aa, with AA and Aa indistinguishable phenotypically. Designate $p = 1 - q$ and let N_{AA}, N_{Aa}, and N_{aa} be the number of AA, Aa, and aa genotypes, respectively. Using the notations above, we have $D = (N_{AA} + N_{Aa})$ and $R = N_{aa}$. To facilitate exposition, let us suppose that $D = 9996$ and $R = 4$.

Since we cannot observe N_{AA} and N_{Aa} directly (they are indistinguishable phenotypically), the two numbers represent incomplete data from a three-category trinomial distribution. The complete data specification is as follows:

$$f(N_{AA}, N_{Aa}, N_{aa} \mid q) = \frac{N!}{N_{AA}! N_{Aa}! N_{aa}!} [p^2]^{N_{AA}} [2pq]^{N_{Aa}} [q^2]^{N_{aa}} \qquad (17)$$

The EM algorithm consists of two steps, the estimation step (or E-step) and the maximization step (or M-step). Let us start by setting $q = 0.1$. For the E-step, we estimate N_{AA} and N_{Aa} as follows (with the subscript in $N_{AA.1}$ and $N_{Aa.1}$ indicating the first E-step):

$$N_{AA.1} = D \frac{p^2}{p^2 + 2pq} = 8178.545455$$

$$N_{Aa.1} = D \frac{2pq}{p^2 + 2pq} = 1817.454545 \qquad (18)$$

Substituting these into Eq. (17), we can obtain q by the maximum likelihood method, that is, taking the derivative of $f(N_{AA}, N_{Aa}, N_{aa} \mid q)$ with respect to q, setting the derivative to 0 and solve the resulting equation for q. This gives

$$q_1 = \frac{N_{Aa} + 2N_{aa}}{2N} = 0.091272727 \qquad (19)$$

where the subscript 1 in q_1 indicates the estimated q in the first M-step. We now repeat the E-step according to the following equations equivalent to Eq. (18)

$$N_{AA.i} = D \frac{p^2}{p^2 + 2pq_{i-1}}$$

$$N_{Aa.i} = D \frac{2pq_{i-1}}{p^2 + 2pq_{i-1}} \qquad (20)$$

$$p = 1 - q_{i-1}$$

and the M-step with q_i obtained from the following equation equivalent to Eq. (19)

$$q_i = \frac{N_{Aa.i} + 2N_{aa}}{2N} \tag{21}$$

Repeating the E-step and M-step will result in q_i asymptotically approaching 0.02, and N_{Aa} and N_{AA} approaching 392 and 9604, respectively.

1.3   MULTIPLE COMPARISONS AND THE METHOD OF FALSE DISCOVERY RATE

The material in this section can be found in several books and papers (e.g., Xia, 2012b; 2013a). It is included purely for reader's convenience.

Modern comparative genomic studies may often involve the functional association of thousands of genes or more. With N genes, there are $N(N - 1)/2$ possible pairwise associations and $N(N - 1)/2$ tests of associations. There are $N(N-1)(N-2)/6$ possible triplet associations. So it is necessary to consider the topic of how to control for error rates in multiple comparisons.

There are two approaches for adjusting type I error rate involving multiple comparisons, one controlling for familywise error rate (FWER) by the Bonferroni method which is known to be overly conservative, and the other controlling for the false discovery rate (FDR) (Nichols and Hayasaka, 2003). While FWER methods are available in many statistical packages and covered in many books, there are few computational tutorials for the FDR in comparative genomics, an imbalance which I will try to compensate below.

The FDR protocol works with a set of p values from individual comparisons. For example, with 10 genes, there are 45 pairwise tests of gene associations, yielding 45 p values. Even if there is no true association among these genes, repeated sampling from a large number of gene pairs will eventually generate a gene pair that would have a p value smaller than 0.05 or 0.01. In such cases, if we reject the null hypothesis of null association, we would have committed a type I error. The conventional Bonferroni correction and the FDR protocol are to reduce the chance of committing such type I error. Both increases the chance of committing a type II error, but the increase in committing a type II error is so large as to be unreasonable. The FDR protocol is to specify a reasonable FDR (typically designated by q) and find a critical p (designated $p_{critical}$) so that a p value that is smaller than $p_{critical}$ is considered as significant, otherwise it is not. The q value is typically 0.05

or 0.01. Two general FDR procedures, Benjamini–Hochberg (BH) and Benjamini–Yekutieli (BY), are illustrated below.

Suppose we have a set of 15 sorted p values from testing 15 different hypotheses (Table A-1). The Bonferroni method uses α/m (where m is the number of p values) as a critical p value ($p_{critical.Bonferroni}$) for controlling for FWER. We have $m = 15$. If we take $\alpha = 0.05$, then $p_{critical.Bonferroni} = 0.05/15 = 0.00333$ which would lead to the rejection of the first three hypotheses with the three smallest p values.

The classical FDR approach (Benjamini and Hochberg, 1995), now commonly referred to as the BH procedure, computes $p_{critical.BH.i}$ for the ith p value (where the subscript BH stands for the BH procedure) as

$$p_{critical.BH.i} = \frac{q \bullet i}{m} \qquad (22)$$

where q is FDR (e.g., 0.05), and i is the rank of the p value in the sorted array of p values (Table A-1). If k is the largest i satisfying the condition of $p_i \leq p_{critical.BH.i}$, then we reject hypotheses from H_1 to H_k. In Table 1, $k = 4$ and we reject the null hypotheses in the first four tests. Note that the fourth hypothesis was not rejected by $p_{critical.Bonferroni}$ but rejected by $p_{critical.BH.4}$. Also note that $p_{critical.Bonferroni}$ is the same as $p_{critical.BH.1}$.

TABLE A-1 Illustration of the BH (Benjamini and Hochberg, 1995) and BY (Benjamini and Yekutieli, 2001) procedures in controlling for FDR.

I	p	$P_{critical.BH.i}$	$P_{critical.BY.i}$
1	0.0001	0.00333	0.00100
2	0.0005	0.00667	0.00201
3	0.0020	0.01000	0.00301
4	0.0094	0.01333	0.00402
5	0.0200	0.01667	0.00502
6	0.0279	0.02000	0.00603
7	0.0295	0.02333	0.00703
8	0.0354	0.02667	0.00804
9	0.0439	0.03000	0.00904
10	0.3239	0.03333	0.01005
11	0.4252	0.03667	0.01105
12	0.5312	0.04000	0.01205
13	0.6228	0.04333	0.01306
14	0.7555	0.04667	0.01406
15	1.0000	0.05000	0.01507

The FDR procedure above assumes that the test statistics are independent. A more conservative FDR procedure has been developed that relaxes the independence assumption (Benjamini and Yekutieli, 2001). This method, now commonly referred to as the BY procedure, computes $p_{critical.BY.i}$ for the ith hypothesis as

$$p_{critical.BY.i} = \frac{q \bullet i}{m \sum_{i=1}^{m} \frac{1}{i}} = \frac{p_{critical.BH.i}}{\sum_{i=1}^{m} \frac{1}{i}} \tag{23}$$

With $m = 15$ in our case, $\Sigma 1/k = 3.318228993$. Now k (the largest i satisfying $p_i \leq p_{critical.BY.i}$) is 3 (Table A-1). Thus, only the first three null hypotheses are rejected. The BY procedure was found to be too conservative and several alternatives have been proposed (Ge et al., 2008). For large m, $\Sigma 1/k$ converges to $\ln(m) + \gamma$ (Euler's constant equal approximately to 0.57721566). Thus, for $m = 10,000$, $\Sigma 1/k$ is close to 10. So $p_{critical.BY}$ is nearly 10 times smaller than $p_{critical.BH}$.

One may also obtain empirical distribution of p values by resampling the data. For studying association between genes or between gene and environmental factors, one may compute the frequencies of states 0 (absence) and 1 (presence) for each gene (designated f_0 and f_1, respectively) and reconstitute each column by randomly sampling from the pool of states with f_0 and f_1. For each resampling, we may carry out the likelihood ratio test shown above to obtain p values. If we have generated 10,000 p values, then the 500th smallest p value may be taken as the critical p value.

References

Adachi, J.; Hasegawa M. Model of Amino Acid Substitution in Proteins Encoded by Mitochondrial DNA. *J. Mol. Evol.* **1996,** *42,* 459–468.

Akaike, H. Information Theory and an Extension of Maximum Likelihood Principle. In *Second International Symposium on Information Theory*; Petrov B. N., Csaki F., Eds.; Akademiai Kiado: Budapest, 1973; pp 267–281.

Akashi, H. Synonymous Codon Usage in Drosophila Melanogaster: Natural Selection and Translational Accuracy. *Genetics* **1994,** *136* (3); 927–935.

Althaus, E.; Caprara, A.; Lenhof, H. P.; Reinert, K. Multiple Sequence Alignment with Arbitrary Gap Costs: Computing an Optimal Solution Using Polyhedral Combinatorics. *Bioinformatics* **2002,** *18 Suppl 2,* S4–S16.

Altschul, S. F.; Gish W.; Miller, W.; Myers, E. W.; Lipman, D. J. Basic Local Alignment Search Tool. *J. Mol. Biol.* **1990,** *215* (3), 403–410.

Argos, P.; Rossmann, M. G.; Grau, U. M.; Zuber, A.; Franck, G.; Tratschin, J. D. Thermal Stability and Protein Structure. *Biochemistry (Mosc.)* **1979,** *18,* 5698–5703.

Ashkenazy, H.; Penn, O.; Doron-Faigenboim, A.; Cohen, O.; Cannarozzi, G.; Zomer, O.; Pupko, T. FastML: A Web Server for Probabilistic Reconstruction of Ancestral Sequences. *Nucleic Acids Res.* **2012,** *40* (Web Server issue), W580–W584.

Auch, A. F.; Henz, S. R.; Holland, B. R.; Goker, M. Genome BLAST Distance Phylogenies Inferred from Whole Plastid and Whole Mitochondrion Genome Sequences. *BMC Bioinformatics* **2006,** *7,* 350.

Barker, D.; Pagel, M. Predicting Functional Gene Links from Phylogenetic-statistical Analyses of Whole Genomes. *PLoS Comput. Biol.* **2005,** *1* (1), e3.

Baron, D.; Cocquet, J.; Xia, X.; Fellous, M.; Guiguen, Y.; Veitia, R. A. An Evolutionary and Functional Analysis of FoxL2 in Rainbow Trout Gonad Differentiation. *J. Mol. Endocrinol.* **2004,** *33,* 705–715.

Beacham, T. D.; Wallace, C.; MacConnachie, C.; Jonsen, K.; McIntosh, B.; Candy, J. R.; Devlin, R. H.; Withlera, R. E. Population and Individual Identification of Coho Salmon in British Columbia Through Parentage-based Tagging and Genetic Stock Identification: An Alternative to Coded-wire Tags. *Can. J. Fish. Aquat. Sci.* **2017,** *74* (9), 1391–1410.

Benjamini, Y.; Hochberg, Y. Controlling the False Discovery Rate: A Practical and Powerful Approach to Multiple Testing. *J. R. Statist. Soc.B* **1995,** *57* (1), 289–300.

Benjamini, Y.; Yekutieli, D. The Control of the False Discovery Rate in Multiple Hypothesis Testing Under Dependency. *Ann. Stat.* **2001,** *29,* 1165–1188.

Bernardi, G. The Organization of the Vertebrate Genome and the Problem of the CpG Shortage. *Prog. Clin. Biol. Res.* **1985,** *198,* 3–10.

Bernardi, G. The Isochore Organization of the Human Genome, *Annu. Rev. Genet.* **1989,** *23,* 637–61.

Bernardi, G. The Vertebrate Genome: Isochores and Evolution. *Mol. Biol. Evol.* **1993,** *10* (1), 186–204.

Bernardi, G. Isochores and the Evolutionary Genomics of Vertebrates. *Gene* **2000,** *241* (1), 3–17.

Bernardi, G.; Mouchiroud, D.; Gautier, C. Compositional Patterns in Vertebrate Genomes: Conservation and Change in Evolution. *J. Mol. Evol.* **1988,** *28* (1-2), 7–18.

Bernardi, G.; Olofsson, B.; Filipski, J.; Zerial, M.; Salinas, J.; Cuny, G.; Meunier-Rotival, M.; Rodier, F. The Mosaic Genome of Warm-blooded Vertebrates. *Science* **1985,** *228* (4702), 953–958.

Bestor, T. H.; Coxon, A. The Pros and Cons of DNA Methylation. *Curr. Biol.* **1933,** *6,* 384–386.

Blackburne, B. P.; Whelan, S. Class of Multiple Sequence Alignment Algorithm Affects Genomic Analysis. *Mol. Biol. Evol.* **2013,** *30* (3), 642–53.

Britten, R. J. Rates of DNA Sequence Evolution Differ Between Taxonomic Groups. *Science* **1986,** *231,* 1393–1398.

Brooks, D. R.; McLennan, D. A. *Phylogeny, Ecology and Behavior: A Research Program in Comparative Biology*; University of Chicago Press: Chicago, 1991.

Bulmer, M. The Selection-mutation-drift Theory of Synonymous Codon Usage. *Genetics* **1991,** *129,* 897–907.

Buonagurio, D. A.; Nakada, S.; Parvin, J. D.; Krystal, M.; Palese, P.; Fitch, W. M. Evolution of Human Influenza A Viruses Over 50 Years: Rapid, Uniform Rate of Change in NS Gene. *Science* **1986,** *232,* 980–982.

Burnham, K. P.; Anderson, D. R. *Model Selection and Multimodel Inference: A Practical Information-Theoretic Approach*; Springer: New York, NY, 2002.

Cao, Y.; Janke, A.; Waddell, P. J.; Westerman, M.; Takenaka, O.; Murata, S.; Okada, N.; Paabo, S.; Hasegawa, M. Conflict Among Individual Mitochondrial Proteins in Resolving the Phylogeny of Eutherian Orders. *J. Mol. Evol.* **1998,** *47* (3), 307–22.

Cardon, L. R.; Burge, C.; Clayton, D. A.; Karlin, S. Pervasive CpG Suppression in Animal Mitochondrial Genomes. *Proc. Natl. Acad. Sci. USA* **1994,** *91,* 3799–3803.

Carullo, M.; Xia, X. An Extensive Study of Mutation and Selection on the Wobble Nucleotide in tRNA Anticodons in Fungal Mitochondrial Genomes. *J. Mol. Evol.* **2008,** *66* (5), 484–493.

Chakraborty, R. Estimation of Time of Divergence from Phylogenetic Studies. *Can. J. Genet. Cytol.* **1977,** *19,* 217–223.

Chambaud, I.; Heilig, R.; Ferris, S.; Barbe, V.; Samson, D.; Galisson, F.; Moszer, I.; Dybvig, K.; Wroblewski, H.; Viari, A. et al. The Complete Genome Sequence of the Murine Respiratory Pathogen Mycoplasma Pulmonis. *Nucleic Acids Res.* **2001,** *29* (10), 2145–2153.

Chang, B. S.; Jonsson, K.; Kazmi, M. A.; Donoghue, M. J.; Sakmar, T. P. Recreating a Functional Ancestral Archosaur Visual Pigment. *Mol. Biol. Evol.* **2002a,** *19* (9), 1483–1489.

Chang, B. S.; Kazmi, M. A.; Sakmar, T. P. Synthetic Gene Technology: Applications to Ancestral Gene Reconstruction and Structure-function Studies of Receptors. *Methods Enzymol.* **2002b,** *343,* 274–294.

Chithambaram, S.; Prabhakaran, R.; Xia, X. Differential Codon Adaptation Between dsDNA and ssDNA Phages in *Escherichia coli. Mol. Biol. Evol.* **2014a,** *31* (6), 1606–1617.

Chithambaram, S.; Prabhakaran, R.; Xia, X. The Effect of Mutation and Selection on Codon Adaptation in *Escherichia coli* Bacteriophage. *Genetics* **2014b,** *197* (1), 301–315.

Cocquet, J.; De Baere, E.; Gareil, M.; Pannetier, M.; Xia, X.; Fellous, M.; Veitia, R. A. Structure, Evolution and Expression of the FOXL2 Transcription Unit. *Cytogenet. Genome Res.* **2003,** *101*, 206–211.

Dalgaard, J. Z.; Garrett, R. A. Archaeal Hyperthermophile Genes. In *The Biochemistry of Archaea (Archaebacteria)*; Kates, M., Kushner, D. J., Matheson, A. T., Eds.; Elsevier: Amsterdam, 1993 .

Darwin, C. The Orgin of Species by Means of Natural Selection, or the Preservation of Favoured Races in the Struggle for Life; John Murray: London, 1859.

Dayhoff, M. O.; Schwartz, R. M.; Orcutt, B. C. A Model of Evolutionary Change in Proteins. In *Atlas of Protein Sequence and Structure*; Dayhoff, M. O., Eds.; National Biomedical Research Foundation: Washington D.C., 1978; pp 345–352.

De Baere, E.; Lemercier, B.; Christin-Maitre, S.; Durval, D.; Messiaen, L.; Fellous, M.; Veitia, R. FOXL2 Mutation Screening in a Large Panel of POF Patients and XX Males. *J. Med. Genet.* **2002,** *39* (8), e43.

Deng, R.; Huang, M.; Wang, J.; Huang, Y.; Yang, J.; Feng, J.; Wang, X. PTreeRec: Phylogenetic Tree Reconstruction Based on Genome BLAST Distance. *Comput. Biol. Chem.* **2006,** *30* (4), 300–302.

Desper, R.; Gascuel, O. Fast and Accurate Phylogeny Reconstruction Algorithms Based on the Minimum-evolution Principle. *J. Comput. Biol.* **2002,** *9* (5), 687–705.

Desper, R.; Gascuel, O. Theoretical Foundation of the Balanced Minimum Evolution Method of Phylogenetic Inference and its Relationship to Weighted Least-squares Tree Fitting. *Mol. Biol. Evol.* **2004,** *21* (3), 587–598.

Drouin, G.; Daoud, H.; Xia, J. Relative Rates of Synonymous Substitutions in the Mitochondrial, Chloroplast and Nuclear Genomes of Secd Plants. *Mol. Phylogenet. Evol.* **2008,** *49* (3), 827–831.

Drummond, A.; Forsberg, R.; Rodrigo, A. G. The Inference of Stepwise Changes in Substitution Rates Using Serial Sequence Samples. *Mol. Biol. Evol.* **2001,** *18* (7), 1365–1371.

Drummond, A.; J.; Pybus, O. G.; Rambaut, A.; Forsberg, R.; Rodrigo, A. G. Measurably Evolving Populations. *Trends Ecol. Evol.* **2003a,** *18* (9), 481–488.

Drummond, A.; Pybus, O. G.; Rambaut, A. Inference of Viral Evolutionary Rates from Molecular Sequences. *Adv. Parasitol.* **2003b,** *54*, 331–358.

Drummond, A.; Rambaut, A. BEAST: Bayesian Evolutionary Analysis by Sampling Trees. *BMC Evol. Biol.* **2007,** *7* (1), 214.

Drummond, A.; Rodrigo, A. G. Reconstructing Genealogies of Serial Samples Under the Assumption of a Molecular Clock Using Serial-sample UPGMA. *Mol. Biol. Evol.* **2000,** *17* (12), 1807–1815.

Edgar, R. C. MUSCLE: Multiple Sequence Alignment with High Accuracy and High Throughput. *Nucleic Acids Res.* **2004,** *32* (5), 1792–1797.

Edgar, R. C.; Batzoglou, S. Multiple Sequence Alignment. *Curr. Opin. Struct. Biol.* **2006,** *16* (3), 368–373.

Efron, B. The Jackknife, the Bootstrap and Other Resampling Plans; Society for Industrial and Applied Mathematics: Philadelphia, Pa, 1982.

Emery, C. Pacific Salmon: The Canada-United States Dispute (BP429E). In Devision, Pa. S. A., Eds.; Government of Canada: Canada, 1997.

Felsenstein, J. Maximum-likelihood and Minimum-steps Methods for Estimating Evolutionary Trees from Data on Discrete Characters. *Syst. Zool.* **1973,** *22*, 240–249.

Felsenstein J. Cases in Which Parsimony and Compatibility Methods will be Positively Misleading. *Syst. Zool.* **1978a,** *27*, 401–410.

Felsenstein, J. The Number of Evolutionary Trees. *Syst. Zool.* **1978b,** *27*, 27–33.

Felsenstein, J. Evolutionary Trees from DNA Sequences: A Maximum Likelihood Approach. *J. Mol. Evol.* **1981,** *17*, 368–376.

Felsenstein, J. Confidence Limits on Phylogenies: An Approach Using the Bootstrap. *Evolution* **1985a,** *39*, 783–791.

Felsenstein, J. Phylogenies and the Comparative Method. *Am. Nat.* **1985b,** *125*, 1–15.

Felsenstein, J. Inferring Phylogenies; Sinauer: Sunderland, Massachusetts, 2004.

Felsenstein, J. *PHYLIP 3.695 (Phylogeny Inference Package)*; Department of Genetics, University of Washington: Seattle, 2014.

Felsenstein, J.; Churchill, G. A. A Hidden Markov Model Approach to Variation Among Sites in Rate of Evolution. *Mol. Biol. Evol.* **1996,** *13* (1), 93–104.

Feng, D. F.; Doolittle, R. F. Progressive Sequence Alignment as a Prerequisite to Correct Phylogenetic Trees. *J. Mol. Evol.* **1987,** *25* (4), 351–360.

Feng, D. F.; Doolittle, R. F. Progressive Alignment and Phylogenetic Tree Construction of Protein Sequences. *Methods Enzymol.* **1990,** *183*, 375–387.

Fitch, W. M. Toward Defining the Course of Evolution: Minimum Change for a Specific Tree Topology. *Syst. Zool.* **1971,** *20*, 406–416.

Fitch, W. M.; Margoliash, E. Construction of Phylogenetic Trees. *Science* **1967,** *155*, 279–284.

Frederico, L. A.; Kunkel, T. A.; Shaw, B. R. A Sensitive Genetic Assay for the Detection of Cytosine Deamination: Determination of Rate Constants and the Activation Energy. *Biochemistry (Mosc.)* **1990,** *29* (10), 2532–2537.

Galtier, N.; Lobry, J. R. Relationships Between Genomic G+C Content, RNA Secondary Structures, and Optimal Growth Temperature in Prokaryotes. *J. Mol. Evol.* **1997,** *44* (6), 632–636.

Gao, L.; Qi, J. Whole Genome Molecular Phylogeny of Large dsDNA Viruses Using Composition Vector Method. *BMC Evol. Biol.* **2007,** *7*, 41.

Gascuel, O.; Steel, M. Neighbor-joining Revealed. *Mol. Biol. Evol.* **2006,** *23* (11), 1997–2000.

Ge, Y.; Sealfon, S. C.; Speed, T. P. Some Step-Down Procedures Controlling The False Discovery Rate Under Dependence. *Stat. Sin.* **2008,** *18* (3), 881–904.

Gillespie, J. H. *The Causes of Molecular Evolution*; Oxford University Press: Oxford, 1991.

Gojobori, T.; Li, W. H.; Graur, D. Patterns of Nucleotide Substitution in Pseudogenes and Functional Genes. *J. Mol. Evol.* **1982,** *18* (5), 360–369.

Golding, G. B. Estimates of DNA and Protein-Sequence Divergence—An Examination of Some Assumptions. *Mol. Biol. Evol. 1* (1), 125–142.

Goldman, N.; Yang, Z. A Codon-based Model of Nucleotide Substitution for Protein-coding DNA Sequences. *Mol. Biol. Evol.* **1994,** *11* (5), 725–736.

Goto, M.; Washio, T.; Tomita, M. Causal Analysis of CpG Suppression in the Mycoplasma Genome. *Microb. Comp. Genomics* **2000,** *5* (1), 51–58.

Gotoh, O. An Improved Algorithm for Matching Biological Sequences. *J. Mol. Biol.* **1982,** *162* (3), 705–708.

Gowri-Shankar, V.; Rattray, M. A Reversible Jump Method for Bayesian Phylogenetic Inference with a Nonhomogeneous Substitution Model. *Mol. Biol. Evol.* **2007**, *24* (6), 1286–1299.

Gramm, J.; Niedermeier, R. Breakpoint Medians and Breakpoint Phylogenies: A Fixed-parameter Approach. *Bioinformatics* **2002**, *18 Suppl 2*, S128–S139.

Grantham, R. Amino Acid Difference Formula to Help Explain Protein Evolution. *Science* **1974**, *185*, 862–864.

Gray, M. W. The Evolutionary Origins of Organelles. *Trends Genet.* **1989a**, *5* (9), 294–299.

Gray, M. W. Origin and Evolution of Mitochondrial DNA. *Annu. Rev. Cell. Biol.* **1989b**, *5*, 25–50.

Gray, M. W. The Endosymbiont Hypothesis Revisited. *Int. Rev. Cytol.* **1992**, *141*, 233–357.

Gray, M. W. Origin and Evolution of Organelle Genomes. *Curr. Opin. Genet. Dev.* **1993**, *3* (6), 884–890.

Gray, M. W. Mitochondrial Evolution. *Cold Spring Harb. Perspect. Biol.* **2012**, *4* (9), a011403.

Grosjean, H.; de Crecy-Lagard, V.; Marck, C. Deciphering Synonymous Codons in the Three Domains of Life: Co-evolution with Specific tRNA Modification Enzymes. *FEBS Lett.* **2010**, *584* (2), 252–264.

Gu, X.; Zhang, J. A Simple Method for Estimating the Parameter of Substitution Rate Variation Among Sites. *Mol. Biol. Evol.* **1997**, *14* (11), 1106–1113.

Guindon, S.; Gascuel, O. A Simple, Fast, and Accurate Algorithm to Estimate Large Phylogenies by Maximum Likelihood. *Syst. Biol.* **2003**, *52* (5), 696–704.

Guindon, S.; Lethiec, F.; Duroux, P.; Gascuel, O. PHYML Online—A Web Server for Fast Maximum Likelihood-based Phylogenetic Inference. *Nucleic Acids Res.* **2005**, *33* (Web Server issue), W557–559.

Gupta, S. K.; Kececioglu, J. D.; Schaffer, A. A. Improving the Practical Space and Time Efficiency of the Shortest-paths Approach to Sum-of-pairs Multiple Sequence Alignment. *J. Comput. Biol.* **1995**, *2* (3), 459–472.

Gusfield, D. Algorithms on Strings, Trees, and Sequences: Computer Science and Computational Biology; Cambridge University Press: Cambridge, 1997.

Hartigan, J. A. Minimum Mutation Fits to a Given Tree. *Biometrics* **1973**, *29* (1), 53–65.

Harvey, P. H.; Pagel, M. D. *The Comparative Method in Evolutionary Biology*; Oxford University Press: Oxford, 1991.

Hasegawa, M.; Kishino, H. Heterogeneity of Tempo and Mode of Mitochondrial DNA Evolution Among Mammalian Orders. *Jpn. J. Genet.* **1989**, *64* (4), 243–258.

Hasegawa, M.; Kishino, H.; Yano, T. Dating of the Human-ape Splitting by a Molecular Clock of Mitochondrial DNA. *J. Mol. Evol.* **1985**, *22* (2), 160–174.

Hein, J. A Unified Approach to Phylogenies and Alignments. *Methods Enzymol.* **1990**, *183*, 625–644.

Hein, J. TreeAlign. *Methods Mol. Biol.* **1994**, *25*, 349–364.

Hendy, M. D.; Penny, D. A Framework for the Quantitative Study of Evolutionary Trees. *Syst. Zool.* **1989**, *38*, 297–309.

Hendy, M. D.; Penny, D. Branch and Bound Algorithms to Determine Minimal Evolutionary Trees. *Math. Biosci.* **1982**, *60*, 133–142.

Henikoff, S.; Henikoff, J. G. Amino Acid Substitution Matrices from Protein Blocks. *Proc. Natl. Acad. Sci. USA* **1992**, *89*, 10915–10919.

Henz, S. R.; Huson, D. H.; Auch, A. F.; Nieselt-Struwe, K.; Schuster, S. C. Whole-genome Prokaryotic Phylogeny. *Bioinformatics* **2005**, *21* (10), 2329–2335.

Herman, J. L.; Challis, C. J.; Novak, A.; Hein, J.; Schmidler, S. C. Simultaneous Bayesian Estimation of Alignment and Phylogeny Under a Joint Model of Protein Sequence and Structure. *Mol. Biol. Evol.***2014**, *31* (9), 2251–2266.

Herniou, E. A.; Luque, T.; Chen, X.; Vlak, J. M.; Winstanley, D.; Cory, J. S.; O'Reilly, D. R. Use of Whole Genome Sequence Data to Infer Baculovirus Phylogeny. *J. Virol.* **2001**, *75* (17), 8117–8126.

Hickson, R. E.; Simon, C.; Perrey, S. W. The Performance of Several Multiple-sequence Alignment Programs in Relation to Secondary-structure Features for an rRNA Sequence. *Mol. Biol. Evol.* **2000**, *17* (4), 530–539.

Higgins, D. G. CLUSTAL V: Multiple Alignment of DNA and Protein Sequences. *Methods Mol. Biol.* **1994**, *25*, 307–318.

Higgs, P. G.; Attwood, T. K. *Bioinformatics and Molecular Evolution*; Blackwell: Malden, 2005.

Higgs, P. G.; Ran, W. Coevolution of Codon Usage and tRNA Genes Leads to Alternative Stable States of Biased Codon Usage. *Mol. Biol. Evol.***2008**, *25* (11), 2279–2291.

Hillis, D. M.; Moritz, C.; Mable, B. K. *Molecular Systematics*; Sinauer Associates, Inc: Sunderland, Massachusetts, 1996.

Hobolth, A.; Christensen, O. F.; Mailund, T.; Schierup, M. H. Genomic Relationships and Speciation Times of Human, Chimpanzee, and Gorilla Inferred from a Coalescent Hidden Markov Model. *PLoS Genet.* **2007**, *3* (2), e7.

Hogeweg, P.; Hesper, A. B. The Alignment of Sets of Sequences and the Construction of Phylogenetic Trees: An Integrated Method. *J. Mol. Evol.* **1984**, *20*, 175–186.

Holmes, I.; Bruno, W. J. Evolutionary HMMs: A Bayesian Approach to Multiple Alignment. *Bioinformatics* **2001**, *17* (9), 803–820.

Hudson, R. R. Gene Trees, Species Trees and the Segregation of Ancestral Alleles. *Genetics* **1992**, *131* (2), 509–513.

Huelsenbeck, J. P.; Bollback, J. P. Empirical and Hierarchical Bayesian Estimation of Ancestral States. *Syst. Biol.* **2001**, *50* (3), 351–366.

Huelsenbeck, J. P.; Larget, B.; Alfaro, M. E. Bayesian Phylogenetic Model Selection Using Reversible Jump Markov Chain Monte Carlo. *Mol. Biol. Evol.* **2004**, *21* (6), 1123–1133.

Hurst, L. D.; Merchant, A. R. High Guanine-cytosine Content is not an Adaptation to High Temperature: A Comparative Analysis Amongst Prokaryotes. *Proc. R. Soc. Lond. B* **2001**, *268*, 493–497.

Ikemura, T. Correlation Between the Abundance of *Escherichia coli* Transfer RNAs and the Occurrence of the Respective Codons in its Protein Genes. *J. Mol. Biol.* **1981a**, *146*, 1–21.

Ikemura, T. Correlation Between the Abundance of *Escherichia coli* Transfer RNAs and the Occurrence of the Respective Codons in its Protein Genes: A Proposal for a Synonymous Codon Choice that is Optimal for the *E coli* Translational System. *J. Mol. Biol.* **1981b**, *151*, 389–409.

Ikemura, T. Correlation Between the Abundance of Yeast Transfer RNAs and the Occurrence of the Respective Codons in Protein Genes. Differences in Synonymous Codon Choice Patterns of Yeast and *Escherichia coli* with Reference to the Abundance of Isoaccepting Transfer RNAs. *J. Mol. Biol.* **1982**, *158* (4), 573–597.

Ikemura, T. Correlation Between Codon Usage and tRNA Content in Microorganisms. In *Transfer RNA in Protein Synthesis*; Hatfield, D. L., Lee, B. J., Pirtle, R. M., Eds.; CRC Press: Boca Raton, 1992; pp 87–111.

Jayaswal, V.; Jermiin, L. S.; Robinson, J. Estimation of Phylogeny Using a General Markov Model. *Evol. Bioinform.* Online **2005**, *1*, 62–80.

Jensen, J. L.; Hein, J. Gibbs Sampler for Statistical Multiple Alignment. *Stat. Sin.* **2005**, *15*, 889–907.

Jin, L.; Nei, M. Limitations of the Evolutionary Parsimony Method of Phylogenetic Analysis. *Mol. Biol. Evol.***1990**, *7*, 82–102.

Johnson, N. L.; Kotz, S. Discrete Distributions; Houghton Mifflin: Boston, 1969.

Jones, D. T.; Taylor, W. R.; Thornton, J. M. The Rapid Generation of Mutation Data Matrices from Protein Sequences. *Comput. Appl. Biosci.* **1992**, *8*, 275–282.

Josse, J.; Kaiser, A. D.; Kornberg, A. Enzymatic Synthesis of Deoxyribonucleic Acid VII. Frequencies of Nearest Neighbor Base-sequences in Deoxyribonucleic Acid. *J. Biol. Chem.* **1961**, *236*, 864–875.

Jukes, T. H.; Cantor, C. R. Evolution of Protein Molecules. In*Mammalian Protein Metabolism*; Munro, H. N., Eds.; New York: Academic Press, 1969; pp 21–123.

Karlin, S.; Burge, C. Dinucleotide Relative Abundance Extremes: A Genomic Signature. *TIG* **1995**, *11* (7), 283–290.

Karlin, S.; Mrazek, J. What Drives Codon Choices in Human Genes. *J. Mol. Biol.* **1996**, *262*, 459–472.

Kass, R. E.; Raftery, A. E. Bayes Factors. *J. Am. Stat. Assoc.* **1995**, *90* (430), 773–795.

Katoh, K.; Asimenos, G.; Toh, H. Multiple Alignment of DNA Sequences with MAFFT. *Methods Mol. Biol.* **2009**, *537*, 39–64.

Katoh, K.; Kuma, K.; Toh, H.; Miyata, T. MAFFT Version 5: Improvement in Accuracy of Multiple Sequence Alignment. *Nucleic Acids Res.* **2005**, *33* (2), 511–518.

Katoh, K.; Toh, H. Parallelization of the MAFFT Multiple Sequence Alignment Program. *Bioinformatics* **2010**, *26* (15), 1899–1900.

Kettleborough, G.; Dicks, J.; Roberts, I. N.; Huber, K. T. Reconstructing (Super)Trees from Data Sets with Missing Distances: Not all is Lost. *Mol. Biol. Evol.* **2015**, *32* (6), 1628–1642.

Kimura, M. Evolutionary Rate at the Molecular Level. *Nature* **1968**, *217*, 624–626.

Kimura, M. Preponderance of Synonymous Changes as Evidence for the Neutral Theory of Molecular Evolution. *Nature* **1977**, *267*, 275–276.

Kimura, M. A Simple Method for Estimating Evolutionary Rates of Base Substitutions Through Comparative Studies of Nucleotide Sequences. *J. Mol. Evol.* **1980**, *16*, 111–120.

Kimura, M. The Neutral Theory of Molecular Evolution; Cambridge Universiy Press: Cambridge, England, 1983.

Kimura, M.; Ohta, T. On the Stochastic Model for Estimation of Mutational Distance Between Homologous Proteins. *J. Mol. Evol.* **1972**, *2*, 87–90.

King, M. C.; Jukes, T. H. Non-Darwinian Evolution. *Science* **1969**, *164*, 788–798.

Kishino, H.; Hasegawa, M. Evaluation of the Maximum Likelihood Estimate of the Evolutionary Tree Topologies from DNA Sequence Data, and the Branching Order in Hominoidea. *J. Mol. Evol.* **1989**, *29*, 170–179.

Kishino, H.; Hasegawa, M. Converting Distance to Time: Application to Human Evolution. *Methods Enzymol.* **1990**, *183*, 550–570.

Kishino, H.; Miyata, T.; Hasegawa, M. Maximum Likelihood Inference of Protein Phylogeny and the Origin of Chloroplasts. *J. Mol. Evol.* **1990**, *31*, 151–160.

Kjer, K. M. Use of Ribosomal-RNA Secondary Structure in Phylogenetic Studies to Identify Homologous Positions—An Example of Alignment and Data Presentation from the Frogs. *Mol. Phylogenet. Evol.* **1995,** *4* (3), 314–330.

Koshi, J. M.; Goldstein, R. A. Probabilistic Reconstruction of Ancestral Protein Sequences. *J. Mol. Evol.* **1996,** *42* (2), 313–320.

Kreutzer, D. A.; Essigmann, J. M. Oxidized, Deaminated Cytosines are a Source of C --> T Transitions In Vivo. *Proc. Natl. Acad. Sci. USA* **1998,** *95* (7), 3578–3582.

Kumar, S.; Filipski, A. Multiple Sequence Alignment: In Pursuit of Homologous DNA Positions. *Genome Res.* **2007,** *17* (2), 127–135.

Kumar, S.; Stecher, G.; Tamura, K. MEGA7: Molecular Evolutionary Genetics Analysis Version 7.0 for Bigger Datasets. *Mol Biol Evol.* **2016** .

Kushiro, A.; Shimizu, M.; Tomita, K. -I. Molecular Cloning and Sequence Determination of the *Tuf* Gene Coding for the Elongation Factor Tu of *Thermus thermophilus* HB8. *Eur. J. Biochem.* **1987,** *170*, 93–98.

Kyte, J.; Doolittle, R. F. A Simple Method for Displaying the Hydropathic Character of a Protein. *J. Mol. Biol.* **1982,** *157*, 105–132.

Lake, J. A. Reconstructing Evolutionary Trees from DNA and Protein Sequences: Paralinear Distances. *Proc. Natl. Acad. Sci. USA* **1994,** *91*, 1455–1459.

Lanave, C.; Preparata, G.; Saccone, C.; Serio, G. A New Method for Calculating Evolutionary Substitution Rates. *J. Mol. Evol.* **1984,** *20* (1), 86–93.

Lane, N.; Martin, W. The Energetics of Genome Complexity. *Nature* **2010,** *467* (7318), 929–934.

Li, C. C. *First Course in Population Genetics*; The Boxwood Press: Pacific Grove, California, 1976.

Li, W. -H. *Molecular Evolution*; Sinauer: Sunderland, Massachusetts, 1997.

Li, W. -H.; Tanimura, M.; Sharp, P. M. Rates and Dates of Divergence Between AIDS Virus Nucleotide Sequences. *Mol. Biol. Evol.* **1988,** *5*, 313–330.

Li, W. -H.; Tanimura, M. The Molecular Clock Runs More Slowly in Man than in Apes and Monkeys. *Nature* **1987,** *326*, 93–96.

Li, W-H.; Wolfe, KH.; Sourdis, J.; Sharp, P. M. Reconstruction of Phylogenetic Trees and Estimation of Divergence Times Under Nonconstant Rates of Evolution. *Cold Spring Harb. Symp. Quant. Biol.* **1987,** *52*, 847–856.

Li, W. H. Unbiased Estimation of the Rates of Synonymous and Nonsynonymous Substitution. *J. Mol. Evol.* **1993,** *36*, 96–99.

Li, W. H.; Wu, C. I. Rates of Nucleotide Substitution are Evidently Higher in Rodents than in Man. *Mol. Biol. Evol.* **1987,** *4* (1), 74–82.

Li, W. H.; Wu, C. I.; Luo, C. C. Nonrandomness of Point Mutation as Reflected in Nucleotide Substitutions in Pseudogenes and its Evolutionary Implications. *J. Mol. Evol.* **1984,** *21* (1), 58–71.

Lin, G. N.; Cai, Z.; Lin, G.; Chakraborty, S.; Xu, D. ComPhy: Prokaryotic Composite Distance Phylogenies Inferred from Whole-genome Gene Sets. *BMC Bioinformatics* **2009,** *10 Suppl 1*, S5.

Lindahl, T. Instability and Decay of The Primary Structure of DNA. *Nature* **1993,** *362*, 709–715.

Lipman, D. J.; Altschul, S. F.; Kececioglu, J. D. A Tool for Multiple Sequence Alignment. *Proc. Natl. Acad. Sci. USA* **1989**, *86* (12), 4412–4415.

Lobry, J. R. Asymmetric Substitution Patterns in the Two DNA Strands of Bacteria. *Mol. Biol. Evol.* **1996a**, *13* (5), 660–665.

Lobry, J. R. Origin of Replication of *Mycoplasma genitalium*. *Science* **1996b**, *272* (5262), 745–746.

Lockhart, P. J.; Steel, M. A.; Hendy, M. D.; Penny, D. Recovering Evolutionary Trees Under a More Realistic Model of Sequence Evolution. *Mol. Biol. Evol.* **1994**, *11*, 605–612.

Lunter, G.; Rocco, A.; Mimouni, N.; Heger, A.; Caldeira, A.; Hein, J. Uncertainty in Homology Inferences: Assessing and Improving Genomic Sequence Alignment. *Genome Res.* **2008**, *18* (2), 298–309.

Maddison, D. R.; Maddison, W. P. *MacClade 4: Analysis of Phylogeny and Character Evolution*; Sinaur: Sunderland, MA, 2000.

Margulis, L. Origin of Eukaryotic Cells; Evidence and Research Implications for a Theory of the Origin and Evolution of Microbial, Plant, and Animal Cells on the Precambrian Earth; Yale University Press: New Haven, 1970.

Margulis, L. Gaia is a Tough Bitch (Chapter 7). In *Third Culture: Beyond the Scientific Revolution* by John Brockman; Simon & Schuster, 1995; p 413 .

Marin, A.; Xia, X. GC Skew in Protein-coding Genes Between the Leading and Lagging Strands in Bacterial Genomes: New Substitution Models Incorporating Strand Bias. *J. Theor. Biol.* **2008**, *253* (3), 508–513.

Martins, E. P.; Hansen, T. F. Phylogenies and the Comparative Method: A General Approach to Incorporating Phylogenetic Information into the Analysis of Interspecific Data. *Am. Nat.* **1997**, *149*, 646–667.

Mereschkowski, C. Über Natur und Ursprung der Chromatophoren im Pflanzenreiche. *Biol Centralbl.* **1905**, *25*, 593–604.

Miyata, T.; Miyazawa, S.; Yasunaga, T. Two Types of Amino Acid Substitutions in Protein Evolution. *J. Mol. Evol.* **1979**, *12* (3), 219–236.

Miyata, T.; Yasunaga, T. Molecular Evolution of mRNA: A Method for Estimating Evolutionary Rates of Synonymous and Amino Acid Substitutions from Homologous Nucleotide Sequences and its Application. *J. Mol. Evol.* **1980**, *16* (1), 23–36.

Moerschell, R. P.; Hosokawa, Y.; Tsunasawa, S.; Sherman, F. The Specificities of Yeast Methionine Aminopeptidase and Acetylation of Amino-terminal Methionine In Vivo. Processing of Altered Iso-1-cytochromes C Created by Oligonucleotide Transformation. *J. Biol. Chem.* **1990**, *265* (32), 19638–19643.

Moriyama, E. N.; Powell, J. R. Codon Usage Bias and tRNA Abundance in Drosophila. *J. Mol. Evol.* **1997**, *45* (5), 514–523.

Muse, S. V.; Gaut, B. S. A Likelihood Approach for Comparing Synonymous and Nonsynonymous Nucleotide Substitution Rates, with Application to the Chloroplast Genome. *Mol. Biol. Evol.* **1994**, 11, 715–724.

Mushegian, A, R.; Koonin, E. V. A Minimal Gene Set for Cellular Life Derived by Comparison of Complete Bacterial Genomes. *Proc. Natl. Acad. Sci. USA* **1996**, *93* (19), 10268–10273.

Nachman, M. W.; Crowell, S. L. Estimate of the Mutation Rate Per Nucleotide in Humans. *Genetics* **2000**, *156* (1), 297–304.

Nakashima, H.; Fukuchi, S.; Nishikawa, K. Compositional Changes in RNA, DNA and Proteins for Bacterial Adaptation to Higher and Lower Temperatures. *J. Biochem. (Tokyo)* **2003,** *133* (4), 507–513.

Needleman, S. B.; Wunsch, C. D. A General Method Applicable to the Search of Similarities in the Amino Acid Sequence of Two Proteins. *J. Mol. Biol.* **1970,** *48*, 443–453.

Nei, M. Relative Efficiencies of Different Tree-making Methods for Molecular Data. In *Phylogenetic Analysis of DNA Sequences*; Miyamoto, M. M., Cracraft, J., Eds.; Oxford University Press: New York, 1991; pp 90–128.

Nei, M. Phylogenetic Analysis in Molecular Evolutionary Genetics. *Annu. Rev. Genet.* **1996,** *30*, 371–403.

Nei, M.; Gojobori, T. Simple Methods for Estimating the Numbers of Synonymous and Nonsynonymous Nucleotide Substitutions. *Mol. Biol. Evol.* **1986,** *3*, 418–426.

Nei, M.; Kumar, S. *Molecular Evolution and Phylogenetics*; Oxford University Press: New York, 2000.

Nichols, T.; Hayasaka, S. Controlling the Familywise Error Rate in Functional Neuroimaging: A Comparative Review. *Stat. MethodsMed. Res.* **2003,** *12* (5), 419–446.

Noah, K., J. Hao, Y. Li, X. Sun, B. T. Foley, Q. Yang and X. Xia. "Major revisions in arthropod phylogeny through improved supermatrix, with support for two possible waves of land invasion by chelicerates." *Evolutionary Bioinformatics* 2020 **(in press)**.

Nomenclature Committee of the International Union of Biochemistry. Nomenclature for Incompletely Specified Bases in Nucleic Acid Sequences. Recommendations 1984. *Eur. J. Biochem.* **1985,** *150*, 1–5.

Notredame, C.; O'Brien, E. A.; Higgins, D. G. RAGA: RNA Sequence Alignment by Genetic Algorithm. *Nucleic Acids Res.* **1997,** *25* (22), 4570–4580.

Nur, I.; Szyf, M.; Razin, A.; Glaser, G.; Rottem, S.; Razin, S. Procaryotic and Eucaryotic Traits of DNA Methylation in Spiroplasmas (Mycoplasmas). *J. Bacteriol.* **1985,** *164* (1), 19–24.

Nussinov, R. Doublet Frequencies in Evolutionary Distinct Groups. *Nucleic Acids Res.* *12*(3), 1749–1763.

O'Brien, J. D.; She, Z. S.; Suchard. M. A. Dating the Time of Viral Subtype Divergence. *BMC Evol. Biol.* **2008,** *8*, 172.

Olsen, G. J.; Matsuda, H.; Hagstrom, R.; Overbeek, R. fastDNAML: ATool for Construction of Phylogenetic Trees of DNA Sequences Using Maximum Likelihood. *CABIO* **1994,** *10* (1), 41–48.

Olsen, G. J.; Woese, C. R. Ribosomal RNA: A Key to Phylogeny. *FASEB J.* **1993,** *7*, 113–123.

Otu, H. H.; Sayood, K. A New Sequence Distance Measure for Phylogenetic Tree Construction. *Bioinformatics* **2003,** *19* (16), 2122–2130.

Page, R. D. M. Introduction. In *Tangled Trees: Phylogeny, Cospeciation and Coevolution*; Page, R. D. M., Eds.; University of Chicago Press: Chicago, 2003; pp 1–21.

Pagel, M. Detecting Correlated Evolution on Phylogenies: A General Method for the Comparative Analysis of Discrete Characters. *Proc. R. Soc. Lond. B. Biol. Sci.* **1994,** *255* (1342), 37–45.

Pagel, M. Inferring Evolutionary Processes from Phylogenies. *Zool. Scr.* **1997,** *26* (4), 331–348.

Pagel, M. Inferring the Historical Patterns of Biological Evolution. *Nature* **1999,** *401* (6756), 877–84.

Pagel, M.; Meade, A.; Barker, D. Bayesian Estimation of Ancestral Character States on Phylogenies. *Syst Biol.* **2004,** *53* (5), 673–684.

Palidwor, G. A.; Perkins, T. J.; Xia, X. A General Model of Codon Bias Due to GC Mutational Bias. *PLoS One* **2010,** *5* (10), e13431.

Pamilo, P.; Bianchi, N. O. Evolution of the ZFX and ZFY Genes: Rates and Interdependence Between the Genes. *Mol. Biol. Evol.* **1993,** *10,* 271–281.

Paterson, A. M.; Gray, R. D.; Wallis, G. P. Of Lice and Men: The Return of the 'Comparative Parasitology' Debate. *Parasitol. Today* **1995,** *11,* 158–160.

Pei, J.; Kim, B. H.; Grishin, N. V. PROMALS3D: A Tool for Multiple Protein Sequence and Structure Alignments. *Nucleic Acids Res.* **2008,** *36* (7), 2295–2300.

Pereira, S. L.; Baker, A. J. A Mitogenomic Timescale for Birds Detects Variable Phylogenetic Rates of Molecular Evolution and Refutes the Standard Molecular Clock. *Mol. Biol. Evol.* **2006,** *23* (9), 1731–1740.

Pevzner, P. A. Computational Molecular Biology: An Algorithmic Approach; The MIT Press: Cambridge, Massachusetts, 2000.

Pinheiro, J. C.; Bates, D. M. Mixed-effects Models in S and S-PLUS; Springer-Verlag: Berlin/Heidelberg, 2000.

Prabhakaran, R.; Chithambaram, S.; Xia, X. *Escherichia coli* and Staphylococcus Phages: Effect of Translation Initiation Efficiency on Differential Codon Adaptation Mediated by Virulent and Temperate Lifestyles. *J. Gen. Virol.* **2015,** *96,* 1169–1179.

Press, W. H.; Teukolsky, S. A.; Tetterling, W. T.; Flannery, B. P. *Numerical Recipes in C: The Art of Scientifi Computing*; Cambridge University Press: Cambridge, 1992.

Raaum, R. L.; Sterner, K. N.; Noviello, C. M.; Stewart, C. -B.; Disotell, T. R. Catarrhine Primate Divergence Dates Estimated from Complete Mitochondrial Genomes: Concordance with Fossil and Nuclear DNA Evidence. *J. Hum. Evol.* **2005,** *48* (3), 237.

Rambaut, A.; Bromham, L. Estimating Divergence Dates from Molecular Sequences. *Mol. Biol. Evol.* **1998,** *15* (4), 442–448.

Ran, W.; Higgs, P. G. Contributions of Speed and Accuracy to Translational Selection in Bacteria. *PLoS One* **2012,** *7* (12), e51652.

Rannala, B.; Yang, Z. Inferring Speciation Times Under an Episodic Molecular Clock. *Syst. Biol.* **2007,** *56* (3), 453–466.

Razin, A.; Razin, S. Methylated Bases in Mycoplasmal DNA. *Nucleic Acids Res.* **1980,** *8* (6), 1383–1390.

Regier, J. C.; Shultz, J. W.; Zwick, A.; Hussey, A.; Ball, B.; Wetzer, R.; Martin, J. W.; Cunningham, C. W. Arthropod Relationships Revealed by Phylogenomic Analysis of Nuclear Protein-coding Sequences. *Nature* **2010,** *463* (7284), 1079–1083.

Reinert, K.; Stoye, J.; Will, T. An Iterative Method for Faster Sum-of-pairs Multiple Sequence Alignment. *Bioinformatics* **2000,** *16* (9), 808–814.

Rideout, W. M. I.; Coetzee, G. A.; Olumi, A. F.; Jones, P. A. 5-Methylcytosine as an Endogenous Mutagen in the Human LDL Receptor and p53 Genes. *Science* **1990,** *249,* 1288–1290.

Ritland, K.; Clegg, M. Optimal DNA Sequence Divergence for Testing Phylogenetic Hypotheses. Molecular Evolution; Alan R. Liss: New York, 1990; pp 289–296.

Rivera, M. C.; Jain, R.; Moore, J. E.; Lake, J. A. Genomic Evidence for Two Functionally Distinct Gene Classes. *Proc. Natl. Acad. Sci. USA* **1998,** *95* (11), 6239–6244.

Rosenberg, M. S.; Kumar, S. Heterogeneity of Nucleotide Frequencies Among Evolutionary Lineages and Phylogenetic Inference. *Mol. Biol. Evol.* **2003,** *20* (4), 610–621.

Rzhetsky, A.; Nei, M. A Simple Method for Estimating and Testing Minimum-evolution Trees. *Mol. Biol. Evol.* **1992,** *9,* 945–967.

Rzhetsky, A.; Nei, M. METREE: A Program Package for Inferring and Testing Minimum-evolution Trees. *CABIO* **1994a,** *10* (4), 409–412.

Rzhetsky, A.; Nei, M. Unbiased Estimates of the Number of Nucleotide Substitutions when Substitution Rate Varies Among Different Sites. *J. Mol. Evol.* **1994b,** *38* (3), 295–299.

Rzhetsky, A.; Nei, M. Tests of Applicability of Several Substitution Models for DNA Sequence Data. *Mol. Biol. Evol.* **1995,** *12* (1), 131–151.

Sachs, G.; Weeks, D. L.; Melchers, K.; Scott, D. R. The Gastric Biology of *Helicobacter pylori. Annu. Rev. Physiol.* **2003,** *65* (1), 349–369.

Saenger, W. Principles of Nucleic Acid Structure; Springer: New York, 1984.

Sagan, L. On the Origin of Mitosing Cells. *J. Theor. Biol.* **1967,** *14,* 225–274.

Saitou, N.; Nei, M. Polymorphism and Evolution of Influenza A Virus Genes. *Mol. Biol. Evol.* **1986,** *3* (1), 57–74.

Saitou, N.; Nei, M. The Neighbor-joining Method: A New Method for Reconstructing Phylogenetic Trees. *Mol. Biol. Evol.* **1987,** *4,* 406–425.

Sanderson, M. J. A Nonparametric Approach to Estimating Divergence Times in the Absence of Rate Constancy. *Mol. Biol. Evol.* **1997,** *14,* 1218–1232.

Sankoff, D. Minimal Mutation Trees of Sequences. *SIAM J. Appl. Math.* **1975,** *28,* 35–42.

Sankoff, D.; Morel, C.; Cedergren, R. J. Evolution of 5S RNA and the Non-randomness of Base Replacement. *Nat. New Biol.* **1973,** *245* (147), 232–234.

Schluter, D.; Price, T. D.; Mooers, A. Ø.; Ludwig, D. Likelihood of Ancestor States in Adaptive Radiation. *Evolution* **1997,** *51,* 1699–1711.

Schwarz, G. Estimating the Dimension of a Model. *Ann. Stat.* **1978,** *6* (2), 461–464.

Shimodaira, H.; Hasegawa, M. Multiple Comparisons of Log-Likelihoods with Applications to Phylogenetic Inference. *Mol. Biol. Evol.* **1999,** *16* (8), 1114–1116.

Sistla, S.; Rao, D. N. S-Adenosyl-L-methionine-dependent Restriction Enzymes. *Crit. Rev. Biochem. Mol. Biol.* **2004,** *39* (1), 1–19.

Smith, A. B.; Pisani, D.; Mackenzie-Dodds, J. A.; Stockley, B.; Webster, B. L.; Littlewood, D. T. Testing the Molecular Clock: Molecular and Paleontological Estimates of Divergence Times in the Echinoidea (Echinodermata). *Mol. Biol. Evol.* **2006,** *23* (10), 1832–1851.

Smith, T. F.; Waterman, M. W. Identification of Common Molecular Subsequences. *J. Mol. Biol.* **1981,** *147,* 195–197.

Sneath, P. H. A. The Construction of Taxonomic Groups. In *Microbial Classification;* Ainsworth, G. C., Sneath, P. H. A., Eds.; Cambridge University Press: Cambridge, 1962; pp 289–332.

Stoebel, D. M. Lack of Evidence for Horizontal Transfer of the lac Operon into Escherichia coli. *Mol. Biol. Evol.* **2005,** *22* (3), 683–690.

Stoye, J.; Moulton, V.; Dress, A. W. DCA: An Efficient Implementation of the Divide-and-conquer Approach to Simultaneous Multiple Sequence Alignment. *Comput. Appl. Biosci.* **1997,** *13* (6), 625–626.

Sved, J.; Bird, A. The Expected Equilibrium of the CpG Dinucleotide in Vertebrate Genomes Under a Mutation Model. *Proc. Natl. Acad. Sci. USA* **1990,** *87*, 4692–4696.

Swofford, D. Phylogenetic Analysis Using Parsimony; Illinois Natural History Survey: Champaign, IL, 1993.

Swofford, D. L. Phylogeentic Analysis Using Parsimony (* and Other Methods); Sinauer: Sunderland, Mass, 2000.

Tajima, F. Unbiased Estimation of Evolutionary Distance Between Nucleotide Sequences. *Mol. Biol. Evol.* **1993,** *10* (3), 677–688.

Tajima, F.; Nei, M. Estimation of Evolutionary Distance Between Nucleotide Sequences. *Mol. Biol. Evol.* **1984,** *1* (3), 269–285.

Takezaki, N.; Nei, M. Inconsistency of the Maximum Parsimony Method When the Rate of Nucleotide Substitution is Constant. *J. Mol. Evol.* **1994,** *39* (2), 210–218.

Takezaki, N.; Rzhetsky, A.; Nei, M. Phylogenetic Test of the Molecular Clock and Linearized Trees. *Mol. Biol. Evol.* **1995,** *12* (5), 823–833.

Tamura, K.; Kumar, S. Evolutionary Distance Estimation Under Heterogeneous Substitution Pattern Among Lineages. *Mol. Biol. Evol.* **2002,** *19* (10), 1727–1736.

Tamura, K.; Nei, M. Estimation of the Number of Nucleotide Substitutions in the Control Region of Mitochondrial DNA in Humans and Chimpanzees. *Mol. Biol. Evol.* **1993,** *10*, 512–526.

Tamura, K.; Nei, M.; Kumar, S. Prospects for Inferring Very Large Phylogenies by Using the Neighbor-joining Method. *Proc. Natl. Acad. Sci. USA* **2004,** *101* (30), 11030–11035.

Tavaré, S. Some Probabilistic and Statistical Problems in the Analysis of DNA Sequences. In *Some Mathematical Questions in Biology—DNA Sequence Analysis*; Miura, R. M., Eds.; American Mathematical Society: Providence; RI, 1986; pp 57–86.

Thompson, J. D.; Higgins, D. G.; Gibson, T. J. CLUSTAL W: Improving the Sensitivity of Progressive Multiple Sequence Alignment Through Sequence Weighting, Positions-specific Gap Penalties and Weight Matrix Choice. *Nucleic Acids Res.* **1994,** *22*, 4673–4680.

Thorne, J. L.; Kishino, H. Freeing Phylogenies from Artifacts of Alignment. *Mol. Biol. Evol.* **1992,** *9* (6), 1148–1162.

Thorne, J. L.; Kishino, H. Estimation of Divergence Times from Molecular Sequence Data. In *Statistical Methods in Molecular Evolution*; Nielsen R., Eds; Springer-Verlag: New York, 2005; pp 233–256.

Tinn, O.; Oakley, T. H. Erratic Rates of Molecular Evolution and Incongruence of Fossil and Molecular Divergence Time Estimates in Ostracoda (Crustacea). *Mol. Phylogenet. Evol.* **2008,** *48* (1), 157–167.

Ugalde, J. A.; Chang, B. S.; Matz, M. V. Evolution of Coral Pigments Recreated. *Science* **2004,** *305* (5689), 1433.

Van de Peer, Y.; Neefs, J. M.; De Rijk, P.; De Wachter, R. Reconstructing Evolution from Eukaryotic Small-ribosomal-subunit RNA Sequences: Calibration of the Molecular Clock. *J. Mol. Evol.* **1993,** *37* (2), 221–232.

Vinci, G.; Xia, X.; Veitia, R. A. Preservation of Genes Involved in Sterol Metabolism in Cholesterol Auxotrophs: Facts and Hypotheses. *PLoS One* **2008,** *3* (8), e2883.

Vlasschaert, C.; Cook, D;.; Xia, X.; Gray, D. A. The Evolution and Functional Diversification of the Deubiquitinating Enzyme Superfamily. *Genome Biol. Evol.* **2017,** *9* (3), 558–573.

Vlasschaert, C.; Xia, X.; Coulombe, J.; Gray, D. A. Evolution of the Highly Networked Deubiquitinating Enzymes USP4, USP15, and USP11. *BMC Evol. Biol.* **2015,** *15*, 230.

Vos, R. A.; Balhoff, J. P.; Caravas, J. A.; Holder, M. T.; Lapp, H.; Maddison, W. P.; Midford, P. E.; Priyam, A.; Sukumaran, J.; Xia, X et al. NeXML: Rich, Extensible, and Verifiable Representation of Comparative Data and Metadata. *Syst. Biol.* **2012,** *61* (4), 675–689.

Waddell, P. J. Statistical Methods of Phylogenetic Analysis: Including Hadamard Conjugations, LogDet Transforms, and Maximum Likelihood. Ph.D. Thesis, Massey University: New Zealand, 1995.

Waddell, P. J.; Steel, M. A. General Time-reversible Distances with Unequal Rates Across Sites: Mixing Gamma and Inverse Gaussian Distributions with Invariant Sites. *Mol. Phylogenet. Evol.* **1997a,** *8* (3), 398–414.

Waddell, P. J.; Steel, M. A. General Time-reversible Distances with Unequal Rates Across Sites: Mixing Lambda and Inverse Gaussian Distributions with Invariant Sites. *Mol. Phylogenet. Evol.* **1997b,** *8* (3), 398–414.

Wakeley, J. Substitution-rate Variation Among Sites and the Estimation of Transition Bias. *Mol. Biol. Evol.* **1994,** *11*, 436–442.

Wang, H. C.; Hickey, D. A. Evidence for Strong Selective Constraint Acting on the Nucleotide Composition of 16S Ribosomal RNA Genes. *Nucleic Acids Res.* **2002,** *30* (11), 2501–2507.

Wang, H. C.; Xia, X.; Hickey, D. A. Thermal Adaptation of Ribosomal RNA Genes: A Comparative Study. *J. Mol. Evol.* **2006,** *63* (1), 120–126.

Wei, Y.; Wang, J.; Xia, X. Coevolution Between Stop Codon Usage and Release Factors in Bacterial Species. *Mol. Biol. Evol.* **2016,** *33* (9), 2357–2367.

Wei, Y.; Xia, X. The Role of +4U as an Extended Translation Termination Signal in Bacteria. *Genetics* **2017,** *205* (2), 539–549.

Wilks, S. S. The Large-Sample Distribution of the Likelihood Ratio for Testing Composite Hypotheses. *Ann. Math. Stat.* **1938,** *9*, 60–62.

Woese, C. R.; Fox, G. E. Phylogenetic Structure of the Prokaryotic Domain: The Primary Kingdoms. *Proc. Natl. Acad. Sci. USA* **1977,** *74* (11), 5088–5090.

Wolfe, K. H.; Li, W. H.; Sharp, P. M. Rates of Nucleotide Substitution Vary Greatly Among Plant Mitochondrial, Chloroplast and Nuclear DNAs. *Proc. Natl. Acad. Sci. USA* **1987,** *84*, 9054–9058.

Wong, K. M.; Suchard, M. A.; Huelsenbeck, J. P. Alignment Uncertainty and Genomic Analysis. *Science* **2008,** *319* (5862), 473–476.

Wu, C. I.; Li, W. H. Evidence for Higher Rates of Nucleotide Substitution in Rodents than in Man. *Proc. Natl. Acad. Sci. USA* **1985,** *82* (6), 1741–1745.

Xia, X. Uncertainty of Paternity Can Select Against Paternal Care. *Am. Nat.* **1992,** *139*, 1126–1129.

Xia, X. A Full Sibling is not as Valuable as an Offspring: On Hamilton's Rule. *Am. Nat.* **1993,** *142*, 174–185.

Xia, X. Revisiting Hamilton's Rule. *Am. Nat.* **1995a,** *145*, 483–492.

Xia X. Body temperature, rate of biosynthesis and evolution of genome size, *Mol Biol Evol.* **1995b,** 12:834–842

Xia, X. Maximizing Transcription Efficiency Causes Codon Usage Bias. *Genetics* **1996,** *144*, 1309–1320.

Xia, X. How Optimized is the Translational Machinery in *Escherichia coli, Salmonella typhimurium* and *Saccharomyces cerevisiae*? *Genetics* **1998a,** *149* (1), 37–44.

Xia, X. The Rate Heterogeneity of Nonsynonymous Substitutions in Mammalian Mitochondrial Genes. *Mol. Biol. Evol.* **1998b,** *15,* 336–344.

Xia, X. Phylogenetic Relationship among Horseshoe Crab Species: The Effect of Substitution Models on Phylogenetic Analyses. *Syst. Biol.* **2000,** *49,* 87–100.

Xia, X. Data Analysis in Molecular Biology and Evolution; Kluwer Academic Publishers: Boston, 2001.

Xia, X. DNA Methylation and Mycoplasma Genomes. *J. Mol. Evol.* **2003,** *57,* S21–S28.

Xia, X. Mutation and Selection on the Anticodon of tRNA Genes in Vertebrate Mitochondrial Genomes. *Gene* **2005,** *345* (1), 13–20.

Xia, X. Topological Bias in Distance-based Phylogenetic Methods: Problems with Over- and Underestimated Genetic Distances. *Evol. Bioinformat.* **2006,** *2,* 375–387.

Xia, X. *Bioinformatics and the Cell: Modern Computational Approaches in Genomics, Proteomics and Transcriptomics*; Springer US: New York, 2007a.

Xia, X. Molecular Phylogenetics: Mathematical Framework and Unsolved Problems. In *Structural Approaches to Sequence Evolution;* Bastolla, U., Porto, M., Roman, H. E., Vendruscolo, M., Eds.; Springer, 2007b; pp 171–191.

Xia, X. The Cost of Wobble Translation in Fungal Mitochondrial Genomes: Integration of Two Traditional Hypotheses. *BMC Evol. Biol.* **2008,** *8,* 211.

Xia, X. Information-theoretic Indices and an Approximate Significance Test for Testing the Molecular Clock Hypothesis with Genetic Distances. *Mol. Phylogenet. Evol.* **2009,** *52,* 665–676.

Xia, X. DNA Replication and Strand Asymmetry in Prokaryotic and Mitochondrial Genomes. *Curr. Genomics* **2012a,** *13* (1), 16–27.

Xia, X. Position Weight Matrix, Gibbs Sampler, and the Associated Significance Tests in Motif Characterization and Prediction. *Scientifica* **2012b,** 15 .

Xia, X. Rapid Evolution of Animal Mitochondria. In *Evolution in the Fast Lane: Rapidly Evolving Genes and Genetic Systems*; Singh, R. S., Xu, J., Kulathinal, R. J., Eds.; Oxford University Press: Oxford, 2012c; pp 73–82

Xia, X. *Comparative Genomics*; Springer, 2013a .

Xia, X. DAMBE5: A Comprehensive Software Package for Data Analysis in Molecular Biology and Evolution. *Mol. Biol. Evol.* **2013b,** *30,* 1720–1728.

Xia, X. Phylogenetic Bias in the Likelihood Method Caused by Missing Data Coupled with Among-Site Rate Variation: An Analytical Approach. In *Bioinformatics Research and Applications*; Basu, M., Pan, Y., Wang, J., Eds.; Springer, 2014; pp 12–23.

Xia, X. A Major Controversy in Codon-Anticodon Adaptation Resolved by a New Codon Usage Index. *Genetics* **2015,** 199, 573–579.

Xia, X. PhyPA: Phylogenetic Method with Pairwise Sequence Alignment Outperforms Likelihood Methods in Phylogenetics Involving Highly Diverged Sequences. *Mol. Phylogenet. Evol.* **2016,** *102,* 331–343.

Xia, X. DAMBE6: New Tools for Microbial Genomics, Phylogenetics, and Molecular Evolution. *J. Hered.* **2017a,** *108* (4), 431–437.

Xia, X. Deriving Transition Probabilities and Evolutionary Distances from Substitution Rate Matrix by Probability Reasoning. *J. Genet. Genome Res.* **2017b,** *3,* 031.

Xia, X. *Bioinformatics and the Cell: Modern Computational Approaches in Genomics, Proteomics and Transcriptomics*, 2nd ed.; Springer: New York, 2018a.

Xia, X. DAMBE7: New and Improved Tools for Data Analysis in Molecular Biology and Evolution. *Mol Biol Evol.* **2018b,** 35, 1550–1552.

Xia X. Imputing Missing Distances in Molecular Phylogenetics. *PeerJ* **2018c,** *6,* e5321.

Xia, X.; Hafner, M. S.; Sudman, P. D. On Transition Bias in Mitochondrial Genes of Pocket Gophers. *J. Mol. Evol.* **1996,** *43,* 32–40.

Xia, X.; Huang, H.; Carullo, M.; Betran, E.; Moriyama, E. N. Conflict Between Translation Initiation and Elongation in Vertebrate Mitochondrial Genomes. *PLoS One* **2007,** *2,* e227.

Xia, X.; Kumar, S. Codon-based Detection of Positive Selection can be Biased by Heterogeneous Distribution of Polar Amino Acids Along Protein Sequences. In *Computational Systems Bioinformatics: Proceedings of the Conference CSB 2006*; Markstein, P., Xu, Y., Eds.; Imperial College Press, 2006; pp 335–340.

Xia, X.; Lemey, P. Assessing Substitution Saturation with DAMBE. In *The Phylogenetic Handbook,* 2nd ed.; Lemey, P., Salemi, M., Vandamme, A. M., Eds.; Cambridge University Press: Cambridge, UK, 2009; pp 615–630.

Xia, X.; Li, W. H. What Amino Acid Properties Affect Protein Evolution? *J. Mol. Evol.* **1998,** *47* (5), 557–564.

Xia, X.; Millar, J. S. Paternal Behaviour by *Peromyscusleucopus* in Enclosures. *Can. J. Zool.* **1988,** *66,* 1184–1187.

Xia, X.; Millar, J. S. Dispersion of Adult Males in Relation to Female Reproductive Status in *Peromyscusleucopus. Can. J. Zool.* **1989,** *67,* 1047–1052.

Xia, X.; Millar, J. S. Genetic Evidence of Promiscuity in *Peromyscus leucopus. Behav. Ecol. Sociobiol.* **1991,** *28,* 171–178.

Xia, X.; Palidwor, G. Genomic Adaptation to Acidic Environment: Evidence from *Helicobacter pylori. Am. Nat.* **2005,** *166* (6), 776–784.

Xia, X.; Wang, H.; Xie, Z.; Carullo, M.; Huang, H.; Hickey, D. Cytosine Usage Modulates the Correlation Between CDS Length and CG Content in Prokaryotic Genomes. *Mol. Biol. Evol.* **2006,** *23* (7), 1450–1454.

Xia, X.; Xie, Z. DAMBE: Software Package for Data Analysis in Molecular Biology and Evolution. *J. Hered.* **2001,** *92* (4), 371–373.

Xia, X.; Xie, Z. Protein Structure, Neighbor Effect, and a New Index of Amino Acid Dissimilarities. *Mol. Biol. Evol.* **2002,** *19* (1), 58–67.

Xia, X.; Xie, Z.; Kjer, K. M. 18S Ribosomal RNA and Tetrapod Phylogeny. *Syst. Biol.* **2003a,** *52* (3), 283–295.

Xia, X.; Xie, Z.; Salemi, M.; Chen, L.; Wang, Y. An Index of Substitution Saturation and its Application. *Mol. Phylogenet. Evol.* **2003b,** *26* (1), 1–7.

Xia, X.; Yang, Q. A Distance-based Least-square Method for Dating Speciation Events. *Mol. Phylogenet. Evol.* **2011,** *59* (2), 342–353.

Xia, X.; Yang, Q. Cenancestor. In *Encyclopedia of Genetics* 2nd ed; Maloy, S., Hughes, K., Eds.; Academic Press: San Diego, 2013; pp 493–494.

Xia, X. H.; Wei, T.; Xie, Z.; Danchin, A. Genomic Changes in Nucleotide and Dinucleotide Frequencies in Pasteurella Multocida Cultured Under High Temperature. *Genetics* **2002,** *161* (4), 1385–1394.

Xu, Z.; Hao, B. CVTree Update: A Newly Designed Phylogenetic Study Platform Using Composition Vectors and Whole Genomes. *Nucleic Acids Res.* **2009,** *37* (Web Server issue), W174–W178.

Yahnke, C. J.; Johnson, W. E.; Geffen, E.; Smith, D.; Hertel, F.; Roy, M. S.; Bonacic, C. F.; Fuller, T. K.; Van Valkenburgh, B.; Wayne, R. K. Darwin's Fox: A Distinct Endangered Species in a Vanishing Habitat. *Conserv. Biol.* **1996,** *10* (2), 366–375.

Yampolsky, L. Y.; Stoltzfus, A. The Exchangeability of Amino Acids in Proteins. *Genetics* **2005,** *170* (4), 1459–1472.

Yang, Z. Maximum Likelihood Phylogenetic Estimation from DNA Sequences with Variable Rates Over Sites: Approximate Methods. *J. Mol. Evol.* **1994,** *39,* 306–314.

Yang, Z. Phylogenetic Analysis by Maximum Likelihood (PAML). Version 3.12. University College: London, 2002.

Yang, Z. Computational Molecular Evolution. Oxford University Press: Oxford, 2006.

Yang, Z.; Kumar, S.; Nei, M. A New Method of Inference of Ancestral Nucleotide and Amino Acid Sequences. *Genetics* **1995,** *141,* 1641–1650.

Yang, Z.; Nielsen, R. Estimating Synonymous and Nonsynonymous Substitution Rates Under Realistic Evolutionary Models. *Mol. Biol. Evol.* **2000,** *17* (1), 32–43.

Yang, Z.; O'Brien, J. D.; Zheng, X.; Zhu, H. Q.; She, Z. S. Tree and Rate Estimation by Local Evaluation of Heterochronous Nucleotide Data. *Bioinformatics* **2007,** *23* (2), 169–176.

Yang, Z.; Yoder, A. D. Comparison of Likelihood and Bayesian Methods for Estimating Divergence Times Using Multiple Gene Loci and Calibration Points, with Application to a Radiation of Cute-looking Mouse Lemur Species. *Syst. Biol.* **2003,** *52* (5), 705–716.

Yoder, A. D.; Yang, Z. Estimation of Primate Speciation Dates Using Local Molecular Clocks. *Mol. Biol. Evol.* **2000,** *17* (7), 1081–1090.

Zhang, D.; Xiong, H.; Shan, J.; Xia, X.; Trudeau, V. Functional Insight into Maelstrom in the Germline piRNA Pathway: A Unique Domain Homologous to the DnaQ-H 3'-5' Exonuclease, its Lineage-specific Expansion/Loss and Evolutionarily Active Site Switch. *Biol. Direct* **2008,** *3,* 48.

Zharkikh, A. Estimation of Evolutionary Distances Between Nucleotide Sequences. *J. Mol. Evol.* **1994,** *39,* 315–329.

Zhu, C.; Byrd, R. H.; Lu, P.; Nocedal, J. Algorithm 778: L-BFGS-B: Fortran Subroutines for Large-scale Bound-constrained Optimization. *ACM Trans. Math. Softw.* **1997,** *23* (4), 550–560.

Zhu, J.; Liu, J. S.; Lawrence, C. E. Bayesian Adaptive Sequence Alignment Algorithms. *Bioinformatics* **1998,** *14* (1), 25–39.

Zuckerkandl, E.; Pauling, L. Evolutionary Divergence and Convergence in Proteins. In *Evolving Genes and Proteins*; Bryson V., Vogel H. J., Eds.; Academic Press: New York, 1965; pp 97–166.

Index

Printed and bound by CPI Group (UK) Ltd, Croydon, CR0 4YY

23/10/2024

01777694-0002